# Equine Respiratory Diseases

# Equine Respiratory Diseases

**Bonnie Rush and Tim Mair**

**Blackwell**
Science

Editorial offices:
Blackwell Science Ltd, 9600 Garsington Road, Oxford OX4 2DQ, UK
  Tel: +44 (0) 1865 776868
Blackwell Publishing Professional, 2121 State Avenue, Ames, Iowa 50014-8300, USA
  Tel: +1 515 292 0140
Blackwell Science Asia Pty Ltd, 550 Swanston Street, Carlton, Victoria 3053, Australia
  Tel: +61 (0) 3 8359 1011

First published 2004 by Blackwell Science Ltd.
Reprinted 2006

ISBN-10: 0-632-05262-7
ISBN-13: 978-0-632-05262-2

Library of Congress Cataloging-in-Publication Data
Rush, Bonnie.
    Equine respiratory diseases / Bonnie Rush
        and Tim Mair.—1st ed.
      p. cm.
    Includes bibliographical references and index.
    ISBN 0-632-05262-7 (pbk. : alk. paper)
    1. Horses—Diseases. 2. Respiratory organs—
        Diseases. I. Mair, Tim S. II. Title.
    SF959.R47.B66 2004
    636.1'08962—dc22
                        2004004234

A catalogue record for this title is available from the British Library

Set in 10/13pt. Sabon
by Data Management, Inc., Cedar Rapids, Iowa, USA
Printed and bound by Replika Press Pvt. Ltd, India

The publisher's policy is to use permanent paper from mills that operate a sustainable forestry
policy, and which has been manufactured from pulp processed using acid-free and elementary
chlorine-free practices. Furthermore, the publisher ensures that the text paper and cover board
used have met acceptable environmental accreditation standards.

For further information on Blackwell Publishing, visit our website:
www.blackwellpublishing.com

# Contents

---

# About the Authors

---

**Bonnie Rush** earned her DVM degree from The Ohio State University in 1989. She completed her internship training at North Carolina State University in 1990, and her internal medicine residency training at The Ohio State University in 1993. She has been awarded the 1996 and 2003 Carl J. Norden Distinguished Teacher Award and the 2002 Pfizer Award for Research Excellence at Kansas State University. Dr. Rush's research interest is equine respiratory disease, particularly respiratory physiology, immunology, and aerosol drug therapy. Her clinical interest is in equine respiratory, neurologic, and immune-mediated disease.

**Tim Mair** graduated from the University of Bristol in 1980. After working in general practice, he returned to the University of Bristol to undertake research into equine respiratory immunology. He earned his PhD in 1986, and then stayed on at Bristol as a lecturer in equine medicine. In 1990 he returned to practice, and is currently a partner at the Bell Equine Veterinary Clinic in Kent, England. He has been editor of Equine Veterinary Education since 1996. His particular interests are in respiratory and gastrointestinal medicine and surgery.

# Introduction

Diseases of the respiratory tract are common in horses of all ages and types. Respiration is a cellular activity, and the respiratory tract is the organ that permits respiration to take place. The requirements placed on the respiratory system by the body's metabolism include the transfer of the precise quantity of oxygen from the inspired air to the arterial blood that the body tissues need, and the removal from venous blood the quantity of carbon dioxide they produce by metabolism. These requirements for respiration increase dramatically during exercise, and the respiratory system of the horse is designed to permit wide fluctuations in the amount of gas exchange taking place within the lungs.

The unique ability of the horse as an athlete is dependent on the integration of the respiratory system with a number of other body systems, including the musculoskeletal, nervous, and cardiovascular systems. Clinical or subclinical dysfunction of any of these systems can result in exercise intolerance, but in the healthy horse it appears to be the respiratory system that is the limiting factor that determines athletic performance.

The horse possesses several unique physiological responses to exercise that allow for an increased capacity for oxygen transport. The maximum oxygen consumption ($VO_2$ max) reached by the Thoroughbred racehorse can exceed 160 ml/kg/min, a value that is about double that of a human athlete. The horse experiences arterial hypoxemia, oxygen desaturation, and hypercapnia during exercise as a result of diffusion limitation and a relative hypoventilation. Any respiratory dysfunction can cause a further decline in ventilation and gas exchange, and therefore respiratory diseases are a major cause of exercise intolerance and poor performance. Respiratory tract diseases are second only to musculoskeletal diseases as the leading cause of wastage in racehorses.

Respiratory disease is rewarding to evaluate and treat for equine clinicians. The respiratory system is highly accessible for diagnostic testing, responds to an extensive armamentarium of drugs, and has a relatively favorable capacity for healing. Techniques used to evaluate the equine respiratory tract include endoscopic examination, radiographic and ultrasonographic imaging, cytologic evaluation and bacterial culture of respiratory secretions, and histopathologic evaluation of respiratory mucosa and pulmonary parenchyma. Advanced imaging techniques, such as computed tomography and magnetic resonance imaging, are also increasingly used in certain diseases, especially diseases affecting the upper respiratory tract.

Unlike the central nervous system, the accessibility of the respiratory system allows clinicians to obtain a definitive diagnosis in most instances. Respiratory disorders typically respond favorably to appropriate medical therapy, and treatment options for bronchodilation, immunomodulation, antimicrobial activity, and reduction of pulmonary inflammation are well-characterized in horses. Surgical therapy for upper respiratory disease is common and results are often favorable. Surgical intervention for treatment of lower respiratory disease is less routine and is typically performed under grave or extreme circumstances.

Disorders of the respiratory system can be classified into 4 basic categories:

- Contagious upper respiratory tract (URT)
- Noncontagious URT
- Infectious lower respiratory tract (LRT)
- Noninfectious LRT disease

Chapters 3 through 22 represent each one of these categories of respiratory disease. Contagious URT pathogens include viral respiratory disease and strangles (*Streptococcus equi*), and are separated in this text from infectious, noncontagious conditions of the URT, such as guttural pouch mycosis and arytenoid chondritis. Noncontagious URT conditions include structural and functional abnormalities of the pharynx, larynx, and nasal passages. Pneumonia and pleuropneumonia are examples of infectious LRT conditions, whereas heaves, inflammatory airway disease, and exercise-induced pulmonary hemorrhage are common noninfectious LRT disease of horses.

Viral respiratory infections are common in horses, and equine herpesvirus type 4 (EHV-4, rhinopneumonitis), equine influenza, and equine viral arteritis are the most notable. Clinical signs of viral respiratory pathogens are often indistinguishable, and include pyrexia, serous nasal discharge, submandibular lymphadenopathy, anorexia, and cough. In addition to respiratory disease, equine herpesvirus type 1 (EHV-1) can cause abortion and neurologic disease. Equine viral arteritis produces respiratory disease, vasculitis, and abortion. Equine herpesvirus type 2, rhinovirus, and reovirus are ubiquitous viral respiratory pathogens, and infection results in minimal clinical disease. Hendra virus is a newly recognized, zoonotic disease of horses identified in Australia. The disease is rapidly fatal in horses, and close contact is necessary for disease transmission.

Secondary bacterial respiratory infections are primarily initiated by viral disease, because viral respiratory infections impair or destroy respiratory defense mechanisms. The most common bacterial organisms associated with pneumonia in horses are opportunistic bacteria originating from the resident microflora of the upper respiratory tract. These bacteria are not capable of primary invasion and require diminished pulmonary defense mechanisms to establish infection. Secondary bacterial disease may result in mucosal bacterial infections (rhinitis and tracheitis), or may produce more serious invasive disease, such as pneumonia and pleuropneumonia.

Clinical evidence of a secondary bacterial infection includes mucopurulent nasal discharge, depression, persistent fever, and abnormal lung sounds. *Streptococcus equi var zooepidemicus* is the most common opportunistic pathogen of the equine lung, although *Actinobacillus equuli, Bordetella bronchiseptica, Escherichia coli, Pasteurella* spp., and *Pseudomonas aeruginosa* are frequently isolated. *Strep. equi var equi,* the causative agent of strangles, is a contagious, primary bacterial pathogen of the URT, and is capable of mucosal invasion without predisposing factors. *Rhodococcus equi* is a primary pathogen of the LRT of foals less than 5 months of age, which produces pulmonary consolidation and abscessation.

Noninfectious LRT diseases are common and typically limit athletic performance. Inflammatory airway disease is characterized by excessive tracheal mucus, airway hyperreactivity, and poor exercise performance in young horses. Reactive airway disease (heaves) is triggered by exposure to organic dusts in older horses (>8 yrs) with a familial allergic predisposition. Small airways are obstructed by bronchoconstriction and excessive mucus production. The severity of clinical signs may range from exercise intolerance to dyspnea at rest. Exercise-induced pulmonary hemorrhage occurs during maximal exercise in short duration events (horseracing, barrel racing); the pathophysiology, impact on performance, and ideal treatment have been extensively studied but are poorly understood.

Diagnostic testing is usually rewarding in horses with respiratory disease. Endoscopic examination allows direct visualization of the upper respiratory tract, guttural pouches, trachea, and mainstem bronchi. Indications for endoscopic examination include URT noise, inspiratory difficulty, poor exercise performance, and nasal discharge. Radiographs of the skull are indicated to investigate facial deformity, abnormalities of the sinus (sinusitis, dental abnormalities, and sinus cyst), guttural pouch (empyema, tympany), and soft tissue structures (epiglottis, soft palate).

The two most important techniques for evaluation of lower respiratory tract secretions are transtracheal wash and bronchoalveolar lavage. Transtracheal wash is indicated to obtain secretions for bacterial and fungal culture of the lower respiratory tract. Bronchoalveolar lavage is indicated for cytologic evaluation of the lower respiratory tract in animals with diffuse, noninfectious pulmonary disease. Nasal/pharyngeal swab culture is inappropriate for investigation of pulmonary infectious disease, but is performed in horses with suspected strangles infection. Thoracic radiography is most useful to identify abnormalities of the pulmonary parenchyma, mediastinum, and diaphragm. Pulmonary consolidation (pneumonia), peribronchial disease, pulmonary abscessation, interstitial disease, and mediastinal masses (neoplasia, abscess, granuloma) are most easily identified via thoracic radiography.

Thoracic ultrasound is the most appropriate technique to evaluate fluid in the pleural space, peripheral pulmonary consolidation, and peripheral pulmonary abscessation. Ultrasonographic examination can identify the volume, location, and character of pleural fluid (pleural effusion) or air (pneumothorax) within the pleural space. Additionally, ultrasound can identify fibrin tags, gas echoes (anaerobic infection), masses, and loculated fluid pockets. Ultrasound cannot penetrate air; therefore, deep pulmonary abscesses and consolidation cannot be detected via ultrasound examination and must be detected via thoracic radiography. Ultrasound examination allows the clinician to determine the most appropriate site for centesis and formulate a prognosis based on the presence of fibrin, gas echoes, and loculated pockets of fluid. Pleurocentesis is performed in animals with accumulation of fluid in the pleural space and should be performed with ultrasound guidance.

Lung biopsy and fine-needle aspirate are invasive procedures and are performed after other diagnostic procedures have been exhausted. Pulmonary neoplasia, pulmonary fibrosis, and interstitial diseases may require lung biopsy to obtain a definitive diagnosis.

Regardless of the type of respiratory disease, environmental factors and supportive care are important to aid the recovery of the horse. A dust- and ammonia-free stable environment prevents further damage to the mucociliary apparatus. Horses with respiratory disease have a variable to poor appetite; therefore, highly palatable feeds are indicated to prevent weight loss and debilitation during the treatment and recovery period. Adequate hydration will decrease the viscosity of respiratory secretions facilitating their removal from the lower respiratory tract. A comfortable and dry environment, maintained at an appropriate temperature will allow the horse to rest, and will minimize the role of the respiratory tract in thermoregulation.

This text is intended to provide diagnostic and therapeutic options for evaluation of horses with respiratory disease. The clinician's primary goal during physical examination of the respiratory tract is to determine the origin (URT vs. LRT) and character (infectious vs. noninfectious) of the respiratory disease affecting the patient to direct diagnostic testing and therapeutic intervention.

# Examination of the Equine Respiratory Tract

The respiratory tract is relatively accessible to physical examination, and a thorough evaluation usually reveals constructive information that will direct subsequent diagnostic testing. Signalment is important to establish, because some respiratory conditions are age-dependent, (e.g., young—anomaly; aged—neoplasia), use-related (e.g., pleuropneumonia—long-distance transport; EIPH—short-burst, maximal exercise), or breed-predisposed (left laryngeal hemiplegia—draft, Thoroughbred). Next, it is essential to identify historical details relating to the primary respiratory complaint. The duration of clinical signs may differentiate infectious (acute to subacute) from noninfectious (chronic) respiratory disease. Traumatic injury to the respiratory tract (rib fracture, tracheal rupture) typically produces acute, severe clinical signs of respiratory distress or subcutaneous emphysema, and external signs of trauma may be obvious. Seasonal incidence of disease increases the suspicion of an allergic or environmental etiology. The rider/driver is carefully questioned regarding details of exercise performance and recovery, such as the presence and character of a respiratory noise (URT), nasal discharge (EIPH, URT infection), coughing (LRT, cardiac), and exercise tolerance. The horse's vaccination status and history of transport will determine susceptibility and exposure to infectious disease; however, the clinician should recognize that a "current" vaccination status does not completely preclude the occurrence of the viral or bacterial respiratory pathogens in horses.

Examination of the equine respiratory tract is performed in a systematic manner, beginning with observation at rest. The rate (normal = 8 to 12 bpm) and effort of respiration is noted prior to physical examination of the horse. Tachypnea does not necessarily indicate a primary respiratory disorder; acidosis, fever, hyperthermia, anxiety, and pain are non-respiratory sources of increased respiratory rate. Conversely, many primary respiratory conditions may present with a normal respiratory rate at rest. Normal breathing in resting horses is characterized by a unique, biphasic, "double effort" of respiration. In most species, inspiration is an active process using the diaphragm and intercostals muscles, and expiration is passively driven by elastic recoil. In horses, expiration is predominately passive, but the final phase is achieved by active abdominal effort. As a consequence, the initial phase of inspiration is passive due to recoil of the thoracic wall, and inspiration is predominately active. The additional abdominal effort of expiration in normal horses may be misinterpreted as low-grade expiratory difficulty.

Clinical signs of respiratory difficulty include flared nostrils, anxious appearance, and extended head and neck. The phase of respiration that is prolonged often indicates the portion and type (obstructive, restrictive) of the respiratory tract impairment. Inspiratory difficulty, particularly associated with inspiratory noise, indicates upper respiratory tract (URT) obstruction. The intra-airway pressures of the URT are subatmospheric during inspiration; therefore, negative pressure during inspiration exacerbates dynamic airway narrowing by drawing soft tissues into the airway. During expiration, intra-airway pressure is positive, which expands the diameter of the upper respiratory tract. A prolonged expiratory phase of respiration, accompanied by excessive abdominal effort, is consistent with obstruction of the lower respiratory tract (LRT). During expiration, intrathoracic pressure is positive, which narrows the diameter of small airways.

Bronchoconstriction and small airway inflammation exacerbate small airway narrowing during expiration, resulting in small airway collapse and air-trapping during expiration. During inspiration, intrathoracic pressure is negative, and small airways are pulled open by parenchymal attachments, minimizing the effects of bronchoconstriction and inflammation. In contrast, restrictive pulmonary disease will produce rapid, shallow respiration with prolonged inspiratory and abbreviated expiratory phases of respiration. Pleural effusion, pneumothorax, and diaphragmatic hernia are examples of extrapulmonary restrictive disorders that prevent pulmonary expansion. Pulmonary fibrosis and granulomatous pneumonitis are intrapulmonary restrictive diseases producing difficult inspiration, exaggerated elastic recoil, and rapid, shallow respiration.

# Examination of the Upper Respiratory Tract

Most clinicians begin physical examination of the respiratory tract at the head of the horse:

- The character, frequency, and lateralization of nasal discharge may reveal the origin.
- Inspiratory noise is a hallmark sign of upper airway obstruction.
- Abnormalities of the maxillary sinus may present with unilateral nasal discharge, facial deformity, and/or epiphora.

The nares are evaluated for nostril flare, nasal discharge, and equivalent airflow. Nostril flare is observed in horses with respiratory distress originating from the upper or lower respiratory tract. As described above, a prolonged phase of inspiration, paired with an inspiratory noise is the hallmark of obstruction of the URT. Respiratory noise can be characterized as stridor, roaring, or snore. Respiratory *stridor* is a high-pitched inspiratory noise associated with pharyngeal obstruction due to retropharyngeal abscess, arytenoid chondritis, bilateral laryngeal paralysis, pharyngeal collapse (hyperkalemic periodic paralysis), or pharyngeal mass. *Roaring* is a specific term referring to the short, low-pitched respiratory noise observed during exercise in horses with left laryngeal hemiplegia (LLH). Horses with "roaring" are exercise-intolerant, but do not demonstrate respiratory noise at rest. *Snoring* is a low-pitched sound observed during inspiration originating from the nasal passages. Nasal septal dysplasia and nasal masses induce a snoring sound during inspiration. Dorsal displacement of the soft palate produces a characteristic guttural, low-pitched fluttering sound during exercise, and is associated with exercise intolerance. In most instances, the origin of noise from the URT can be identified by endoscopic examination.

3

Nasal discharge is characterized as serous, mucoid, purulent, hemorrhagic, or feed contaminated. Serous nasal discharge is observed in horses with viral respiratory infections and allergic rhinitis. Mucoid to purulent discharge indicates increasing evidence of a primary or secondary bacterial respiratory infection. Fresh blood may originate from the URT (guttural pouch mycosis, trauma) or LRT (EIPH). Brown (old hemorrhage), mucoid, malodorous discharge occurs in horses with necrotizing pneumonia and ruptured pulmonary abscess, both of which carry a poor prognosis. Copious nasal discharge (saliva) contaminated with feed indicates an inability to swallow due to mechanical (choke) or functional (neurogenic) obstruction. Low-volume mucoid nasal discharge that is discolored with feed material is consistent with low-grade dysphagia and chronic aspiration (pharyngeal dysfunction). Unilateral nasal discharge indicates that the origin of exudate is rostral to the caudal aspect of the nasal septum, and is most commonly observed in horses with unilateral sinusitis or a nasal/ethmoidal mass. The guttural pouch openings drain into the abaxial nasopharynx. Therefore, owners report nasal discharge to be predominately unilateral, with occasional observation of exudate from the contralateral nostril. Exudate originating from the guttural pouch is often observed during grazing or after exercise. Bilateral nasal discharge may originate from the LRT or bilateral URT infection. It is important to recognize that tracheal exudate is often coughed up and swallowed in horses; therefore, the presence of nasal discharge is inconsistent in horses with pneumonia. The origin of discharge can be definitively determined via endoscopic examination of the upper respiratory tract.

Equivalent airflow through the nasal passages is detected by placing the palms of your hands in front of the nares. Nasal masses (ethmoid hematoma) are the most common cause of unequal airflow. The visible portion of the nasal septum should be examined for fungal granulomas or amyloid plaques. Horner's syndrome produces poor to absent airflow ipsilateral to the ophthalmologic signs, due to vascular dilation and mucosal edema associated with the loss of sympathetic tone to mucosal blood vessels. Airflow obstruction due to Horner's syndrome may be performance-limiting for athletic horses.

The maxillary and frontal sinuses are evaluated by gentle percussion over the maxillary and frontal sinus areas. The maxillary is the largest sinus cavity of the horse and the most likely to be diseased. The dorsal margin of the maxillary sinus is a line drawn from the medial canthus of the eye to the nasoincisive notch, and the rostral limit is the rostral aspect of the facial crest. The caudal limit of the maxillary sinus is defined by an imaginary line drawn from the middle of the orbit to the facial crest, and the ventral limit is parallel and slightly ventral to the facial crest. The rostral limit of the frontal sinus is defined by an imaginary line drawn at right angles from the midline to midway between the medial canthus of the eye and the infraorbital foramen. The caudal limit of the frontal sinus is at the level of the temporomandibular joint. The lateral limit is a line drawn from the medial canthus to the nasoincisive notch. Dull, hyporesonant percussion, pain, and/or unilateral nasal discharge are consistent with sinusitis, sinus cyst, or neoplasia. Characteristic malodorous discharge is observed in horses with sinusitis secondary to tooth root abscess. Sinus cyst and neoplasia may produce facial deformity, exophthalmia, and ipsilateral epiphora (obstruction of the nasolacrimal duct). Patency of the nasolacrimal duct can be determined by retrograde lavage of the nasolacrimal duct, or observation of fluorescein at the nasolacrimal opening after fluorescent stain is placed in the eye (Jones test).

Submandibular lymph nodes are readily palpable in horses less than 24 months of age, but are difficult to detect in adult horses. Lymphadenopathy, characterized by palpably discrete, firm, and moderately painful lymph nodes, is observed in horses with viral respiratory disease. Markedly enlarged, coalescing, painful submandibular lymph nodes should be considered suspect *Streptococcus equi* infection, until proven otherwise. The abscessed lymph nodes may have a palpable soft area, indicating impending rupture, or there may be evidence that some lymph nodes have ruptured already. Markedly enlarged, solid (homogenous via ultrasound, nonproductive aspiration) submandibular lymph nodes are observed in rare cases of multisystemic lymphoma and mycobacterial or fungal infection of the URT.

Palpation of the larynx, pharynx, and proximal trachea is a relatively insensitive measure (compared to endoscopic examination) for detection of abnormalities of these structures. Nonetheless, careful palpation of the cricoid cartilage and muscular process of the larynx may identify atrophy of the cricoarytenoideus dorsal muscle in horses with left laryngeal hemiplegia. The "slap test" may provide additional evidence of LLH. This test is performed by having the examiner palpate the left arytenoid cartilage, while an observer firmly "slaps" the withers on the right side of the horse. The anticipated response is adduction of the contralateral (left) arytenoid. In addition to LLH, fourth branchial arch defect can also be detected by laryngeal palpation. An abnormally wide gap can often be palpated between the caudal margin of the thyroid and the rostral edge of the cricoid; in the normal larynx the two structures overlap. Detection of this palpable abnormality indicates additional investigation via endoscopic and radiographic examination.

Digital compression of the proximal trachea will elicit a cough in horses with tracheal inflammation or irritation (inducible cough). Horses normally have a high cough threshold and will not respond to this procedure. Inducible or spontaneous coughing is a nonspecific response, and is observed in horses with infectious and noninfectious respiratory disease. Paroxysmal coughing is particularly common in horses with influenza. Influenza replicates within respiratory epithelial cells, denuding the mucuciliary apparatus and exposing irritant receptors in the submucosa. Auscultation of the trachea will reveal a "tracheal rattle" in horses with exudate in the lumen of the trachea. Because horses expectorate exudate, it is important for the clinician to detect tracheal exudate via tracheal auscultation, rather than relying on the appearance of nasal discharge.

# Examination of the Lower Respiratory Tract

2

Physical examination of the lower respiratory tract provides diagnostic clues:

- Crackles are short, explosive sounds consistent with excessive exudate, whereas wheezes are long, musical sounds indicative of bronchoconstriction.
- Rebreathing procedure is performed to accentuate abnormal lung sounds and identify lung borders.
- Thoracic pain may manifest as rapid, shallow respiration, abducted elbows, or avoidance/objection to thoracic auscultation.

Physical examination of the lower respiratory tract relies primarily on thoracic auscultation. The caudal borders of the lung correspond to the following landmarks: 17th intercostal space (ICS) at tuber coxae, 16th ICS at the tuber ischii, 13th ICS at mid-thorax, 11th ICS at the point of the shoulder, and the 5th ICS at the point of the elbow. Horses should be examined at rest to detect abnormal lung sounds, expanded pulmonary fields, or diminished pulmonary fields. Abnormal lung sounds include crackles, wheezes, and pleural friction rubs. *Crackles* are short, explosive sounds produced by airflow bubbled through airway secretions (exudates), or sudden opening of a collapsed small airway. *Wheezes* are long, musical sounds generated by oscillation of bronchial and bronchiolar walls in patients with bronchoconstriction. *Pleural friction rubs* are less commonly observed in horses compared to cattle. The sound originates from rubbing of inflamed visceral and parietal pleura during the respiratory cycle. Horses typically produce effusion in response to inflammation; therefore, pleural friction rubs are observed prior to formation of significant effusion (peracute disease) or after drainage of the pleural cavity.

Expanded pulmonary fields are observed in horses with small airway obstructive disease (particularly heaves), due to their strategy to breathe at high lung volumes to maximize airway caliber. Diminished pulmonary borders are observed in horses with numerous conditions, including (but not limited to) pleural effusion, pneumothorax, pulmonary abscess, pulmonary consolidation, atelectasis, and diaphragmatic hernia. Detection of borboygmi during thoracic auscultation is common, and does not necessarily indicate the presence of a diaphragmatic hernia. Thoracic percussion and ultrasonographic examination is indicated in horses with diminished pulmonary borders to differentiate these conditions.

A rebreathing procedure is performed to increase the rate and depth of respiration, accentuate abnormal lung sounds, or detect altered pulmonary borders. The procedure is performed by placing a large (40 L) plastic bag over the entire muzzle of the horse, allowing the horse to rebreathe expired air, thereby increasing $PCO_2$ and respiratory drive. In addition to auscultation during the procedure, the clinician should subjectively evaluate time necessary for recovery and induction of cough. Horses with normal respiratory function rapidly recover from a rebreathing procedure by taking 3 or 4 deep breaths. Rebreathing is contraindicated in horses with respiratory difficulty or distress.

Thoracic percussion is performed using a large spoon and a rubber reflex hammer. The clinician begins in the dorsal lung field, holding the convex surfaced of the spoon firmly against the surface of the horse in an intercostal space. The hammer is tapped against the concave surface of the spoon, and the clinician listens for a resonant sound generated by air-filled lung. Hyporesonance indicates an absence of air-filled lung. The examiner progresses ventrally along a single ICS, and the process is repeated at each ICS throughout all pulmonary fields. The goal is to identify a region of hyporesonance indicating a pulmonary or pleural abnormality. In horses with pleural effusion, thoracic percussion can often identify a fluid line. Thoracic percussion should not be performed in horses with pleural pain (pleurodynia). Horses with pleural pain may stand with abducted elbows and demonstrate rapid, shallow respiration. These horses may object to thoracic auscultation (bite, pin ears) or perform evasive maneuvers to attempted auscultation.

Horses with pleuropneumonia demonstrate many of the clinical signs presented above, including pleural pain, diminished pulmonary fields, and a fluid line on thoracic percussion. In addition, horses with pleural effusion (septic or nonseptic) may have a plaque of edema in the ventral pectoral region due to the weight of the fluid within the thoracic cavity. Cardiac sounds may be absent or radiating in horses with extensive pleural effusion.

Synchronous diaphragmatic flutter ("thumps") is an uncommon respiratory pattern in which respiration is triggered by cardiac contraction. Thumps is often observed in horses with moderate to severe derangement of acid-base and serum electrolyte concentrations, specifically hypocalcemia, hypochloremia, and metabolic alkalosis. The phrenic nerve travels over the base of the right atrium. Electrolyte imbalance is hypothesized to produce irritability of the phrenic nerve, resulting in excitation of the nerve from cardiac stimulation. The condition is observed in horses after long-distance, strenuous exercise (endurance racing, competitive trail, cross-country phase 3-day eventing) due to electrolyte loss in sweat, blister beetle toxicity (marked hypocalcemia), and hypocalcemic tetany.

# Noncontagious Diseases of the Upper Respiratory Tract

Noncontagious respiratory diseases rank second only to musculoskeletal diseases as a cause of poor performance or exercise intolerance in horses. Many horses have problems involving more than one body system, and this makes the determination of the relative importance of different conditions even more complicated. Although upper respiratory tract conditions are common causes of exercise intolerance in all breeds and types of performance horses, the frequency of specific diseases and the degree to which each disease limits performance can vary with breed, use, and age.

# Diseases Causing Airway Obstruction in the Horse

3

Although many diseases of the upper respiratory tract will produce obvious clinical signs at rest, many other conditions resulting in a functional obstruction of the airway will be apparent only at exercise. Accurate diagnosis of some of these functional airway obstructions can be extremely difficult, and may require examination of the horse during fast exercise. Racehorses have the highest requirements for airflow, and, therefore, often show significant exercise intolerance with functional lesions that may not be apparent at rest. On the other hand, horses that perform less strenuous work tend to require a greater degree of airway obstruction before performance is affected, and these diseases are more likely to be apparent at rest.

## PATHOPHYSIOLOGY

The horse is an obligatory nasal breather. The conchal scrolls of the nasal chambers are anatomically simple, and the nasal meati are streamlined. Despite these features, the upper airway accounts for the majority of the total airway resistance during exercise. The resistance to airflow is inversely related to the diameter of the airway, and small reductions in airway size lead to large increases in airway resistance. Any increase in airway resistance requires an increase in the work of breathing to generate the same airflow.

The movement of air through the respiratory tract is achieved by the creation of pressure gradients during inspiration and expiration. During inspiration, the pressure within the lumen of the airways is lower than that within the tissues of the walls of the tract and the external environment; this produces a collapsing force on the airway wall. During expiration the gradients are reversed. The greater the work of breathing, the greater are the collapsing forces

13

applied to the walls of the upper respiratory tract, such that during inspiration at exercise a collapsing force as high as 40 cm $H_2O$ is present.

During quiet breathing, the upper respiratory tract, principally the nostrils and larynx, provides 70–85% of the total resistance, but when required this can be reduced to under 50% by the active dilation of the nares and larynx and by straightening the airway. The structural rigidity provided by the conchal cartilages and the tracheal rings provides stability through much of the upper respiratory tract, but in three important areas of the airway—the nostrils, pharynx and larynx—resistance to collapse is provided by active muscular dilation. These three areas are the sites at which much of the resting airway resistance occurs, and it is suggested that relatively minor lesions or dysfunction at these sites of high resistance may significantly increase total resistance to airflow. During exercise, full abduction of the rima glottidis (by the action of the intrinsic laryngeal musculature) is sustained through all phases of the respiratory cycle and continues during the immediate post-exercise recovery period. Failure of this function—for example, in laryngeal hemiplegia—leads to dynamic collapse of the flaccid structures into the airway during inspiration, with resultant restriction of airflow. Dynamic dysfunction at the level of the pharynx and larynx accounts for the majority of cases of obstructive dyspnea in athletic horses.

The horse is designed to be an obligatory nose-breathing animal and never to breathe through its mouth. It has an intranarial larynx whereby the cartilages of the larynx are locked into the caudal wall of the nasopharynx by the palatopharyngeal arch, which acts as an airtight seal. The palatal arch has to disengage momentarily for deglutition, but at all other times the larynx remains in its intranarial position.

## RESPIRATION AND LOCOMOTION

At the walk, the trot, and when pacing, there is no fixed relationship between locomotion and respiration. However, at the canter and gallop, a one-to-one relationship exists, such that one respiratory cycle is completed in the time taken for one stride. At these paces, inspiration occurs during the extensor phase of the forelimbs. Conversely, expiration occurs during the weight-bearing phase of the forelimbs.

Horses may need to swallow during exercise, and respiration cannot continue through deglutition; it is suspended after the inspiratory phase, and resumes with expiration on completion of swallowing. For horses at the canter and gallop, deglutition must be completed exactly in the time taken for a whole number of strides, usually one.

## RESPIRATORY NOISE

When horses are exercised, the process of inspiration should be silent to the unaided human ear. In contrast, vibrant sounds generated by the alar folds frequently make expiration a noisy process—"high blowing." Airway obstructions lead to the generation of increased noise as a result of tissue vibration and turbulent airflow. Thus, the identification of an abnormal noise during exercise suggests that an airway obstruction is present, and it increases the likelihood that airway obstruction is responsible for exercise intolerance. Noise generated only during inspiration suggests a dynamic obstruction that occurs only during the negative pressures generated on inspiration. These negative inspiratory pressures promote airway collapse, vibration, and noise. During expiration, in contrast, positive pressures tend to dilate the airway, moving the obstruction out of the way; the noise will therefore be less or absent during expiration. In contrast, a fixed obstruction is likely to limit airflow during both inspiration and expiration, resulting in noise during both phases of respiration. The level of exercise needed to generate the abnormal noise, and the duration or persistence of noise can also provide valuable information. A noise that suddenly appears and suddenly disappears, for example, suggests a transient obstruction.

## DIAGNOSIS OF AIRWAY OBSTRUCTIONS

Horses are presented for respiratory assessment at pre-purchase examinations and because of nasal discharge, abnormal respiratory noises, acute and chronic coughing, prolonged post-exercise tachypnea, fatigue at exercise, and poor performance.

### History
In the context of poor performance, it is important to discover whether the performance is unproven and may result from an inherent lack of ability, or whether the patient has been an effective athlete but is no longer successful.

Prior to commencing an examination of the upper respiratory tract the bodily condition of the patient should be noted. Overweight, unfit horses are inclined to produce "stuffy" respiratory noises resulting from pharyngeal flaccidity. Vital parameters should be obtained, nasal discharge noted, and regional lymph nodes palpated for evidence of current upper respiratory infections.

### Palpation tests
During the examination at rest, the larynx is palpated to detect for cartilaginous abnormalities, atrophy of the intrinsic musculature, and evidence of previous surgery. The slap test and arytenoid depression test are performed during laryngeal palpation. The trachea is palpated to detect disruption of the normal ring architecture by previous trauma or surgery. Congenitally flattened rings may also be detected.

### Endoscopy at rest
An endoscopic examination should be performed in the unsedated horse in a systematic manner, and a standard routine is recommended. The examination

should include both nasal chambers, the nasopharynx, guttural pouches, epiglottis, soft palate, larynx, and trachea. Apart from the overall conformation of the lumen of the airway, the relationships between structures such as the soft palate and epiglottis should be noted, and the resting movements of the larynx observed. The vocal cords and saccules are examined for evidence of previous surgery. Note is made of the presence, character (serous, mucoid, purulent, serosanguinous), and origin (unilateral, bilateral, submandibular) of discharge. During the examination, the patient is stimulated to swallow on several occasions in order to provide the best opportunity to identify anomalies that may not be consistently visible, such as epiglottal entrapment and small subepiglottic cysts. Normal swallowing causes a quick maximal abduction of the arytenoids, and the epiglottis is maintained dorsal to the soft palate at the conclusion of a swallow. The endoscope is passed into the trachea to determine the presence of discharge or aspirated food material. It is common for the horse to have its palate displaced when the endoscope is retrieved from the trachea into the pharynx, giving the examiner the opportunity to assess the free edge of the palate. However, the horse should replace the palate quickly by swallowing when the endoscope is back in the pharynx.

Manual occlusion of the nostrils forces the horse to create more negative inspiratory pressures in the airway, and this may aid in the identification of dynamic airway collapse. The duration of occlusion is variable, and is often dependent on the temperament of the horse. Young horses and fatigued horses will easily and frequently displace their palates. Some clinicians favor the administration of lobeline (0.3 mg/kg, IV) to stimulate increased respiratory effort as a means of assessing laryngeal and pharyngeal function more fully.

## Radiographic examination

Radiographic examination of the upper respiratory tract can provide additional diagnostic information, particularly to reveal structures obscured from endoscopic view, such as the tissues ventral to a permanently displaced soft palate.

## Exercise tests

All ridden and lunged exercise tests to detect respiratory sounds should include a canter in both directions in a confined area. A ridden test is preferred, because in a collected canter the poll is flexed and the resultant curvature of the airway exaggerates untoward respiratory noises. Any adventitious noises can be timed with respect to the phase of the respiratory cycle—i.e., inspiratory versus expiratory.

## Treadmill endoscopy

Dynamic obstructive lesions of the upper respiratory tract may not be apparent at rest, and endoscopic examination during exercise on a high-speed treadmill is necessary to achieve the diagnosis. Comparison of the results of resting endoscopy and findings during exercise suggests that diagnosis at rest yields a significantly inaccurate result in as much as 50% of cases. Treadmill exercise also gives the opportunity for simultaneous physiological tests, not only to assess whether the anomalies observed endoscopically are compromising respiratory function but as the means to test the efficacy of surgical methods of correction.

## Spectrum analysis of respiratory sounds

There is renewed interest in the spectral analysis of respiratory sounds recorded in the exercising horse by a microphone suspended in front of the horse's nose or strapped over the trachea. Certain airway abnormalities may produce characteristic sound bands or formants.

## FURTHER READING

Davidson, E.J., and Martin, B.B. 2003. Diagnosis of upper respiratory tract diseases in the performance horse. *Vet Clinics N Am Equine Pract* 19:51–62.

Embertson, R.M. 1998. Evaluation of the young horse upper airway: What is normal, and what is acceptable. In *Proc 44th Ann Conv Am Assoc Equine Pract*, pp 34–38.

Franklin, S.H., Usmar, S.G., Lane, J.G., Shuttleworth, J., and Burn, J.F. 2003. Spectral analysis of respiratory noise in horses with upper airway disorders. *Equine Vet J* 35:264–268.

Lane, J.G. 1998. Disorders of the ear, nose and throat. In *Equine Medicine, Surgery and Reproduction.* T. Mair, S. Love, J. Schumacher, and E. Watson, eds. London: W.B. Saunders, pp 81–117.

Parente, E.J. 2003. Endoscopic evaluation of the upper respiratory tract. In *Current Therapy in Equine Medicine,* 5th ed. N.E. Robinson, ed. Philadelphia: W.B. Saunders, pp 366–369.

# The Nasal Cavity and Paranasal Sinuses

4

Besides serving as a conduit for airflow, the primary functions of the nasal cavity and paranasal sinuses are to warm, humidify, and remove particulate debris from inspired air prior to exposure to the lower respiratory tract. In addition, the mucosal surface of the nasal passages and paranasal sinuses provides the first line of immunologic defense against inspired pathogens. Consequently, these structures are a complicated network of discrete, communicating chambers designed to maximize the mucosal surface area of the upper respiratory tract.

## Nasal cavity

The nasal cavity is the first segment of the respiratory tract, and along with the paranasal sinuses, is encased within the facial bones of the skull. It is separated from the mouth ventrally by the palate. The external nares (nostrils) represent the rostral limit of the nasal cavity, and the caudal limit is the posterior nares or choanae that communicate with the pharynx.

The widely spaced nostrils are supported medially by the alar cartilages. The nostrils contribute more than 50% to the total resistance to flow of the entire upper respiratory tract during quiet breathing. This can be reduced considerably by active dilation during exertion. The C-shaped alar cartilages, back-to-back at the midline, provide rigidity for the otherwise soft structures of the external nares. Dilation of the nostril margins is achieved through the action of the nasolabialis muscles, which receive their motor supply through the dorsal buccal branches of the facial nerves. The alar folds, which attach to the ventral conchus, mark the dorsal margin of the airway through the nasal vestibule. Dorsal to the alar fold there is a blind cutaneous pouch called the "false nostril" (or nasal diverticulum).

The nasal cavity is divided into two halves by the nasal septum and vomer bone. The nasal septum is composed of hyaline cartilage that merges with the ethmoid bone at the caudal end of the nasal cavity. The nasal septum extends from the rostral limit of the nasal cavity to the ethmoidal labyrinth. Its ventral border rests in a groove in the vomer bone caudally, and on the palatine processes of the incisive bones rostrally. Its dorsal margin is attached to the frontal and nasal bones. The septum is covered by respiratory epithelium, and in the ventral part there is an abundant venous plexus.

The two nasal conchae or turbinates arise from the lateral walls of the nasal cavity and divide the cavity into the dorsal, middle, and ventral nasal meati. The conchae are composed of delicate scrolls of bone that coil in opposite directions medially toward the midline. The conchae occupy much of the volume of the nasal cavity. The dorsal concha is larger, and its caudal part communicates with the frontal sinus. The rostral part of the dorsal concha is divided by septa into several independent cavities or cells, each of which has a separate opening into the middle nasal meatus. The ventral concha is smaller, and its caudal part is in direct communication with the rostral maxillary sinus. The rostral part of the ventral concha is also divided into separate cavities or cells. At the level of the first cheek tooth, the rostral ends of both conchae are attached to prominent and highly vascular folds of mucous membrane.

The ventral nasal meatus is the largest of the three meati, and is the preferred route for passage of a nasogastric tube or endoscope. The ventral nasal meatus leads directly to the nasopharynx through the choanae. Each choana is a horizontal opening caudal to the caudal edge of the hard palate and separated from the other choana by the vomer bone.

The ethmoidal labyrinth projects rostrally into the nasal cavity from the cribiform plate. The labyrinth is made up of numerous, delicate scroll-like bones, called the ethmoturbinates or ethmoidal conchae.

The mucous membrane of the nasal cavity is lined by a pseudostratified columnar epithelium with numerous goblet cells. Rostrally, this epithelium merges with the skin of the nostrils and vestibule. Numerous mucoserous glands lie within the mucous membrane. The caudodorsal parts of the nasal cavity are covered by a thicker olfactory epithelium.

## Paranasal sinuses

The paranasal sinuses are extensive air-filled spaces lined by a respiratory epithelium. Goblet cells and mucus glands are abundant. The normal removal of mucus is a dynamic process depending on mucociliary flow to the drainage ostia that do not lie at the lowest points in the sinuses. Once the nasal meati are reached, mucus is lost by a combination of evaporation and further mucociliary flow toward the nasopharynx.

There are five main paired paranasal sinuses (Fig. 4.1):

1. Frontal/conchofrontal
2. Caudal maxillary

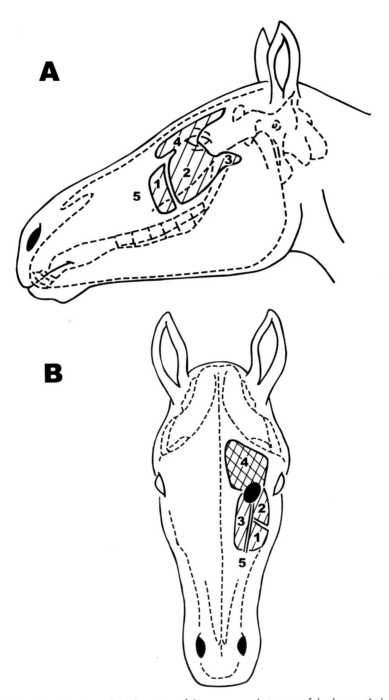

**Fig. 4.1.** Line drawing of the location of the paranasal sinuses of the horse. A. Lateral projection: 1 = rostral maxillary sinus; 2 = caudal maxillary sinus; 3 = sphenopalatine sinus; 4 = frontal sinus; 5 = infraorbital foramen. B. Dorsal projection outlining access to paranasal sinuses for percutaneous centesis: 1 = rostral maxillary sinus; 2 = caudal maxillary sinus; 3 = dorsal conchal sinus; 4 = frontal sinus; 5 = infraorbital foramen, from which the infraorbital canal projects between the maxillary sinus and the dorsal conchal sinus; black oval = frontomaxillary opening.

3. Rostral maxillary
4. Ethmoidal
5. Sphenopalatine

The frontal sinus has a large communication at its rostral end with the dorsal conchal sinus, and it combines with the dorsal conchal sinus to form the conchofrontal sinus. Drainage takes place through the frontomaxillary foramen into the caudal maxillary sinus. The two frontal sinuses are separated along the midline by a bony septum. The rostral limit of the frontal sinus is at a line drawn at right angles from the midline to midway between the medial canthus of the eye and the infraorbital foramen. This corresponds to the point at which the nasal bones lose their parallel course and diverge toward the orbit. The caudal limit of the frontal sinus is at the level of the temporomandibular joint. The lateral limit is a line drawn from the medial canthus to the nasoincisive notch. The ethmoidal labyrinth projects into the floor of the frontal sinus between the orbits.

The maxillary sinus is divided into the rostral maxillary sinus and the caudal maxillary sinus. These cavities represent the largest paranasal sinus in the horse. The dorsal margin of the maxillary sinus is a line drawn from the medial canthus of the eye to the nasoincisive notch. The rostral limit is at the level of the rostral end of the facial crest. The caudal limit is at a line drawn from the middle of the orbit to the facial crest. The ventral limit is parallel and slightly ventral to the facial crest. In young horses (less than 5 years of age), the maxillary sinuses are largely filled with the reserve crowns of the 3rd to 6th cheek teeth (4th premolar, and 1st, 2nd, and 3rd molars). As the horse ages and the cheek teeth become shorter, so the maxillary sinus enlarges and its rostral limit approaches the infraorbital foramen. The position of the bony septum between the rostral and caudal maxillary sinuses is variable, but it is usually directed obliquely across the roots of the 4th and 5th cheek teeth, about 5 cm from the rostral end of the facial crest. The dorsal part of the septum is formed by the caudal bulla of the ventral conchal sinus.

The rostral maxillary sinus is divided into a lateral bony and a medial turbinate portion within the ventral conchus (ventral conchal sinus). They are separated by the infraorbital canal and a sheet of bone joining it ventrally to the roots of the cheek teeth. In the young horse the lateral bony compartment is largely occupied by the roots of the cheek teeth, and regardless of age, the ventral conchal sinus is not easily accessible for surgery other than via the floor of the conchofrontal sinus. The long slit-like communication between the lateral compartment and the ventral conchal sinus is called the conchomaxillary opening. The rostral maxillary sinus has an independent narrow drainage ostium that merges with the drainage aperture from the caudal maxillary sinus into the middle nasal meatus. The roots of the 3rd cheek tooth form the rostral wall of the rostral maxillary sinus.

The caudal maxillary sinus is larger than the rostral maxillary sinus. It has a large opening into the sphenopalatine sinus caudal and medial to the infraorbital canal. It also has a small opening into the middle conchal sinus. Dorsally, the caudal maxillary sinus communicates with the frontal sinus through the frontomaxillary opening; this is a large oval opening measuring approximately 4 x 3 cm. The nasomaxillary opening is a compressed passageway between the caudal maxillary sinus and the middle nasal meatus. It is situated between the rostral edge of the frontomaxillary opening and the caudal bulla of the ventral conchal sinus; this corresponds to the level of the medial canthus of the eye. The ethmoidal and sphenopalatine sinuses also drain via the caudal maxillary sinus into the middle nasal meatus.

The sphenopalatine sinus is a diverticulum of the caudal maxillary sinus. It lies beneath the ethmoidal labyrinth. Several vessels and nerves course through the sphenopalatine sinus, including the optic nerve.

Blood flow to the frontal sinus is mainly from the ethmoidal artery. The maxillary sinus is supplied by the sphenopalatine artery.

## Function
The major functions of the nasal cavity are airflow, warming, moistening and filtration of air, and olfaction. The horse is an obligate nasal breather, and is normally unable to breathe through the mouth. Up to 80–90% of total airway resistance is located within the nasal cavity, most of which is at the level of the nostrils. Airflow through the meati may be enhanced by vasoconstriction of vessels in the ventral conchae and nasal septum.

## EXAMINATION OF THE NASAL CAVITY AND PARANASAL SINUSES

Examination of the nasal cavity and paranasal sinuses can include observing common presenting signs; obtaining an accurate history; physical, endoscopic, and radiographic examinations; computed tomography (CT) and magnetic resonance imaging (MRI); nuclear scintigraphy; percutaneous centesis, and surgical exploration and biopsy.

### Common presenting signs
The clinical signs of nasal and paranasal sinus diseases almost invariably include a nasal discharge, which may be mucoid, purulent, hemorrhagic, or a combination of these. There may also be facial swelling and obstructive dyspnea. Some expansive lesions in this area will displace orbital tissues resulting in exophthalmos but it is exceptional for a sinus disorder to extend caudally into the cranium to provoke central nervous signs. The intranasal structures are richly vascular; therefore, traumatic injury and invasive conditions frequently produce epistaxis.

### History
An accurate history, including the duration of the problem, previous surgery or trauma, previous treatments and effects of the condition on exercise toler-

ance should be obtained. Note should be made of possible contact with contagious respiratory disease. It is unusual for sinusitis to be bilateral, and it is logical that the discharge will be largely unilateral when its origin lies proximal to the caudal limit of the midline septum. When a horse is presented with unilateral epistaxis, inquiries should be made regarding associations with exercise to eliminate a diagnosis of exercise-induced pulmonary hemorrhage. Epistaxis due to guttural pouch mycosis may be acute and, even if episodic, the course of the history is unlikely to exceed 3 weeks. A diagnosis of progressive ethmoidal hematoma is more likely to be correct when episodes of epistaxis span a longer period, especially if the blood is not fresh. A fetid nasal discharge indicates suppuration, but this could arise from a wide range of chronic nasal or sinus lesions.

## Physical examination

The nostrils and external parts of the nasal passages are viewed from directly in front of the horse to determine asymmetry of size or shape, and asymmetry of movement (especially after exercise). Discharge is noted, and airflow at each nostril compared to assess obstruction of the nasal meati. Each nostril can be obstructed in turn to assess airflow on the other side. The nostrils, alar fold, and alar cartilages should be palpated. The facial bones are inspected for evidence of deformity of the supporting bones through swelling or trauma. Percussion of the walls of the paranasal sinuses is an unreliable technique, but increased resonance may be perceived when the walls become thin, or dullness may develop when the sinuses are completely filled by fluid or soft tissue. Percussion is performed by sharply tapping the fingers of one hand against the overlying bone. The corresponding area on the opposite side is immediately percussed afterwards for comparison. If the horse's mouth is held open simultaneously, resonance increases and abnormalities may be easier to detect.

## Endoscopic examination

Endoscopic examination of the nasal area can be performed by conventional passage of the instrument into the nasal meati and, if indicated, direct inspection of the paranasal sinus contents through small trephine holes. Endoscopy is best performed on the standing horse because orientation is straightforward; nasal tissues of the recumbent animal become discolored and engorged.

The nasal meati are examined for evidence of narrowing, conchal distension, or abnormal masses. The region of the sinu-nasal drainage ostium in caudal middle meatus is assessed for evidence of discharge. The ethmoidal labyrinth is examined for evidence of an abnormal mass that might be indicative of progressive ethmoidal hematoma. The mucous membranes of the conchae are examined for evidence of mycotic plaques, ulceration, hemorrhage, or necrosis.

Direct sinus endoscopy can be performed via a trephine hole using a flexible endoscope or an arthroscope. Abnormalities that can be identified by this technique include empyema, dental periapical reactions, mycosis, and progressive ethmoidal hematoma. A small trephine hole can be made into the fronto-conchal sinus (50–60% of the distance between the midline and the medial canthus of the eye) or into the caudal maxillary sinus (2.5–3.0 cm dorsal to the facial crest, 2.5–3.0 cm rostral to the orbit) to allow entry of the endoscope (see Fig. 4.1). A second portal can be made to allow insertion of biopsy forceps or a Ferris-Smith rongeur, which is used to create an opening into the ventral conchal sinus. Thus, introduction of the endoscope into the frontal sinus provides access to the ventral conchal or rostral maxillary sinus. The procedure of direct sinus endoscopy is limited in cases where the sinus is filled with exudate or blood.

## Radiographic examination

The contrast provided between bone and air renders the nasal chambers and paranasal sinuses excellent candidates for radiographic diagnosis. Lateral, lateral oblique, lesion-oriented oblique, and ventro-dorsal views can be obtained. The typical radiographic signs of nasal and paranasal sinus disease include

- Free fluid interfaces in the sinuses (Fig. 4.2)
- Loss of normal air contrast through substitution by fluid or soft tissue
- Depression or elevation of the supporting bones of the face
- Distortion of normal structures, such as the tooth roots, sinus walls, midline septum, and infraorbital canals

## Computed tomography (CT) and magnetic resonance imaging (MRI)

Computed tomography and MRI provide considerable additional diagnostic information regarding the nasal and paranasal sinus diseases. Multiplanar im-

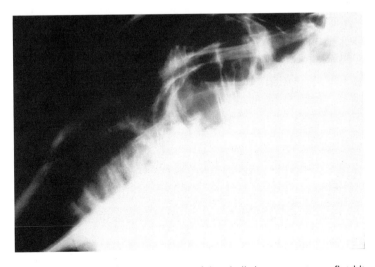

**Fig. 4.2.** Lateral radiographic projections of the skull demonstrating a fluid line in the caudal maxillary sinus above the 6th upper cheek tooth.

ages, without superimposition of overlying structures, allow the clinician to view the exact location, extent, and condition of adjacent structures in horses with masses, infection, or trauma to the nasal passages and paranasal sinuses (Fig. 4.3). However, the expense, necessity for general anesthesia, and lack of availability of this technology limits its use to referral facilities.

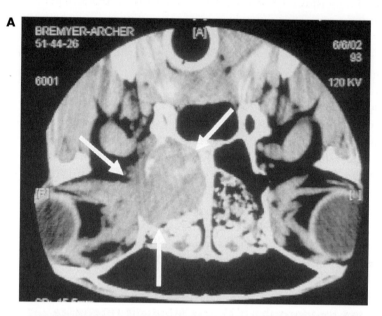

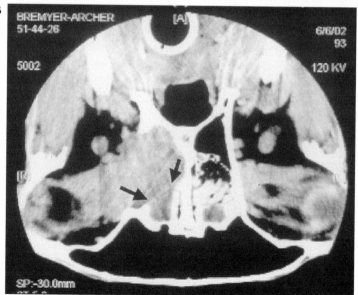

**Fig. 4.3.** Computed tomographic images of a horse with a retrobulbar neoplastic mass invading the ethmoidal conchae and the calvarium at the level of the frontal lobe. The extent of the sinus mass is denoted by the white arrows (A), and invasion of the calvarium is denoted by the black arrows (B).

### Nuclear scintigraphy

The diagnosis of dental periapical disease and determination of which tooth root is involved is not always straightforward. Radiographic changes may be subtle, and the superimposition of other structures on standard views makes the interpretation of radiographs difficult, especially in early dental disease. Because many disorders are associated with pathological change in adjacent bone, nuclear scintigraphy can be helpful in confirming the presence of dental disease and in determining which tooth root is diseased. Often the combination of results of both radiography and scintigraphy are necessary.

### Percutaneous centesis

Fluid samples may be obtained from the frontal or maxillary sinuses of standing horses, using local anesthesia. Following aseptic skin preparation, a 1 cm long incision is made in the skin and subcutaneous tissues, and a sterile 2–4mm diameter Steinmann pin attached to a Jacob's chuck is used to penetrate the thin bone plate overlying the sinus cavity. A small sterile catheter can then be passed into the sinus to permit aspiration of a sample of fluid. Lavage with a small volume of sterile saline may be necessary to obtain an adequate sample in cases where the fluid is very viscous. The fluid sample can be used for cytological examination, Gram stain, bacteriological culture, and sensitivity testing. The same technique can be used to permit flushing of the sinus; as long as the nasomaxillary drainage aperture is patent, instillation of large volumes of fluid into the sinus will result in drainage out of the nose.

   If the horse has long-standing sinus disease and facial swelling, the overlying bone plate is frequently very thin and a 16 gauge needle may be used to penetrate the bone without prior drilling. The sites for centesis are determined by clinical and radiographic findings, but in general they are similar for those used for direct sinus endoscopy. For the caudal maxillary sinus, a site 2.5–3 cm dorsal to the facial crest and 2.5–3 cm rostral to the medial canthus is used. If the rostral maxillary sinus is to be sampled, a site 3 cm dorsal to the facial crest and approximately 3 cm caudal to the infraorbital foramen is selected (see Fig. 4.1).

### Surgical exploration and biopsy

Even after full endoscopic and radiographic investigations, surgical exploration may be required before a specific diagnosis can been made. Suspect tissues may be biopsied to differentiate neoplastic disorders from other disease processes.

## TREATMENT OBJECTIVES IN NASAL AND SINUS DISEASE

The treatment objectives for horses with nasal cavity and paranasal sinus disease can be summarized as follows:

1. Accurate diagnosis of the primary disorder and removal of diseased tissue
2. Restoration of the normal drainage mechanisms or the creation of alternative drainage through a sinu-nasal fistula
3. Adequate visibility within the sinuses and nasal meati for accurate diagnosis and surgery
4. Control hemorrhage during surgery and recovery
5. A secured airway during surgery and recovery
6. Facilities for topical postoperative treatments and monitoring progress
7. Early return to exercise
8. An esthetic cosmetic outcome

## MEDICAL MANAGEMENT

Nonsurgical treatments for sinusitis include antibiotics, mucolytics, steam inhalations, volatile inhalations, and controlled exercise. The objective is the return of normal mucociliary clearance. Most cases of simple primary sinusitis will be resolved either naturally or with minimal veterinary assistance, provided that the necessary supportive management is instituted promptly.

## TREPHINATION OF THE PARANASAL SINUSES

Trephination allows limited access to the paranasal sinuses. The procedure can be performed in the standing, sedated horse to allow direct endoscopic examination, aspiration, lavage, biopsy, and limited surgical procedures. In cases of maxillary sinusitis, the bony septum between the rostral and caudal maxillary sinuses can be broken down via trephine holes, and this improves drainage from and between the sinus cavities. Irrigation and topical antibiotic infusions are used to help clearance of stagnant mucus and eliminate secondary infection. Indwelling balloon catheters provide a means for daily irrigation until discharge to the nostril ceases. Tooth repulsion can be performed through a trephine hole with the horse placed under general anesthesia.

For generalized sinusitis, a trephine hole can be placed into the frontal sinus at a point midway between the medial canthus of the eye and the dorsal midline of the skull (see Fig. 4.1). For specific trephination of the frontal portion of the frontal sinus, the landmarks are 4 cm from midline on a line joining the supraorbital processes. For the conchal portion of the frontal sinus, a site 5 cm from the midline at a level 3–4 cm caudal to the rostral end of the facial crest can be used. The preferred site for trephination is into the caudal maxillary sinus in the angle formed between the margin of the bony orbit and the facial crest. The rostral maxillary sinus is less available for simple trephination, especially in young horses where the lateral compartment is largely occupied by the roots and reserve crowns of the 3rd and 4th cheek teeth. A point 2.5 cm caudal and 3.5 cm dorsal to the rostral limit of the facial crest allows access to the rostral maxillary sinus in older horses. In young horses, a site at the level of the infraorbital foramen and 2 cm caudal to the end of the facial crest allows access to the ventral conchal sinus over the infraorbital canal.

Following routine skin preparation, the chosen site for trephination is infiltrated subcutaneously with local anesthetic solution. A circle of skin is marked with the trephine and excised with a scalpel, along with the subcutaneous tissue and fascia. The trocar point of the trephine is used to drill a small hole in the bone that stabilizes the trephine as it is rotated to cut through the bone. The plug of bone is removed, thereby allowing direct access to the sinus cavity. The trephine hole will heal by granulation, and usually closes within 21–30 days. To prevent premature closure, the hole can be plugged with a rolled plug of sterile gauze.

## BONE FLAP SURGERY

Bone flap techniques allow greater access to the sinus cavities than can be achieved via trephine holes. Frontonasal or maxillary flap surgery is required for extensive excisional procedures, such as the removal of sinus cysts, progressive ethmoidal hematomas, and selected tumors, as well as for the relief of chronic sinusitis. In the face of chronic sinusitis, sinus cyst, and progressive ethmoidal hematoma, the natural drainage system of the sinuses may be physically obstructed. Fistulae can be made to improve drainage in such cases. These include removal of the floor of the conchofrontal sinus and the medial wall of the ventral conchal sinus so that there is free communication between the sinus cavities and the nasal meati. Additional drainage from the caudal maxillary sinus is achieved by removal of the septum, dividing it from the rostral maxillary sinus. The bulla of the rostral maxillary sinus may bulge caudally into the caudal maxillary sinus when it is inflated by purulent exudate, and it can easily be broken down. In older horses, a secondary fistula through the bone plate ventral to the infraorbital canal provides communication between the lateral bony compartment and the ventral conchal sinus.

A variety of different surgical techniques for bone plate surgery have been described, but basically the surgical choice is between a fronto-nasal flap and a lateral (maxillary) flap (Fig. 4.4). Lesser decisions relate to the size and shape of the bone flap, the direction in which the skin/periosteal flap is raised, and whether to reject or preserve the bone flap. A frontonasal flap approach allows access to the conchofrontal and caudal maxillary sinuses; additional dissection will allow access to the rostral maxillary sinus and ventral conchal sinus. The lateral approach into the maxillary sinuses provides limited access, and it should be reserved for those instances where the disease process is restricted to the maxillary compartments; older horses are most suitable.

Although bone flap surgery is most commonly performed under general anesthesia, a fronto-nasal flap approach has been described in the standing

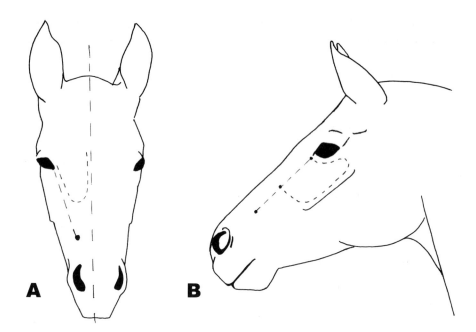

**Fig. 4.4.** Examples of different bone flap configurations, showing the line from the medial canthus of the eye to the nasoincisive notch: caudally-based frontal flap (A) and maxillary "up flap" (B).

horse. One advantage of performing this surgery in the standing patient is a reduction in the amount of hemorrhage.

Incisions are made through skin and periosteum in the same plane before the periosteum is peeled away from the underlying bone. The bone flap is best fashioned with an oscillating saw, but handsaws or a series of trephine holes can also be used. Once the sinus contents are exposed, the disease focus is identified and removed. Pressure packing of the sinus cavities and nasal chambers is essential to control hemorrhage on completion of the surgery and during the initial recovery period. Sock-and-bandage packing consisting of lengths of cotton bandage packed into tubular stockinette socks is suitable. The open end of the stockinette is led to the nostril. Closure of the incision can be achieved with a single layer of mattress sutures, but accurate alignment is required for the best cosmetic result in horses with natural facial markings.

Temporary bilateral carotid occlusion can reduce hemorrhage and improve visibility during the intraluminal stages of sinus flap surgery. The advantages in terms of hemorrhage control must be weighed against the disadvantages of prolonging the surgery and the risk of iatrogenic damage to the vagosympathetic trunks. A cuffed endotracheal tube is essential to protect the lower airways from the inhalation of blood, purulent exudate, surgical debris, and irrigation fluids during surgery.

A Foley balloon catheter implanted into the frontal or caudal maxillary sinuses offers a convenient route for postsurgical irrigation and medication.

Blood clots and devitalized tissue are inevitably left after facial flap surgery, and opportunistic infections, frequently mycoses, are likely. Balloon catheters are therefore recommended as a routine to permit physical displacement of debris by irrigation. The topical medication should include an antimycotic agent.

## FURTHER READING

Freeman, D.E. 1991. Paranasal sinuses. In *Equine Respiratory Disorders*. J. Beech, ed. Philadelphia: Lea & Febiger, pp 275–303.

Freeman, D.E. 2003. Diagnosis of sinus diseases. In *Current Therapy in Equine Medicine*, 5th ed. N.E. Robinson, ed. Philadelphia: W.B. Saunders, pp 369–374.

Freeman, D.E. 2003. Sinus disease. *Vet Clinics N Am Equine Pract* 19:209–243.

Lane, J.G. 1998. Disorders of the ear, nose and throat. In *Equine Medicine, Surgery and Reproduction*. T. Mair, S. Love, J. Schumacher, and E. Watson, eds. London: W.B. Saunders, pp 81–117.

Ruggles, A.J., Ross, M.W., and Freeman, D.E. 1991. Endoscopic examination of normal paranasal sinuses in horses. *Vet Surg* 20:418–423.

Weller, R., Livesey, Maierl, J., Nuss, K., Bowen, I.M., Cauvin, E.R., Weaver, M., Schumacher, J., and May, S.A. 2001. Comparison of radiography and scintigraphy in the diagnosis of dental disorders in the horse. *Equine Vet J* 33:49–58.

# Congenital and Developmental Malformations of the Nasal Cavity

Congenital and developmental malformations of the nasal cavity include wry nose, nasal septal deviation, and choanal atresia/stenosis.

## WRY NOSE

Wry nose is a congenital deformity of the nose resulting from gross foreshortening of the premaxilla on one side. There is deviation of the maxilla, nasal bone, incisive bone, and nasal septum to one side. There may be a corresponding, but milder, deviation of the mandible. Malocclusion of the incisor teeth, and sometimes premolar teeth, is present, and there may be an abnormal respiratory noise. Nursing may or may not be affected. The deformity is not thought to be genetically transmitted but may be due to abnormal fetal positioning in utero.

In very mild cases, some spontaneous improvement can be expected with time. In severe cases, surgical treatment can be considered. However, even radical surgery is unlikely to render the horse capable of serious exercise. Surgical correction generally involves at least two procedures. The first stage is aimed at correcting maxillary alignment by performing an osteotomy in the premaxilla; Steinmann pins or an external fixator is used to stabilize the repair. A bone graft may be used to repair the gap left in the maxilla. The second surgery involves realignment of the nasal bone and nasal resection if necessary. The nostrils can also be enlarged as necessary.

## NASAL SEPTAL DEVIATION

Congenital deviation of the nasal septum is invariably present in cases of wry nose but may also occur as an independent entity. It may not come to light until the horse commences training and investigations into the cause of abnormal respiratory noise take place. Permanent damage to the nasal septum has also been recognized in foals where the halter has not been replaced and the nose has outgrown the noseband. Occasionally deviation and damage to the nasal septum may result from external trauma.

Clinical signs include stertorous breathing and dyspnea during exercise, usually in young horses. The abnormal respiratory noise is usually loudest during inspiration.

Digital palpation may indicate an abnormality of the rostral end of the nasal septum. There may be a history of difficulty in passing a nasogastric tube through one nasal passage. Although a diagnosis of septal deviation may be suggested by endoscopy, the diagnosis can be confirmed only by radiography in the ventro-dorsal plane showing that the septum is deviated away from the midline position and/or abnormally thickened.

Septal resection is a feasible treatment for septal disorders in horses. Hemorrhage is profuse with this surgery, and a compatible blood donor should be available. The nasal cavity is packed following resection of the septum, so a temporary tracheotomy must be provided. The standard surgical technique involves creating a trephine hole into the nasal cavity in the dorsal midline immediately rostral to the frontal sinus (at the level where the nasal bones diverge from a parallel course toward the medial canthus of the eye). The nasal septum is grasped with forceps inserted through the trephine hole. The rostral end of the nasal septum is then incised in a vertical direction, and a guarded chisel used to sever the dorsal and ventral attachments back to the level of the forceps. The septum is then cut with a chisel along the line of the forceps, and the freed septum is retrieved through the nostrils. The nasal cavity is then packed with sterile gauze. Modifications of this technique involve cutting the caudal part of the septum at an oblique angle to remove a greater part of the caudal septum, and using obstetrical wire to make the horizontal cuts in the septum.

An alternative technique involves resection of the septum via a bone flap. A rectangular bone flap the same size as the portion of septum to be removed is created. The dorsal attachments of the septum are cut with a saw. Forceps are placed at the rostral and caudal limits of the portion of septum to be removed, and vertical incisions made at these levels with a chisel. The ventral attachments of the septum are then broken by rocking the septum back and forth.

Postoperatively, the packing is removed after 48–72 hours. The nasal cavity is lavaged through the trephine hole to remove blood and debris. The tracheotomy tube can be removed at the same time.

## CHOANAL ATRESIA/STENOSIS

Choanal atresia or stenosis is a congenital obstruction or narrowing of the airways at the level where the nasal meati meet the nasopharynx. This site corresponds with location of the bucconasal membrane in the developing fetus. This membrane should perforate and retract well before term so that the foal can commence nose breathing immediately after birth. Persistence of the bucconasal membrane usually occurs as a membranous septum, and can be uni- or bilateral. The membrane causes severe obstruction to nose-breathing with no air movement through the diseased side. Bilateral cases may asphyxiate rapidly, or the foal may learn to mouth-breathe.

Diagnosis is achieved by physical examination (lack of airflow through the nostril on the affected side) and endoscopic examination. Contrast radiography can also be used to delineate the deformity. Affected horses show limited athletic capacity. Although surgical removal of the occluding membrane via a frontonasal bone flap has been described, it is unlikely that the animal will be capable of intense exercise. Stents may be placed for 6–8 weeks after surgery to maintain patency of the airway. Repeated bougienage has also been suggested as a possible treatment. Some affected foals will have other, concurrent, congenital abnormalities, and a careful evaluation should be performed prior to considering surgical treatment.

## FURTHER READING

Freeman, D.E. 1991. Nasal passages. In *Equine Respiratory Disorders*. J. Beech, ed. Philadelphia: Lea & Febiger, pp 253–273.

Goring, R.L., Campbell, M., and Hillidge, C.J. 1984. Surgical correction of congenital bilateral choanal atresia in a foal *Vet Surg* 13:211–216.

McKellar, G.M.W., and Collins, A.P. 1993. The surgical correction of a deviated anterior maxilla in a horse. *Aust Vet J* 70:112–114.

Richardson, J.D., Lane, J.G., and Day, M.J. 1994. Congenital choanal restriction in 3 horses. *Equine Vet J* 26:162–165.

Sullivan, E.K., and Parente, E.J. 2003. Disorders of the pharynx. *Vet Clinics N Am Equine Pract* 19:159–167.

Tulleners, E.P., and Raker, C.W. 1983. Nasal septum resection in the horse. *Vet Surg* 12:41–47.

Valdez, H., McMullen, W.C., Hobson, H.P. 1978. Surgical correction of a deviated nasal septum and premaxilla in a colt. *J Am Vet Med Assoc* 173:1001–1004.

# Diseases Affecting the Nostrils (External Nares)

## HYPERTROPHY OF ALAR FOLDS/REDUNDANT ALAR FOLDS

It is normal for the alar folds that form the floor of the false nostril to vibrate during exhalation. This is the origin of the vibrant expiratory noise known as "high blowing." Occasionally, horses will produce a similar vibrant sound during inspiration; this is considered to be abnormal. Excessive or thickened alar folds, or a functional problem involving the transversus nasi muscle (which normally elevates the alar cartilages and closes the nasal diverticulum during exercise) have been proposed as causes.

Clinical signs include a biphasic harsh whistling or snoring noise during exercise. The expiratory noise is louder than the inspiratory noise. In most cases there is no obvious effect on exercise tolerance, but in a few cases the flaccid alar folds can cause a partial obstruction and increase upper airway resistance. Confirmation that the origin of the noise lies at the alar folds is achieved by placing full thickness mattress sutures from the skin at the dorsal aspect of the nose across the openings of the false nostrils. The technique is performed under local anesthesia so that the noise can be compared before and after suture placement.

Treatment of hypertrophied or redundant alar folds consists of bilateral resection of the fold. The surgery is performed under general anesthesia. Although the surgery can be performed through the external nares, the procedure is more easily performed after incision of the lateral wall of the external nares (i.e., via a rhinotomy). The alar fold is incised at its junction with the lamina of the alar cartilage and dissected caudally to the caudal limit of the nasal diverticulum. A second incision is made caudally from the medial attachment of the alar fold to meet the previous incision. This results in resection of a portion of the cartilage of the ventral concha (medial accessory cartilage). Copius hemorrhage is expected. The incision is sutured using a simple continuous pattern with an absorbable suture material.

## EPIDERMAL INCLUSION CYST ("ATHEROMA") OF THE FALSE NOSTRIL

Epidermal inclusion cysts are fluid-filled cystic structures located at the caudal aspect of the nasal diverticulum. They are painless and can usually be seen at the dorsal aspect of the nose, rostral to the naso-maxillary notch (Fig. 6.1). Although the swellings can be sizable, they do not obstruct respiration and are of cosmetic significance only. They are usually unilateral.

Cysts may be treated by drainage or surgical removal. However, treatment is required only for cosmetic reasons. The cyst can be lanced through the nasal diverticulum and allowed to heal by secondary intention. The cyst cavity may also be thoroughly swabbed with a counterirritant, such as 2% tincture of iodine. Recurrence is common following these treatments. Surgical excision of

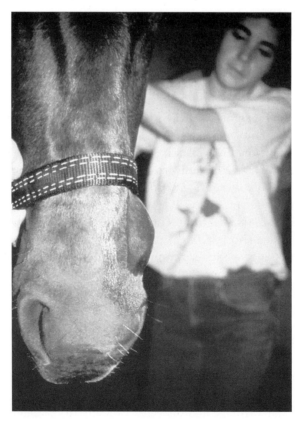

**Fig. 6.1.** Epidermal inclusion cyst (atheroma) located at the caudal aspect of the nasal diverticulum (false nostril).

the cyst can be performed in the standing horse using local anesthetic infiltration or an infraorbital nerve block. The cyst is carefully dissected out via a longitudinal dorsal skin incision. Alternatively, the cyst can be removed via a ventral approach inside the nasal diverticulum. Recurrence is improbable after surgical excision.

## LACERATIONS AND WOUNDS OF THE NOSTRILS

Wounds to the nostrils are common. Wherever possible, first intention healing should be the primary aim of treatment. Wounds are debrided and wound edges carefully apposed. Failure to achieve first intention healing may lead to significant scarring and stenosis of the nostril. This is likely to have a significant effect on upper airway resistance and may result in exercise intolerance. Treatment to enlarge a stenotic nostril can be attempted using a double apposing Z-plasty.

## ALAR CARTILAGE NECROSIS

Neglected penetration injuries of the alar cartilages may be followed by the extension of suppuration into the cartilage matrix. Careful resection of the diseased tissue is required but loss of mechanical stability at this location represents a serious complication.

## PARALYSIS OF THE NOSTRILS

The facial nerve (cranial nerve VII) is predominantly motor innervating the muscles of facial expression. It innervates the muscles that retract the walls of the nostrils and collapse the nasal diverticulum. Damage to this nerve therefore results in an inability to dilate the nostril during exercise and deep inspiration. Facial paralysis is generally recognized as a drooping of the ear and lips, ptosis of the upper eyelid, retraction of the nose toward the unaffected side, and protrusion of the tongue out of the affected side. Facial nerve paralysis can have numerous causes, and may occur as a result of either central or peripheral damage. The prognosis depends on the underlying cause. In cases of permanent paralysis, improvement of airflow and exercise tolerance can be achieved by surgical resection of the skin over the nostrils along the edges of the nasoincisive notch and removing the alar folds.

## FURTHER READING

Bowman, K.F., Swaim, S.F., and Vaughan, J.T. 1982. Double opposing Z-plasty for correction of stenotic naris in a horse. *J Am Vet Med Assoc* 180:772.

Foerner, J.J. 1971. The diagnosis and correction of false nostril noises. In *Proc 23rd Ann Conv Am Assoc Equine* Pract, pp 315–327.

Freeman, D.E. 1991. Nasal passages. In *Equine Respiratory Disorders*. J. Beech, ed. Philadelphia: Lea & Febiger, pp 253–273.

Nickels, F.A., and Tulleners, E.P. 1992. Nasal passages. In *Equine Surgery*. J.A. Auer, ed. Philadelphia: W.B. Saunders, pp 433–446.

Stashak, T.S. 1991. *Equine Wound Management*. Baltimore: Williams and Wilkins, pp 89–144.

# Diseases of the Nasal Cavity and Paranasal Sinuses

## PRIMARY AND SECONDARY SINUSITIS AND SINUS EMPYEMA

Sinusitis may be primary (associated with stagnation of mucus due to defective mucociliary clearance) or secondary (most commonly due to dental periapical disease):

- Clinical signs include a unilateral mucopurulent or purulent nasal discharge, which may be malodorous.
- Facial swelling and nasal occlusion may occur.
- Diagnosis is made on the basis of the clinical signs, endoscopy, and radiography.
- Early cases of primary sinusitis may respond to antibiotic therapy.
- Established cases of primary sinusitis require irrigation of the sinuses via a catheter implanted through a trephine hole.
- Chronic cases may require facial bone flap surgery to permit evacuation of inspissated pus, and fistulation to aid drainage into the nasal cavity.
- The primary disease must be treated (usually tooth extraction) in secondary sinusitis.

Primary sinusitis and empyema result from the stagnation of mucus in the sinuses due to damage to the dynamic mucociliary clearance system. Most commonly, this is initiated by infection with upper respiratory tract viral agents or *Streptococcus* spp. Initially the dependent portions of the sinuses fill with mucus that passively spills through the drainage ostia into the nasal meati. Secondary bacterial infection follows, exacerbating the mucosal inflammation and leading to purulent exudation. Hyperplasia of the sinus lining is a feature of sinusitis; this narrows the drainage ostia and further impedes mu-cociliary clearance. Inspissation of purulent exudate develops in the later stages, which further occludes the ostia. The conchal walls of the sinuses are not rigid, and in the face of obstructed drainage there is a tendency for them to expand and to obstruct the nasal airways.

Secondary (dental) sinusitis is a sequel to dental periapical suppuration. The roots of the 3rd to 6th maxillary cheek teeth lie within the maxillary sinuses and are covered by a thin layer of alveolar bone and mucosa. Whenever these teeth are devitalized by fracture or infundibular necrosis there is the possi-bility of secondary sinusitis. Older ponies with Cushing's disease appear to be predisposed to chronic or recurrent sinusitis, either as a consequence of periodontitis and/or associated with immunosuppression due to hyperadreno-corticism.

## Clinical signs

In the acute stages, primary sinus empyema produces a mucoid-based, unilat-eral nasal discharge. As the condition becomes more chronic, the discharge be-comes more purulent and malodorous. The discharge of secondary (dental) sinusitis is invariably purulent and often malodorous. It is generally less pro-fuse than with primary empyema. Occasionally, sinus tracts can extend from the involved cheek teeth to the overlying skin.

Primary and secondary sinusitis are rarely bilateral conditions. The dis-charge is occasionally blood-flecked and is often more profuse after exercise. Facial swelling, over the maxillary sinuses, and nasal obstruction are later fea-tures of primary empyema, but rarely occur with secondary empyema. Exer-cise intolerance and abnormal respiratory noises at exercise may occur in chronic empyema. Submandibular lymphadenopathy is sometimes present, and epiphora is occasionally seen with or without facial deformity.

Neurological signs associated with extension of infection from the frontal sinus through the cribiform plate to cause meningoencephalitis occur rarely. Severe infections involving the sphenopalatine sinus can result in blindness, ex-ophthalmos, strabismus, pituitary abscess, and meningitis (Fig. 7.1).

## Diagnosis

The diagnosis of sinusitis is often based on history and clinical signs. The pres-ence and nature of nasal discharge and facial deformity should be noted. The airflow at the external nares is compared; reduced airflow suggests obstruction of the meati which may be caused by distension of the conchal sinuses. Percussion may reveal loss of resonance if the sinus spaces are filled by puru-lent exudate, but this technique is unreliable when filling is incomplete. An oral inspection is performed to evaluate the cheek teeth for fractures, displace-ment, infundibular necrosis, or periodontal disease.

Endoscopic examination may show a flow of discharge from the caudal re-gion of the middle nasal meatus where the sinus drainage ostium is located. Conchal enlargement and narrowing of the meati may also be identified.

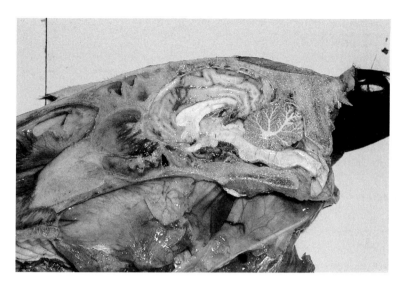

**Fig. 7.1.** Sagittal section of the head of a horse with chronic sinusitis involving the sphenopalatine sinus. The infection has extended into the pituitary gland, causing focal meningitis and disruption of the endocrine function of the pituitary.

Radiography is used to demonstrate free horizontal gas/fluid interfaces (see Chapter 4, Fig. 4.2) or, when the sinuses are full, total loss of air contrast. Mineralization of the sinus contents may be appreciated in chronic cases. Primary sinusitis usually involves all sinus cavities and causes diffuse fluid opacification. In some cases, it can be confined to the ventral conchal sinus, where it forms an abscess that can be difficult to see radiographically. It is important to assess the possibility of dental suppuration as the cause of secondary sinusitis, and oblique views and/or intraoral views are recommended. The teeth most commonly involved, in decreasing order of frequency, are the 4th cheek tooth (first molar), 3rd cheek tooth (4th premolar) and 2nd cheek tooth (3rd premolar).

## Treatment

Early cases of primary sinusitis can be treated nonsurgically using systemic antibiotics, volatile or steam inhalations, and continued light exercise. Those which do not respond to conservative measures should be managed by the implantation of a catheter into the appropriate sinus compartment(s) via a trephine hole, but this usually means the caudal maxillary sinus, which communicates with all of the sinuses except for the rostral maxillary sinus. The catheter is used for topical antibiotic infusion in addition to physical irrigation. A free flow of lavage to the nostrils implies that the drainage ostia are clear, and this is an optimistic sign.

Refractory cases, typically where there is poor drainage during irrigation and a putrid nasal discharge, are candidates for facial flap surgery. Endoscopic and radiological re-assessments are performed to confirm the location of empyema and to determine which technique to use. The objectives of surgery in the management of chronic sinusitis are to break down intercompartmental barriers, thus converting sinuses into a common air space, and to create generous fistulae into the nasal meati.

The treatment of secondary sinusitis involves removal of the diseased tooth or other primary disease process, followed by treatment of the chronic sinusitis as described above. Unsuccessful treatment or recurrence of sinusitis indicates the persistence of diseased tissue, including dental fragments, sequestrae, or osteitis/osteomyelitis.

## Prognosis

The prognosis for primary sinusitis is generally good. Only a minority of cases of sinus empyema require surgical intervention, and of those which do, the overwhelming majority are resolved by simple trephination and catheterization. The prognosis for secondary empyema and chronic empyema with bony involvement is less favorable. Repeated surgical procedures are not infrequently required to remove all diseased tissue.

## PROGRESSIVE ETHMOIDAL HEMATOMA

Progressive ethmoidal hematomas are non-neoplastic masses that usually arise from the nasal or sinus surfaces of the ethmoidal labyrinth:

- Repeated low-grade epistaxis is the most common presenting sign.
- Diagnosis is aided by endoscopic and radiographic examination.
- Treatment options include surgical resection, cryogenic ablation, laser ablation, and chemical ablation with intralesional formalin.

Progressive ethmoidal hematomas are slowly progressive, expansive, non-neoplastic masses that arise beneath the mucosa in the caudal nasal cavity or paranasal sinuses. The etiology of the lesions is not known, but a congenital or acquired hemangiomatous lesion has been proposed. It appears that repeated submucosal hemorrhages cause these expanding lesions to develop on the surface of the ethmoidal turbinate labyrinth. Lesions may arise on the nasal or sinus aspects of the ethmoidal labyrinth, or occasionally elsewhere in the sinuses. The mucosal capsule splits intermittently, releasing a bloody discharge. The expanding mass may compromise sinus drainage, resulting in a secondary retention of mucus. Alternatively, the nasal airways may become obstructed causing dyspnea. In extreme cases the mass may be extruded at the nares. Lesions occur bilaterally in about 15% of cases.

The lesions are composed of a thick fibrous capsule covered with respiratory epithelium. The fibrous stroma is filled with recent and old hemorrhage. There is an inflammatory infiltrate composed of plasma cells, lymphocytes, neutrophils, and eosinophils. Some areas show necrosis.

## Clinical signs

Progressive ethmoidal hematomas occur in all age groups, but predominantly in horses over 4 years of age, with the incidence increasing with age. All breeds can be affected, but there may be an increased prevalence in Arabians and Thoroughbreds, and decreased prevalence in Standardbreds. Females appear to be at greater risk than males.

The most consistent clinical sign is repeated low-grade epistaxis or a non-odorous sero-hemorrhagic discharge from one nostril. The blood is not fresh and epistaxis is not related to exercise. Between episodes of hemorrhage, unilateral nasal discharge may be present.

Varying degrees of nasal obstruction occur. An adventitious respiratory noise may be present at exercise, and in severe cases a stertorous noise and respiratory distress may be present at rest. Facial swelling is unusual, but may occur as a late feature. Large masses may extend as far as the nasopharynx and cause dysphagia. Rarely the mass can cause pressure on, or infiltrate through, the cribriform plate (typically ventrally) resulting in central nervous signs including blindness. Other less common signs that have been noted in cases of progressive ethmoidal hematomas include coughing, purulent nasal discharge, exophthalmos, and headshaking. The lesion rarely extends along the nasal cavity to become visible at the nares (Fig. 7.2).

## Diagnosis

Diagnosis of progressive ethmoidal hematoma is based on the clinical history, physical examination, endoscopic examination, and radiography. Percussion of the sinuses may identify increased resonance if the walls are becoming thin. Endoscopic examination per nasum will reveal those progressive ethmoidal hematomas arising from the nasal surfaces of the eth-

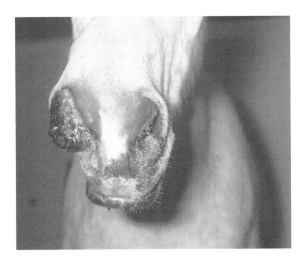

**Fig. 7.2.** Ethmoidal hematoma projecting out of the right nostril from a 15-year-old Arabian gelding. The gelding had loss of airflow from the affected nostril for more than one year.

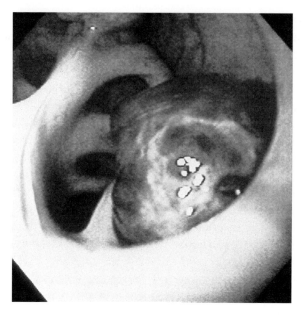

**Fig. 7.3.** Ethmoidal hematoma viewed from the middle meatus and positioned adjacent to the greater ethmoid turbinate.

moidal labyrinth. The lesion usually appears as a smooth walled mass pushing forward from the caudal nasal region (Fig. 7.3). There may be surface hemorrhages and it may appear to be ulcerated. Sometimes, fungal plaques are present on the surface of the lesion. The color of the lesions is variable ranging from yellow/orange to grey/green. A large ethmoidal hematoma may extend caudally around the nasal septum into the contralateral nasal cavity and obscure the contralateral ethmoidal labyrinth. Such a lesion may initially give the impression that there are bilateral hematomas present. Both nasal cavities should be examined in all cases because of the possibility of bilateral involvement. Lesions that arise in the sinuses are usually not visible per nasum; however, a stream of blood may be seen emerging from the sinus drainage ostium. Occasionally, a sinus-based lesion will erode into the nasal cavity or protrude into the nasal cavity through the nasomaxillary aperture. Direct sinus endoscopy through the caudal maxillary or frontal sinuses is often required for a definitive diagnosis of lesions within the sinuses.

Radiographic examination in the standing position (lateral projection) usually reveals a soft tissue mass extending rostral or dorsal to the ethmoidal labyrinth into the caudal maxillary sinus or frontal sinus respectively. Fluid lines may be present due to secondary infection or hemorrhage into the sinuses. Small lesions, especially those within the ethmoidal labyrinth may be obscured by superimposition of the eyes and ethmoidal labyrinth. On the dorsoventral view, a mass may be seen in the nasal passages impinging on the nasal septum. A hematoma confined to the sphenopalatine sinus will not be visible on radiographs or on endoscopy per nasum; diagnosis can be achieved by direct sinus endoscopy in such cases. Computed tomographic scanning or MRI is helpful if available.

## Treatment

Treatment options include surgical ablation, laser photoablation, cryogenic ablation, snare excision, and intralesional injection of formalin, or a combination of these. The choice of treatment modality is dependent on the size, position, and accessibility of the lesion, and available equipment.

Ablation via a frontonasal facial flap can be used for lesions within the sinus or within the nasal cavity. Lesions within the sinuses are easily accessible, but nasal lesions require removal of the floor of the conchofrontal sinus. The lesions are rarely withdrawn without rupture of the mucosal sac, but the basal area should be subjected to thorough curettage. Severe intraoperative hemorrhage is likely, and intravenous isotonic fluid therapy is advisable during surgery. Facilities for a blood transfusion are recommended.

Cryogenic ablation of small ethmoidal hematomas on the nasal side of the ethmoidal labyrinth can be performed under endoscopic guidance, with the horse standing, using liquid nitrogen spray. This treatment can be used to augment surgical debulking of the mass, by ablating the base of the lesion intraoperatively. Control of hemorrhage is necessary before the latter technique can be applied. Care must be taken not to freeze the cribiform plate.

Nd:YAG laser ablation is suitable for small lesions on the nasal portion of the ethmoidal labyrinth, less than about 5 cm in diameter. The horse is sedated, and topical local anesthetic solution applied to the lesion and nasal passage. A non-contact technique is generally used. Multiple treatments at 7-day intervals are usually required. Laser excision can also be used in conjunction with conventional surgery via a frontonasal bone flap. The attachment of the origin of the lesion is severed with the laser.

Intralesional injection of 10% buffered formalin solution (i.e., 4% aqueous solution of formaldehyde gas) can be performed through a flexible endoscope. This method avoids the hemorrhage associated with many of the other treatment options. With the horse standing and sedated, 10–20 ml of formalin can be injected via a catheter passed through the endoscope until the solution is seen leaking out of the mass. With large lesions, more than 20 ml of formalin may be required. This treatment results in necrosis and sloughing of the mass over a period of 2–3 weeks. Repeated treatments are necessary every 3–4 weeks until the lesion has resolved. A lesion in the sinus can also be treated in this way via an endoscope inserted through a trephine hole. Nonsteroidal antiflammatory therapy is recommended following formalin treatment. Fatal neurologic complication has been reported after intralesional formalin administration, whereby the ethmoidal hematoma had been longstanding and invaded the cribiform plate. Neurologic signs were evident 15 minutes after intralesional injection of the mass, and the horse was euthanized within 24 hours.

## Prognosis

The prognosis following treatment is guarded to good. Reported recurrence rates after surgical excision have ranged from 14–45%. Recurrence often occurs within 18 months. Repeated endoscopic examinations (6 monthly) after treatment are recommended to identify recurrence at an early stage. A higher risk of recurrence is present in horses with bilateral lesions. Recurrence may be due to regrowth of the original lesion, due to incomplete removal, or a new lesion may develop.

## PARANASAL SINUS CYSTS

Paranasal sinus cysts occur in young horses (<1 year) or older horses (>4 years):

• A fluid-filled cystic lesion develops in the maxillary or ventral conchal sinus.
• Clinical signs include facial swelling and nasal obstruction.
• Diagnosis is based on history, clinical findings, endoscopic examination, and radiographic examination.

Paranasal sinus cysts are single- or multiloculated fluid-filled structures with an epithelial lining that usually develop in the maxillary sinus or ventral concha. They can extend into the frontal sinus. The etiology of sinus cysts is not known, but they appear to have features common with progressive ethmoidal hematomas because the two conditions may occur concurrently and both show evidence of repeated hemorrhage. Cysts typically contain vivid yellow fluid indicative of blood pigment degradation. Sinus cysts usually arise in the region of the drainage ostium so that expansion either occurs into the sinus or into the nasal meati.

## Clinical signs

Sinus cysts tend to occur either in the first year of life or in horses over 4 years old. Nasal obstruction and facial swelling are typical presenting signs. Facial swelling generally occurs over the conchofrontal or maxillary sinuses, but a small number of cases have midline frontal distension. Nasal discharge may or may not be present and, rarely, proptosis may be observed.

## Diagnosis

The presenting signs, physical examination, endoscopic examination, and radiography provide necessary diagnostic information. Sinus cysts are large space-occupying lesions and can easily be confused with a neoplastic disease. However, cysts are more common in horses than nasal tumors.

Physical examination may reveal considerable swelling over the facial region with or without obstruction to nasal airflow. Increased resonance on percussion can be expected if there is thinning of the nasal bones. Cysts that have expanded in a nasal direction can be seen via endoscopy as discrete rounded masses, typically in the middle meatus. Those that are confined to the sinuses cause diffuse narrowing of the nasal airways to the point where passage of the endoscope to the nasopharynx is obstructed. Needle aspiration of the cyst provides definitive confirmation of the diagnosis by the release of characteristic vivid yellow fluid.

Radiographic evaluation reveals a homogeneous soft tissue density with relatively well-demarcated margins. On lateral standing projections, free gas/fluid lines may be observed, which indicate impeded sinus drainage. There may be dental distortion and displacement, flattening of the tooth roots, and soft tissue mineralization. Ventrodorsal projections demonstrate the limits of the lesion in a rostrocaudal dimension, as well as the extent of any nasal septum or vomer bone deviation. Computed tomographic scanning or MRI may provide additional information if available.

### Treatment
Frontonasal flap surgery is generally effective. The cyst wall is peeled away from the inside of the sinuses. In the event of incomplete ablation, small areas of residual cyst tissue do not appear to cause complications.

### Prognosis
The prognosis for successful surgical ablation is excellent and recurrence is not likely. Facial deformity often resolves following surgery, especially in young horses.

## FUNGAL RHINITIS AND SINUSITIS

Fungal infections of the upper respiratory tract include primary infections by specific fungal species, such as cryptococcosis, rhinosporidiosis, phycomycosis, and coccidioidomycosis. These are rare and have a distinct geographical distribution. Some may have a zoonotic potential. Mycotic rhinitis caused by *Aspergillus* spp. infection has a wider geographical distribution, and in many cases, is considered to be a secondary opportunistic infection.

### Cryptococcosis
*Cryptococcus neoformans* can infect the upper respiratory tract causing granulomas and an invasive rhinitis and sinusitis, often accompanied by draining tracts through the facial bones. A mucopurulent, foul-smelling, blood-tinged unilateral nasal discharge is produced. Infection can be diagnosed by histology of biopsies, cytology, and culture.

### Rhinosporidiosis
*Rhinosporidium seeberi* has been described as a cause of granuloma formation around the nares and nasal septum. Granulomatous polyps may reach sufficient size to cause obstructive dyspnea. Surgical removal of the masses is frequently followed by recurrence.

## Phycomycosis

Phycomycosis includes infection by *Pythium insidiosum* or *Entomophthora coronata* (*Conidiobolus coronatus*). *Entomophthora coronata* has a high affinity for the tissues around the nares and lips, causing a condition called rhinophycomycosis. The lesions include granulomatous and ulcerated masses with cores of necrotic material known as "leeches" or "kunkers." Lesions occur around the rostral nasal cavity, nares, and lips. They are often pruritic, resulting in self-trauma. The lesions may expand into the oral cavity, resulting in dysphagia and weight loss. Surgical excision coupled with topical treatment with amphoteracin B is often successful.

## Coccidioidomycosis

*Coccidioides immitis* appears to be endemic in some semiarid areas of North and South America. Infection can result in a generalized disease or localized granuloma formation. Lesions often develop in the caudal nasal cavity resulting in mucopurulent nasal discharge, epistaxis, abnormal respiratory noise, and exercise intolerance. Diagnosis is made by endoscopic examination and biopsy. The extent of the granulomatous mass may be identified by radiographic examination. Surgical excision may be possible in some cases, but should be followed by ketoconazole or intraconazole therapy.

## Aspergillosis

Although *Aspergillus sp* infection is common after nasal surgery or secondary to other suppurative conditions, such as dental periapical abscessation, horses are encountered where these infections arise on the sinu-nasal tissues without obvious underlying disease. The etiology is not known but the infection consists of a destructive rhinitis/sinusitis, occasionally producing sinu-nasal fistulae.

Horses with *Aspergillus* infections in the nasal region usually show a low-grade unilateral purulent discharge, which may be malodorous or sero-sanguinous. The presence of mycotic plaques can be identified via endoscopy either per nasum or directly into the caudal maxillary sinus.

Topical medication with enilconazole provides an effective and simple remedy. A Foley balloon catheter is placed into the caudal maxillary sinus, and the sinus cavity acts as a reservoir for the medication, which is infused twice daily. Resolution may require prolonged treatment for up to 6 weeks.

## SINUS AND NASAL NEOPLASIA AND POLYPS

Primary tumors of the sinus and nasal regions are rare in the horse:

- Neoplasia of the nasal cavity and paranasal sinuses is rare.
- Clinical signs can include putrid nasal discharge, epistaxis, and nasal obstruction.

- Diagnosis is aided by radiographic, endoscopic, and histopathologic examination.
- Nasal polyps are benign growths that often arise secondary to dental disease.

Squamous cell carcinoma, adenocarcinoma, fibroma, chondroma, lymphoma, mast cell tumor, hemangiosarcoma, osteoma, and osteosarcoma have been reported. Odontogenic tumors (i.e., tumors derived from the tooth-forming tissues) are rarely encountered in young horses. Polyps (i.e., pedunculated inflammatory proliferations enclosed in mucous membrane) sometimes arise as a complication of dental periapical disease.

## Clinical signs

The clinical signs may be similar to those of a chronic primary sinus empyema, cyst, or progressive ethmoidal hematoma—i.e., a putrid nasal discharge possibly mixed with blood, nasal obstruction, and facial swelling. In addition there may be proptosis when the tumor has infiltrated the bony orbit and displaced the globe outward. Some tumors and nasal polyps protrude to the nostrils.

## Diagnosis

Diagnosis is achieved by physical examination, endoscopic, radiographic, and histopathologic examination of biopsy specimens. Computed tomographic scanning provides additional information regarding the location and extent of the mass and the damage/invasion of adjacent structures (see Chapter 4, Fig. 4.3). In horses with proptosis, transocular ultrasonography is used to assess the integrity of the bony orbit. Attempts to aspirate fluid from the lesion will fail to produce exudate or fluid, but needle aspiration can be a means to obtain biopsy material—for example, after exploratory trephination.

Radiographic examination may identify a solid mass with an outline less well-demarcated than with a cyst or empyema. Identifiable mineralized dental tissue may be evident in cases of well-differentiated odontogenic tumors. In cases of suspected polyp, the dental arcade should be reviewed via radiographic examination and oral inspection.

## Treatment

Frontonasal flap surgery may be used on an exploratory basis, and this may or may not permit surgical excision. Nasal polyps can be treated by excision. Electrosurgical excision offers advantages in terms of hemostasis. Small polyps may be removed by snare, transendoscopic electrosurgery, or transendoscopic laser ablation. Any underlying dental disorder should also be treated.

## Prognosis

The prognosis for sinu-nasal tumors in horses is highly variable, and each case must be treated on its merits. Well-circumscribed benign lesions often lend themselves to successful removal by frontonasal flap surgery, and the size of the lesion need not be a deterrent. The prognosis for nasal polyps is generally good, but recurrence following surgical removal may occur.

## AMYLOIDOSIS

Amyloidosis is a rare disease that involves the deposition of amyloid (a glycoprotein) as a result of some form of chronic antigenic stimulation. The upper respiratory tract appears to be a common site of amyloid deposition in the horse. Amyloid deposition in the nasal cavity may occur alone or in association with amyloid deposition in the skin. Deposits can occur on the nostrils, alar folds, nasal septum, and conchae; occasionally, they may occur in the nasopharynx and guttural pouches.

Clinical signs include nasal discharge, epistaxis, nasal obstruction, abnormal respiratory noise, and exercise intolerance. Weight loss may be evident as a result of an underlying primary disease. Diagnosis is achieved by identification of the raised, hemorrhagic nodules at the nostrils or in the nasal cavity. Confirmation of the diagnosis is achieved by biopsy. Treatment should be aimed at identifying and treating any underlying primary disease. Local excision or laser ablation can be used to treat individual deposits.

## CONCHAL NECROSIS AND METAPLASIA

Metaplastic calcification of the conchal cartilages usually occurs as an end stage of dental suppuration that has extended into the nasal tissues. Alternatively, the condition can arise secondary to chronic infection in the ventral conchal sinus. Horses afflicted with this condition present with a fetid nasal discharge; signs directly referable to an underlying dental disease may or may not be evident. Endoscopy shows necrotic debris on the surfaces of the conchal scrolls. Radiography provides the definitive diagnosis in the form of turbinate "coral" formation and loss of the normal turbinate pattern. Treatment involves removal of necrotic and diseased tissue followed by lavage. In addition, underlying dental disease is treated to resolution.

## INTRANASAL FOREIGN BODIES

Intranasal foreign bodies are uncommon. Foreign bodies—such as grass seeds, twigs, and thorns—can occasionally lodge in the nasal cavity. The sudden onset of acute nasal discomfort with intense sneezing and facial rubbing are the likely signs, particularly if there has been recent epistaxis. Some foreign bodies are visible as soon as the alar margins are raised, but others are identified only during endoscopic examination. Radiographic examination may be used in the diagnosis of larger or metallic foreign bodies.

## FACIAL AND SINUS TRAUMA

Facial trauma is common. Traumatic injury can arise as a result of kicks, falls, collisions, and competition injuries, and both open and closed injuries are observed.

Closed depression fractures over the paranasal sinuses frequently result in epistaxis. Initially there may be surprisingly little deformation of the profile of the face because the space between the depressed fracture and the skin fills with blood. However, as healing progresses a depression in the facial profile may result. In nondisplaced fractures, organization of the hematoma and the fracture callus may leave a firm swelling at the site.

Diagnosis is made by a combination of history, physical examination, radiographic examination, and ultrasonographic examination. Radiographic examination can document sinus fractures, but it can provide only a two-dimensional image, and therefore limited information about the extent of the fracture. Treatment in the acute stage should be aimed at control of hemorrhage and preservation of vital functions. Subsequently, treatment directed toward anatomical restoration may be attempted for functional or cosmetic reasons. Depressed fracture fragments may be elevated, and, if necessary, sutured in place. Occasionally sinusitis develops after trauma, in which case antibiotic therapy and irrigation procedures are necessary to eliminate infection. In cases of healed depression fractures with facial deformity, fluorocarbon polymer and carbon fiber can be used to restore the facial contour. Alternatively, a healed fragment can be cut with a saw and elevated into a normal position.

## SUBCUTANEOUS EMPHYSEMA

The presence of air in the subcutaneous tissues suggests one of three events:

- Leakage of air from within the respiratory tract
- Repeated entrapment of air in an external wound
- The presence of gas-forming organisms

Trauma and surgery of the upper respiratory tract—including the paranasal sinuses, larynx, and trachea—may lead to air being forced between the skin and the underlying layers. Emphysema typically arises when the air cannot move freely to the nares during expiration and is therefore forced through a defect in the wall of the tract into the subcutaneous tissues. Edema and spasm after laryngeal surgery and nasal packing after frontonasal surgery are examples of iatrogenic causes of emphysema. Wounds in the axillary region frequently cause progressive entrapment of air with each movement of the forelimb. Clostridial (gas gangrene) infections typically stem from the deep inoculation of the infective agent and, unless identified promptly, are rapidly fatal.

The objectives in treatment of subcutaneous emphysema are to prevent further air entering the subcutaneous space by closure of the defect, or to allow the air to escape more easily by an alternative route. Facilities for emergency tracheotomy or laryngotomy should be readily available in establishments where airway surgery is performed. Neglected subcutaneous emphysema can lead to pneumothorax and fatal pulmonary collapse if air enters the thoracic cavity by way of the mediastinum.

## FURTHER READING

Bell, B.T.L., Baker, J.G., and Foreman, J.H. 1993. Progressive ethmoid haematoma: background, clinical signs, and diagnosis. *Comp Cont Educ Pract Vet* 15:1101–1111.

Bell, B.T.L., Baker, J.G., and Foreman, J.H. 1993. Progressive ethmoid haematoma: characteristics, cause and treatment. *Comp Cont Educ Pract Vet* 15:1391–1399.

Cannon, J.H., Grant, B.D., and Sande, R.D. 1976. Diagnosis and surgical treatment of cyst-like lesions of the equine paranasal sinuses. *J Am Vet Med Assoc* 169:610–613.

Colbourne, C.M., Rosenstein, D.S., Steficek, B.A., Yovich, J.V., and Stick, J.A. 1997. Surgical treatment of progressive ethmoidal hematoma aided by computed tomography in a foal. *J Am Vet Med Assoc* 211:335–338.

Cook, W.R., and Littlewort, M.C. 1974. Progressive haematoma of the ethmoid region in the horse. *Equine Vet J* 6:101–107.

Dixon, P.M., and Head, K.W. 1999. Equine nasal and paranasal sinus tumours: Part 1: Review of literature and tumour classification. *Vet J* 157:261–278.

Dixon, P.M., and Head, K.W. 1999. Equine nasal and paranasal sinus tumours: Part 2: A contribution of 28 case reports. *Vet J* 157:279–294.

Freeman, D.E. 1991. Nasal passages. In *Equine Respiratory Disorders*. J. Beech ed. Philadelphia: Lea & Febiger, pp 253–273.

Freeman, D.E. 2003. Sinus disease. *Vet Clinics N Am Equine Pract* 19:209–243.

Gibbs, C., and Lane, J.G. 1987. Radiographic examination of the facial, nasal and paranasal sinus regions of the horse. II. Radiological findings. *Equine Vet J* 19: 474–479.

Greet, T.R.C. 1981. Nasal aspergillosis in three horses. *Vet Rec* 184:487–489.

Greet, T.R.C. 1992. Outcome of treatment in 23 horses with progressive ethmoidal haematomas. *Equine Vet J* 24:468–471.

Hanselka, D.V. 1972. Equine nasal phycomycosis. *Vet Med Small Anim Clin* 72:253–269.

Hutchins, D.R., and Johnston, K.G. 1972. Phycomycosis in the horse. *Aust Vet J* 48:269–278.

Jakob, W. 1971. Spontaneous amyloidosis of mammals. *Vet Pathol* 8:292–306.

Lane, J.G. 1993. Equine head and hindlimb medicine and surgery. In *Proceedings of the Fifteenth Bain-Fallon Memorial Lectures:* Australian Equine Veterinary Association, Artarmon, NSW.

Lane, J.G. 1993. The management of sinus disorders in the horse. *Equine Vet Educ* 5:5–9.

Lane, J.G. 1998. Disorders of the ear, nose and throat. In *Equine Medicine, Surgery and Reproduction*. T. Mair, S. Love, J. Schumacher, and E. Watson, eds. London: W.B. Saunders, pp 81–117.

Lane, J.G., Longstaffe, J.A., and Gibbs, C. 1987. Equine paranasal sinus cyst: a report of 15 cases. *Equine Vet J* 19:537-544.

Levine, S.B. 1979. Depression fractures of the nasal and frontal bones of the horse. *J Equine Med Surg* 3:186–190.

Myers, D.D. 1964. Rhinosporidiosis in a horse *J Am Vet Med Assoc* 145:345–347.

Reed, S.M., Boles, C.L., and Dade, A.W. 1979. Localized equine nasal coccioidomycosis granuloma. *J Equine Med Surg* 3:119–123.

Roberts, M.C., Sutton, R.H., and Lovell, D.K. 1981. A protracted case of cryptococcal nasal granuloma in a stallion. *Aust Vet J* 57:287–291.

Rothaug, P.G., and Tulleners, E.P. 1999. Neodymium:yttrium aluminium garnet laser-assisted excision of progressive ethmoid haematomas in horses: 20 cases (1986–1996). *J Am Vet Med Assoc* 214:1037–1041.

Schumacher, J., and Honnas, C.M. 2003. Progressive ethmoid hematoma. In *Current Therapy in Equine Medicine*, 5th ed. N.E. Robinson, ed. Philadelphia: W.B. Saunders, pp 375–378.

Schumacher, J., Yarbrough, T., Pascoe, J., Woods, P., Meagher, D., and Honnas, C. 1998. Transendoscopic chemical ablation of progressive ethmoidal hematomas in stranding horses. *Vet Surg* 27:175–181.

Scott, E.A., Duncan, J.R., and McCormack, J.E. 1974. Cryptococcosis involving the postorbital area and frontal sinus in a horse. *J Am Vet Med Assoc* 165:626–627.

Shaw, D.P., Gunson, D.E., and Evans, L.H. 1987. Nasal amyloidosis in four horses. *Vet Pathol* 24:183.

Smith, H.A., and Frankson, M.C. 1961. Rhinosporidiosis in a Texas horse *Southwestern Vet* 15:22–24.

Stashak, T.S. 1991. *Equine Wound Management*. Baltimore: Williams and Wilkins, pp 89–144.

Stich, K.L., Rush, B.R., and Gaughan, E.M. 2001. Progressive ethmoid hematoma in horses. *Comp Cont Educ Pract Vet* 23:1094–1103.

Tremaine, W.H., and Dixon, P.M. 2001. A long-term study of 277 cases of equine sinonasal disease. Part 1. Details of horses, historical, clinical and ancillary diagnostic findings. *Equine Vet J* 33:274–282.

Tremaine, W.H., and Dixon, P.M. 2001. A long-term study of 277 cases of equine sinonasal disease. Part 2. Treatments and results of treatments. *Equine Vet J* 33:283–289.

# The Gutteral Pouches

Diseases of the guttural pouches are relatively uncommon, but they are important differentials for horses with signs of upper respiratory tract disease, cranial nerve dysfunction, predominantly (not exclusively) unilateral discharge, and spontaneous epistaxis.

## ANATOMY AND FUNCTION OF THE GUTTURAL POUCHES

The guttural pouches are the balloon-like caudoventral diverticulae of the eustachian tubes (auditory tubes). Guttural pouches are present in perissodactyls, including all equids. They are located between the base of the cranium dorsally and the pharynx and esophagus ventrally. The two pouches do not communicate, but contact each other medially, being separated rostrally only by a thin layer of areolar tissue; caudally they are separated by the rectus capitis ventralis and longus capitis muscles. The stylohyoid bone divides each pouch into a small lateral and a larger medial compartment (Fig. 8.1). Each guttural pouch has a capacity of about 300–500 ml. The stylohyoid bone travels in a caudodorsal direction to the temporohyoid joint; the distal opening of the eustachian tube opens just lateral to this joint.

The pharyngeal drainage ostia are obliquely directed slit-like openings that lie on the dorso-lateral wall of the pharynx, rostroventral to the pharyngeal recess. A plate of fibrocartilage is located in the mucosa of the flap-like medial wall of each ostium. The pharyngeal drainage ostia are located at the dorsal aspect of the pouches, and thus drainage from the pouch is poor unless the head is lowered. The two ostia lie close to each other, so, although discharge from one pouch may produce a predominantly unilateral nasal discharge,

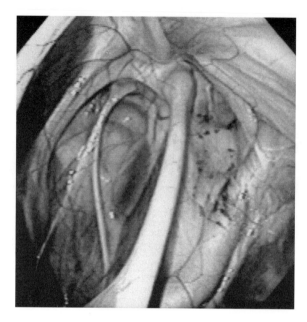

**Fig. 8.1.** Endoscopic view of melanosis of the left guttural pouch. Note the black discolored masses over the external carotid artery and the caudodorsal aspect of the lateral guttural pouch. The stylohyoid bone separates the lateral from medial compartments, and the internal carotid artery can be seen coursing through the caudal aspect of the medial guttural pouch. *(See also color section.)*

more copious discharge from one pouch may cause a bilateral nasal discharge. The pharyngeal orifice of the guttural pouch is a funnel-shaped vestibule that is wider rostrally than caudally. The caudal narrowing is due to a transverse fold of mucous membrane, the plica salpingopharyngea, which connects the medial wall of the eustachian tube to the lateral wall of the pharynx.

The mucosal lining of the guttural pouches is composed of ciliated pseudo-stratified columnar epithelium. Mucus-producing goblet cells and seromucous glands produce a mixture of mucus and surface-active agents that form a protective layer over the mucosa. A dynamic clearance system removes mucus and particulate debris. Aggregates of lymphoid cells lie in the subepithelial tissues.

Each pouch is in contact with the base of the skull, and those structures that enter and leave the cranium through the foramen lacerum cross the pouch. A fold of mucous membrane that extends from the roof of the guttural pouch along the caudal aspect of the medial compartment contains the internal carotid artery, cervical sympathetic trunk, cranial cervical ganglion, and cranial nerves IX (glossopharyngeal), X (vagus), XI (accessory), and XII (hypoglossal). The pharyngeal branch of the vagus nerve (X) and the cranial laryngeal nerve lie in the ventral aspect of the medial compartment. The retropharyngeal lymph nodes also lie beneath the mucosa on the floor of the medial compartment. The facial nerve (VII) emerges from the stylomastoid foramen and courses in the submucosa of the lateral compartment caudodorsally before passing between the mandible and parotid gland. The mandibular nerve (branch of the trigeminal nerve, V) emerges from the foramen lacerum and passes rostrally along the roof of the lateral compartment. The external carotid artery passes rostrally along the ventral surface of the lateral compartment, accompanied in part of its course by cranial nerves IX (glossopharyngeal) and XII (hypoglossal) (see Fig. 8.1). It then turns dorsally to continue as the internal maxillary artery, which is accompanied by the maxillary vein and crosses the wall of the lateral compartment. The maxillary artery gives off the caudal auricular artery and the superficial temporal artery in this area; here, the pouch lies beneath Viborg's triangle.

The precise functions of the guttural pouches remain uncertain. The eustachian tube is believed to equalize air pressure on both sides of the tympanic membrane. The pharyngeal drainage ostia dilate during swallowing, and there is an exchange of air during respiration. Ventilation of the pouch results in a cooling of the blood within the internal carotid artery, and it has been proposed that this may represent a brain-cooling device to dissipate heat produced by muscular activity. Other proposed functions include a resonating chamber for vocalization and a flotation device.

## SIGNS OF GUTTURAL POUCH DISEASES

The major presenting signs of diseases of the guttural pouches result from either compression of adjacent organs when the pouches become distended, or damage to the structures which lie in their walls. Swellings of the guttural pouches may be visible externally at the parotid region, or may partially obstruct the pharynx leading to dyspnea and/or dysphagia. Erosion of the internal carotid artery causes spontaneous hemorrhage to the nares (epistaxis) which can result in fatal exsanguination. Guttural pouch disorders provide potential for a wide range of neuropathies, including paralysis of cranial nerves VII, IX, X, XI, and XII, and Horner's syndrome.

## EXAMINATION OF THE GUTTURAL POUCHES

Examination of the gutteral pouches can include several approaches, including palpation, endoscopic examination, radiographic examination, cytology, advanced diagnostic imaging techniques, and surgical exploration.

### Palpation
External palpation in the parotid area may detect swelling produced by tympany, empyema, abscessation of adjacent lymph glands or neoplasia. The guttural pouch lies in close contact with the auricular cartilage, and palpation deep to the base of the ear may cause pain, especially in cases of guttural pouch mycosis that have resulted in damage to the head of the stylohyoid bone or the temporohyoid articulation.

## Endoscopic examination

The guttural pouches are amenable to direct endoscopic examination using flexible fibreoptic- or video-endoscopes. Once the endoscope is passed into the nasopharynx, the pharyngeal drainage ostia should be inspected for evidence of blood or exudate draining from the pouch (Fig. 8.2). A small quantity of clear mucus draining from the pouch is not abnormal, especially after exercise.

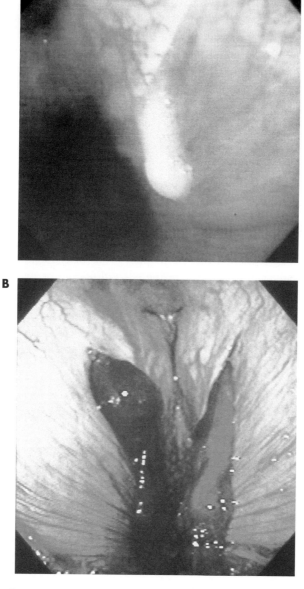

**Fig. 8.2.** Endoscopic view of the guttural pouch openings in a horse with unilateral purulent exudate (empyema)(A) and bilateral hemorrhage originating from the guttural pouch openings (B). *(See also color section.)*

The simplest way to pass an endoscope into the pouch is by using a wire leader passed through the biopsy channel of the endoscope. This channel is usually eccentric, and thus, the wire can be used to raise the cartilage flap before advancing the endoscope into the duct beyond. Alternatively, a stiff metal or plastic catheter can be inserted into the guttural pouch under endoscopic control and used to open the ostium to permit entry of the endoscope. The endoscope can be passed via each ipsilateral nostril to examine the pouches. Alternatively, both pouches may be examined with the endoscope introduced through the same nostril. The normal guttural pouch has a thin, translucent mucosa that allows inspection of the underlying structures. In addition to inspection within the guttural pouches, endoscopic examination should include assessment of cranial nerve function, particularly laryngeal and pharyngeal function. Depression of the roof of the nasopharynx at the pharyngeal recess, and an obscured view of the larynx may result from distension of the guttural pouch (Fig. 8.3).

## Radiographic examination

The guttural pouches are normally air-filled, and radiographic examination can be helpful to identify abnormalities within one or both pouches. Radiography is particularly useful in cases where endoscopic examination is unhelpful (e.g., where discharge within the pouch obscures the endoscopic view). The lateral projection is most commonly used to provide information regarding the dimensions and content of the guttural pouches. Radiographic abnormalities in disease may include distension by air/gas, gas-fluid interfaces, and loss of air contrast through replacement by inspissated pus or soft tissue substitution. Complete obliteration of the normal gas density of a pouch can

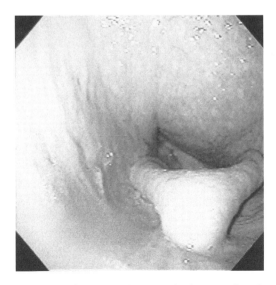

**Fig. 8.3.** Endoscopic view of the nasopharynx of a horse with right unilateral guttural pouch empyema, showing depression of the roof of the nasopharynx caused by distension of the affected pouch.

occur in cases of chronic empyema or chondroid formation. Masses impinging on the guttural pouch and fractures/exostoses of the stylohyoid bone can be detected.

Arteriography can be used to identify the affected vessel in cases of guttural pouch mycosis. The common carotid artery or selected branches can be assessed by injecting 20–30 ml of warmed contrast agent as a bolus with the horse under general anesthesia.

## Cytology

Differential nucleated cell counts of guttural pouch lavages may be helpful in some situations. Less than 5% neutrophils is considered normal, and more than 25% neutrophils is associated with infection.

## Other diagnostic imaging techniques

Diagnostic ultrasonography via the parotid region may identify lymphadenopathy and neoplastic masses in the retropharyngeal area and lateral wall of the guttural pouch. Advanced diagnostic imaging modalities, including CT scanning and MRI, can also provide anatomical detail and orientation of abnormalities within and surrounding the guttural pouch.

## Surgical approaches to the guttural pouches

The complex anatomy of the guttural pouches and surrounding tissues make surgical treatment difficult. Iatrogenic damage to one or more of the neurovascular structures can have serious and life-threatening consequences. Surgical access to the guttural pouch may be required for removal of purulent material, chondroids, mycotic plaques, and foreign bodies, or to establish drainage. The following surgical approaches can be used (Fig. 8.4):

### Hyovertebrotomy

A 10 cm incision is made parallel and 2 cm cranial to the wing of the atlas. The dense fascia is incised, and the parotid salivary gland and overlying parotidoauricularis muscle are reflected forward. The fascia and second cervical nerve are reflected caudally. An endoscope introduced into the guttural pouch per nasum serves to illuminate the membranous lining deep in the surgical site once the loose connective tissue has been bluntly separated. The lining of the guttural pouch can be grasped and punctured with the closed tips of scissors or a hemostat. This site is close to the internal carotid artery, the hypoglossal and glossopharyngeal nerves, and the cranial laryngeal and pharyngeal branches of the vagus nerve, so extreme care must be taken when making the opening in the pouch lining. Following completion of the surgery, the hyovertebrotomy incision can be closed or left partly open to provide access for ingress and egress of lavage fluids. However, drainage from the hyovertebrotomy incision is relatively poor, so an additional opening into the pouch via Viborg's triangle can be helpful.

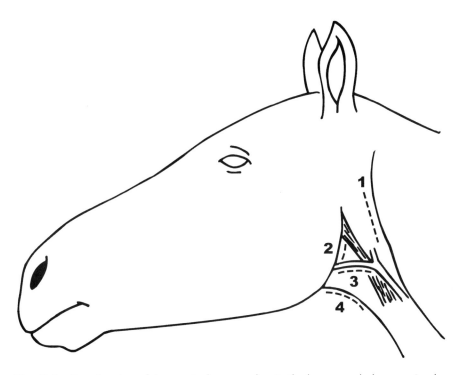

**Fig. 8.4.** Line drawing of the surgical approaches to the larynx and pharynx. 1 = hy-overtebrotomy; 2 = Viborg's triangle defined by the tendon of the sternocephalicus muscle, the ramus of the mandible, and the linguofacial vein; 3 = modified Whitehouse approach; 4 = Whitehouse approach.

## Viborg's triangle

Viborg's triangle is the area bounded by the tendon of the sternocephalicus muscle, the linguofacial vein, and the vertical ramus of the mandible. Access to the guttural pouch by this approach is very restricted except in conditions where there has been stretching of the tissues through distension of the pouch, which increases the overall size of Viborg's triangle. A vertical or horizontal incision is made, taking care to avoid the parotid duct and branches of the vagus nerve along the floor of the pouch. The incision is usually left open to heal by secondary intention.

## Paralaryngeal (Whitehouse) approach

With the horse in dorsal recumbency, a ventral midline incision is made over the larynx. The dissection is continued through the sternohyoideus and omo-hyoideus muscles, and passes lateral to the larynx, trachea, and cricopharynx to reach the pouch ventro-medially. Entry to the guttural pouch is made medial to the stylohyoid bone, the external carotid artery, the glossopharyngeal nerve, and the hypoglossal nerve. The pharyngeal branch of the vagus and cranial laryngeal nerves is close to the incision, and must be avoided. The depth of incision limits the value of this approach.

## Modified Whitehouse approach

Although the surgery is again performed with the patient in dorsal recumbency, the site of the incision corresponds to that used for prosthetic laryngoplasty— i.e., it lies ventral to the linguo-facial vein and then follows the same route to enter the pouch. This approach avoids the necessity to divide the sternohyoideus and omohyoideus muscles.

The Whitehouse approaches are advocated because they allow access to the roof of the guttural pouch, the possibility to explore the lateral compartment digitally, and access to both guttural pouches through the same incision. They also provide good ventral drainage. However, both approaches require deep dissection, and there is believed to be a higher rate of complications, such as dysphagia.

## TOPICAL TREATMENT OF THE GUTTURAL POUCHES

Topical treatments of guttural pouch diseases are commonly employed either as the sole treatment, or, more commonly, as an adjunct to other (surgical) treatments. A 35 cm or longer 30 ml Foley balloon catheter offers a suitable indwelling device for repeated topical infusion of medication. Alternatively, commercial guttural pouch catheters are available. The catheter is passed up the ventral nasal meatus using a metal stylet, slightly bent at the leading end. This is rotated 180° under the cartilage flap of the ostium, which lies on the lateral pharyngeal wall at the same level as the eye. The catheter can be passed blindly or under endoscopic guidance. It should be noted that long-term catheterization can lead to weakening of the ostium and erosion of the cartilage flap.

Irrigation of the pouch with isotonic crystalloid solutions can be used to dislodge and remove purulent exudate, debris, and inflammatory mediators. Infusions can be repeated once or twice a day as necessary. The horse should be sedated for the first infusion so that the head is lowered, and the risk of aspiration of fluid is reduced. Irritating solutions, such as hydrogen peroxide or concentrated antiseptics, should not be used because they can result in serious neuritis of the cranial nerves in the guttural pouch.

## GUTTURAL POUCH TYMPANY

Guttural pouch tympany is an infrequently encountered condition where there is excessive accumulation of air in the guttural pouch:

- It is seen predominantly in foals.
- The cause is a congenital dysfunction of the pharyngeal opening of the pouch.
- Clinical signs include swelling, dyspnea, and dysphagia.

- Diagnosis is made by physical examination, endoscopy, and radiography.
- Treatments include chronic catheterization of the affected pouch, fistulation of the median septum between the two pouches, or enlargement of the pharyngeal drainage ostium.

Guttural pouch tympany involves the accumulation of a large quantity of air within a guttural pouch, probably as a result of a malfunction of the pharyngeal drainage ostium. It has been suggested that air may enter the pouch normally during expiration, but then cannot leave because the plica salpingopharyngea acts as a one-way valve and collapses across the pharyngeal orifice as air is expelled. In most cases there is no obvious anatomical abnormality of the guttural pouch ostium, and a functional rather than a structural abnormality is involved. The condition occurs most commonly as a congenital abnormality in young foals. Inflammation from an upper airway infection, persistent coughing, and muscle dysfunction have been proposed as alternative causes.

## Clinical signs and diagnosis

This is a condition of foals that usually manifests itself within a few days of birth, although occasionally the condition may arise in older foals up to 20 months of age. The disorder appears to be more common in fillies than colts, and is usually unilateral. Rarely, guttural pouch tympany may occur as an acquired disorder of the mature horse.

Air accumulates in the pouch and produces tympanitic swelling in the parotid region, which is initially nonpainful and noninflammatory. The degree of swelling is variable. Most affected foals appear clinically normal apart from the swelling, but in some cases the size of the swelling may cause stertorous or stridorous breathing and dyspnea. Coughing, dysphagia, and aspiration may occur, and there may be nasal return of milk or food. Established cases invariably show evidence of opportunistic infection, because a mucopurulent nasal discharge is generally present by the time afflicted foals are submitted for corrective surgery. The laxity of the medial septum between the guttural pouches may lead to swelling on the normal side, and hence false diagnosis of bilateral tympany may be made.

Lateral radiographs show an enlarged, gas-filled guttural pouch (Fig. 8.5) that may extend beyond the second cervical vertebra. The opposite normal pouch may be visible, or it may be too compressed to be identified. The distended pouch may cause compression of the nasopharynx, and the larynx and proximal trachea may be displaced. Air-fluid interfaces in the guttural pouch compartments may be visible in cases with accumulation of milk or exudate in the guttural pouch. Ventro-dorsal views can be useful to differentiate unilateral and bilateral cases.

Endoscopy usually reveals a normal-appearing pharyngeal drainage ostium. The dorsal roof of the nasopharynx may appear collapsed. Catheterization of the guttural pouches using a Foley catheter or Chambers' urinary catheter de-

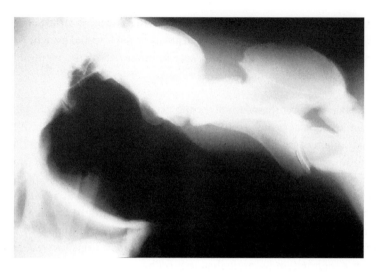

**Fig. 8.5.** Lateral radiographic projection of a 6-month-old Standardbred foal with unilateral guttural pouch tympany. Note the dorsal compression of the pharynx and the caudal extension of the guttural pouch to the level of the $C_2$–$C_3$ articulation.

flates the affected pouch, and this helps determine which pouch is involved. Alternatively, percutaneous centesis may be used to confirm a unilateral disorder. A needle can be inserted percutaneously at the point of greatest distension; there is some risk of iatrogenic damage to the nerves and blood vessels in the pouch with this procedure. Endoscopy should include examination of the trachea in foals that have a history of coughing or dysphagia to ascertain whether there has been aspiration of milk or feed material.

## Treatment
Temporary alleviation of tympany can be achieved by catheterization of the affected pouch or percutaneous needle centesis. Concurrent use of antibacterial and anti-inflammatory drugs is recommended. However, the guttural pouch rapidly refills when these measures are discontinued.

The choice of treatment is determined by whether the condition is unilateral or bilateral, and by the equipment and expertise available. Treatment options include

1. Dilation of the pharyngeal ostium on the affected side
2. The creation of a fistula between the normal and distended pouches by the removal of a section of the medial septum
3. Fistulation between the guttural pouch and the pharyngeal recess

Dilation of the pharyngeal ostium can be achieved by excising a 2.5 cm x 1.5 cm segment of the medial lamina within the guttural pouch orifice (via an approach through Viborg's triangle) or excising the excess plica salpingopharyngea. A simpler conservative technique to remedy the disorder consists of the long-term implantation of an indwelling Foley catheter placed through the defective pharyngeal ostium per nasum and left in place for up to 8 weeks.

The purpose of the medial wall fistulation technique is to facilitate the egress of air from the tympanitic guttural pouch through the pharyngeal ostium of the normal side. The procedure can be performed via an approach through Viborg's triangle or a modified Whitehouse approach. During surgery, passage of an endoscope into the opposite pouch transilluminates the medial septum and makes the identification of an area free of vessels or nerves easier. A 2 cm$^2$ section of septum is removed. Minimally invasive surgical techniques (transendoscopic laser surgery or electrosurgery) can also be used to perform fenestration of the medial septum. These techniques can also be used to create a fistula between the tympanitic pouch and the pharyngeal recess. A site just dorsal and caudal to the nasopharyngeal drainage ostium is chosen for this technique. An indwelling Foley catheter should be placed in the fistula for 14 days postoperatively to prevent closure of the fistula.

If both pouches are tympanitic, fenestration of the medial septum can be combined with resection of one nasopharyngeal drainage ostium.

## Prognosis

The prognosis for guttural pouch tympany is usually favorable regardless of whether the catherization or fistulation technique is used. Secondary infections of the pouch usually resolve spontaneously following successful treatment. The medial wall fistulation technique can fail if the hole seals over or if the condition is bilateral. Resection of the mucosal fold can fail if swelling and inflammation occludes the pharyngeal orifice. Recurrence of tympany is reported to occur in 10–30% of foals following surgical treatment.

## DIVERTICULITIS OF THE GUTTURAL POUCH

A variety of different conditions associated with inflammation of the mucous membrane lining of the guttural pouches can occur, which can loosely be termed "diverticulitis." They include strangles abscessation in the lymphoid tissue of the walls of the pouches, empyema, chondroid formation, and chronic diverticulitis:

- Diverticulitis of the guttural pouch may occur during strangles infection.
- Chronic diverticulitis and empyema of the pouch occur because of a chronic defect of mucociliary clearance, usually secondary to an upper airway infection.
- Swelling of the pouch can cause dyspnea and an abnormal respiratory noise.
- A bilateral mucopurulent nasal discharge is usually present.
- Diagnosis is achieved by physical, endoscopic, and radiographic examination.
- Treatment involves drainage and lavage of the affected pouch.

- Chronic empyema may result in the accumulation of caseous inspissated exudate or concretions (chondroids) that may require surgical removal.
- Chronic diverticulitis results in chronic inflammation of the pouch lining and potentially cranial neuropathies.

A mild self-limiting catarrhal inflammation of the guttural pouch mucosa probably accompanies most upper respiratory tract bacterial and viral infections. Guttural pouch tympany is also commonly accompanied by inflammatory changes.

## Strangles

This is an infectious condition of horses caused by *Streptococcus equ var equii* that consists of a suppurative lymphadenitis of the lymph nodes associated with the upper respiratory tract, including the retropharyngeal lymph nodes in the wall of the guttural pouch. Rupture of retropharyngeal lymph nodes commonly occurs into the guttural pouch, resulting in infection and inflammation of the pouch. Chronic empyema and chondroid formation may ensue (see below). Occasionally the free movement of air through the drainage ostia of the guttural pouches is obstructed by the physical presence of the lymphadenopathy, and a variable degree of tympany and empyema may result. Temporary tracheotomy is indicated for those horses that show life-threatening airway obstruction. Strangles is discussed in greater detail in Chapter 14.

## Chronic guttural pouch empyema and chondroids

Empyema refers to the accumulation of exudate within the guttural pouch. Empyema occurs when mucus and/or purulent exudate accumulates within the pouches because it is failing to drain satisfactorily. The primary etiological factor in guttural pouch empyema is a dysfunction of mucociliary clearance followed by stagnation of mucus, opportunist bacterial infection, and finally purulent exudation. There is a possible etiological association with tympany. Guttural pouch empyema may occur in horses of all ages, but is most common in young horses. Many cases follow an upper respiratory tract infection, especially those associated with ß–hemolytic streptococci and strangles. In view of the association between strangles and chronic empyema, all cases of guttural pouch empyema should be considered as potentially contagious for *Streptococcus equi* until the results of culture are available.

Regardless of the precise etiology of empyema, purulent exudate that is stagnant within the pouch eventually becomes inspissated and progressively leads to the formation of solid concretions called chondroids (Fig. 8.6).

The clinical signs of empyema include a bilateral purulent nasal discharge, with or without swelling of the parotid region and fever. Distension of the affected pouch into the pharynx may produce obstructive dyspnea and an abnormal respiratory noise. Nasal discharge is commonly white and mucoid, and is usually nonodorous (Fig. 8.7). It may be intermittent or continuous. Occasionally, blood may be mixed with the discharge. Although it is usually bilat-

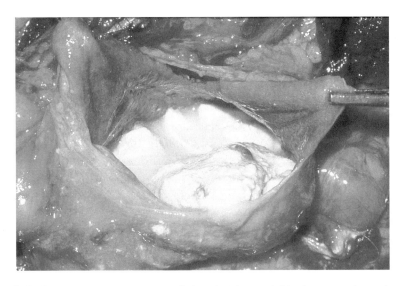

**Fig. 8.6.** Post-mortem examination of chondroid material in the guttural pouch.

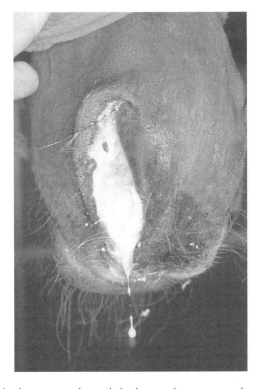

**Fig. 8.7.** Typical white, mucoid nasal discharge due to guttural pouch empyema.

eral, the discharge is frequently more voluminous at the nostril on the same side as the affected pouch. The discharge is greatest when the head is lowered, and may be increased when external pressure is applied to the parotid region on the affected side. In chronic cases, the exudate may become inspissated ("cottage cheese" consistency), which fails to drain, resulting in greater distension of the pouch, more external swelling, and adoption of an extended head carriage. Compression of the nasopharynx by the distended guttural pouch may result in dyspnea, stridor, and dysphagia. In chronic cases, cranial nerve involvement may occur, resulting most commonly in dysphagia.

Endoscopic examination frequently demonstrates mucopurulent exudate draining from the pharyngeal drainage ostium of the affected pouch (see Fig. 8.2A). However, absence of such a finding does not preclude the diagnosis of empyema. Distension of the pouch may cause compression of the nasopharynx on the affected side (see Fig. 8.3). Drainage from the pouch may be promoted by passing a catheter or the endoscope into the pouch. Endoscopic examination of the internal aspects of the pouch may be impeded by the presence of exudate. However, following drainage of liquid exudate, the inflamed and thickened mucosa lining can be examined. If the exudate is inspissated and caseous in nature, transendoscopic lavage will not be successful. A nested basket may be used to remove chondroid material from the guttural pouch in instances where 1/3 of the pouch or less is filled with chondroid material. Both pouches should be examined endoscopically, because bilateral disease is not uncommon. The pharyngeal drainage ostia should be carefully assessed for the presence of adhesions or deformity which might predispose to empyema, and which might complicate treatment. To confirm obstruction of the drainage ostium, manipulation of the flap and vestibule of the pouch may be performed using a Chambers mare catheter or similar instrument passed through the opposite nasal passage while viewing the area endoscopically.

Lateral radiographs confirm the loss of air contrast within the guttural pouch, and if the purulent material is still fluid, an air/fluid interface will be demonstrable. If the affected pouch is completely filled with exudate, there will be loss of the normal air contrast of the pouch. Because both pouches overlie each other in the lateral projection, oblique views or the instillation of a radiographic contrast agent into one pouch may be required to determine which pouch is diseased.

Samples of exudate can be submitted for bacterial culture and sensitivity. Lavage of the pouch can be performed if fluid exudate cannot be retrieved. Samples can also be obtained by percutaneous centesis, but the risk of neurovascular damage needs to be considered.

Treatment of guttural pouch empyema can be achieved in most cases by the insertion of an indwelling self-retaining Foley balloon catheter into the pouch via the pharyngeal drainage ostium. Alternatively a catheter with a coiled distal end (in the pouch) can be sutured to the alar fold. Irrigation with 500–1000 ml of normal saline or very dilute antiseptic solution (e.g., 1% povidone-iodine) should be performed once or twice a day for 7–10 days. More concentrated antiseptic solutions must not be used, because they are irritant and can cause nerve damage. Sedation is used to lower the head and reduce the risk of aspiration during lavage. Care must be taken if *Streptococcus equi* is cultured from the discharge to prevent environmental contamination. Systemic antibiotics (e.g., penicillin) are usually administered concurrently, although the efficacy or necessity of this treatment is undefined. If the horse is dysphagic, antibiotics are indicated to prevent or treat aspiration pneumonia. Feeding should be performed on the ground to allow drainage from the pouch.

The removal of inspissated caseous exudate is difficult using conservative means, and surgery may be required, especially to extirpate chondroids. Lavage with 20–60 ml of 20% (w/v) acetyl cysteine solution can sometimes be effective at breaking up viscous discharges and inspissated concretions, but treatment four times a day for many weeks is often required. Acetyl cysteine solutions are irritating, and assessment of cranial nerve function should be performed for the duration of treatment with this drug. Endoscopic removal of chondroids may also be possible using basket forceps, but the quantity of material accumulated in the pouch may make this procedure difficult and time-consuming. Recently, the use of a memory-helical polyp retrieval basket through the biopsy channel of the endoscope has proved to be a more effective nonsurgical treatment option.

Surgical drainage may be indicated for the evacuation of chondroids and in cases where there is loss of patency of the drainage ostium. Surgery is generally performed via a hyovertebrotomy or a modified Whitehouse incision. All purulent material should be removed; otherwise, recurrence of the problem may occur. Intraoperative endoscopic examination is helpful to check that complete removal of all chondroids has been attained. A spoon or curette is used to gently remove the inspissated material. Damage to the walls of the pouch and the neurovascular structures must be avoided. If the empyema is bilateral, a ventral Whitehouse approach is preferred so that both pouches can be entered through the same incision.

Fistulation of the guttural pouch to the nasopharynx dorsal and caudal to the pharyngeal drainage ostium should be considered in horses with impaired drainage due to loss of patency of the ostium. Laser or electrosurgery can be used to create the fistula. Alternatively, the cartilaginous flap can be resected through a modified Whitehouse approach. An indwelling Foley catheter should be placed into the fistula for about 14 days post-surgery to prevent it from healing over.

The prognosis for guttural pouch empyema is generally good. If the horse is dysphagic due to cranial nerve damage, nutritional support may be required.

## Chronic diverticulitis

Chronic diverticulitis without the presence of empyema may occur, possibly associated with a previous episode of strangles. Clinically, it presents as a collection of neuropathies where any combination of deficits of the glossopharyngeal, vagus, facial, spinal accessory, and sympathetic nerves may be present. It is assumed that the nervous pathways are damaged as an extension of the in-flammatory process in the guttural pouch walls.

The diagnosis is established by a functional assessment of the cranial nerves mentioned, combined with the endoscopic identification of a roughened thick-ening of the guttural pouch lining.

The nervous form of diverticulitis carries a poor prognosis, especially if the horse presents with dysphagia associated with damage to the glossopharyngeal or vagus nerves. Treatment includes antimicrobial and anti-inflammatory ther-apy coupled with lavage of the affected pouch(es), and supportive treatment.

## GUTTURAL POUCH MYCOSIS

Guttural pouch mycosis is a fungal infection of the wall of the guttural pouch:

- Mycotic plaques form on the wall, usually over the internal or external carotid arteries.
- Epistaxis can occur due to invasion of the arterial wall, and fatal hemor-rhage may result.
- Other potential signs include cranial neuropathies, especially pharyngeal paralysis, and Horner's syndrome.
- Diagnosis is achieved by endoscopic examination.
- Treatment involves arterial occlusion to prevent hemorrhage.
- The prognosis for horses with pharyngeal paralysis is poor.

There is no apparent age, gender, breed or geographical predisposition for guttural pouch mycosis, although the condition appears to most commonly af-fect stabled horses during the warmer months of the year. *Aspergillus* spp. are usually involved. The lesions consist of diphtheritic plaques of variable size, composed of necrotic tissue, cell debris, bacteria, and fungal mycelia. The plaques are closely attached to the underlying tissues. They are typically brown, yellow, or black and white, and vary from a small focal nodule to an extensive lesion covering a large part of the lining of the pouch (Fig. 8.8). The fungal plaques are usually found in one of two characteristic sites:

- The majority are on the roof of the medial compartment, caudal and me-dial to the temporohyoid articulation.
- Others occur on the lateral wall of the lateral compartment.

There is a close association between the predilection sites and the underly-ing internal carotid artery, and the external carotid or maxillary arteries, re-spectively.

On histopathological examination, fungal mycelia are found throughout the diphtheritic plaque but also invading the underlying wall of the guttural pouch and associated structures (including arteries and nerves). Erosion of the

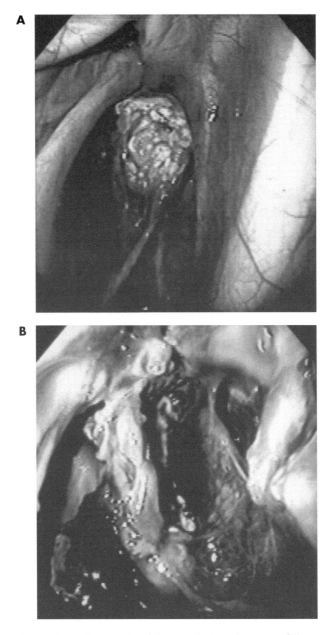

**Fig. 8.8.** Guttural pouch mycosis of the caudodorsal aspect of the medial compart-ment of the right guttural pouch over the internal carotid artery (A). Note the stylohy-oid bone to the left of the mycotic plaque. The endoscopic image in (B) demonstrates blood clots interspersed with the mycotic plaque from a horse with an extensive my-cotic plaque involving the entire pouch. *(See also color section.)*

wall of the internal carotid artery can result in aneurysmal dilation and even-tual rupture. The underlying bone may also be affected, resulting in exostoses. Erosion and fistula formation may occur in the median septum between the two guttural pouches, and into the nasopharynx.

The precise cause of guttural pouch mycosis is unknown. *Aspergillus* spp are likely to be opportunist invaders rather than primary pathogens. An underlying lesion of the arterial wall, such as an aneurysmal dilatation, has been suggested as a predisposing factor. However, aneurysms may also occur secondary to the mycosis.

Most cases of guttural pouch mycosis are unilateral, although bilateral cases can occasionally occur. The mycosis may erode through the median septum and invade the opposite pouch in chronic cases.

## Clinical signs

The development of an invasive fungal plaque on the mucosal wall of the guttural pouch can result in a variety of signs with consequences ranging from occult to fatal. The major presenting signs relate to arterial and neurological damage.

Spontaneous epistaxis at rest is the most frequently observed sign. Often this consists of a small quantity of fresh blood at one nostril in the first instance. Mucus and dark changed blood may continue to appear at the affected nostril for several days following the episode of epistaxis as blood that has accumulated in the pouch slowly drains out. A number of further minor hemorrhages may follow but, if untreated, a severe episode of bilateral epistaxis and exsanguination may follow. It is unusual for the first episode of epistaxis to be fatal, but the course of the disease from first to final hemorrhage rarely spans more than 3 weeks.

Pharyngeal paralysis is the most frequent neuropathy that accompanies guttural pouch mycosis. This results in dysphagia and the presence of ingesta in the nasal discharge. Coughing and free return of water out of the nostrils while drinking may be noted. Endoscopic evidence of pharyngeal paralysis includes persistent dorsal displacement of the palatal arch, the presence of saliva and ingesta in the nasopharynx, weak pharyngeal contractions and a failure of one or both of the pharyngeal ostia of the guttural pouches to dilate during deglutition.

Laryngeal hemiplegia is the next most frequent cranial nerve deficit encountered in horses with guttural pouch mycosis. However, this is unlikely to produce overt clinical signs noted by the owner.

Guttural pouch mycosis may produce a wide range of other signs referable to the head and upper neck. These include facial paralysis and Horner's syndrome, reluctance to lower the head to the ground and stiffness in the upper neck, parotid pain, otorrhea, epiphora, and photophobia. An abnormal head posture may be associated with pain in the atlanto-occipital joint when the mycosis has extended into this joint. Rarely, inflammation or mycotic infection may spread to the brain resulting in central defects such as blindness and ataxia.

## Diagnosis

Diagnosis of guttural pouch mycosis is made on the basis of the clinical signs, history, and endoscopic examination. Clinical signs are not specific, but whenever a horse is presented with spontaneous epistaxis, the possibility of guttural pouch mycosis should be considered, because delayed treatment may result in a fatal outcome.

Endoscopic examination usually reveals blood or mucus draining from the pharyngeal ostium of the affected pouch (see Fig. 8.2B). A definitive endoscopic diagnosis of a mycotic plaque inside the guttural pouch is not always straightforward. It must be recognized that the stress of handling the horse may precipitate a fatal hemorrhage. In addition, endoscopic visibility within the affected pouch may be poor after a recent hemorrhage (see Fig. 8.8B), and accurate location of the lesion may not be possible. Care is required when examining the internal aspects of the guttural pouch, because dislodging a blood clot could result in further hemorrhage. If the epistaxis has been recent, it is sufficient to identify the stream of blood flowing from the pharyngeal drainage ostium. In all cases of mycosis, the contralateral pouch should be checked for extension of the disease through the medial septum and for concurrent bilateral mycosis. A full endoscopic assessment of laryngeal and pharyngeal function is required for an accurate prognosis.

In cases where surgical occlusion of the affected artery is to be undertaken, an attempt should be made to determine which artery is involved (i.e., internal carotid or external carotid/maxillary arteries). Endoscopic examination may permit this assessment. The mycotic plaque or the adjacent inflammatory reaction in the mucosa is identified.

Radiographic examination of the guttural pouches may show partial or complete filling of the affected pouch by fluid. Although radiographs are not required for diagnosis, occasionally a mycotic plaque can be visualized radiographically. Bony exostoses or lysis of the stylohyoid bone may also be identified. Angiography can be used to demonstrate aneurysms of the internal or external carotid arteries; this procedure must be performed under general anesthesia and is necessary only if the source of hemorrhage (i.e., which artery is involved) cannot be determined by other means prior to surgical intervention.

## Treatment

Both medical and surgical treatments for guttural pouch mycosis can be used. The response to topical medication is usually very slow, and in view of the risk of fatal hemorrhage, surgical occlusion of the affected artery is generally recommended. However, medical treatment may be attempted in cases where there is no apparent imminent risk of hemorrhage. Topical antimycotic medication (itraconazole) can be administered via a catheter placed into the pouch in the same way as treatment for guttural pouch empyema. Direct placement of the medication on the lesions via endoscopic guidance is the preferred method of administration. Topical antifungal medication is frequently used as an adjunct to arterial occlusion. If topical medical therapy alone is to be attempted, treatment for several months is likely to be necessary. Systemic antifungal treatment may also be effective, but the treatment is usually very expensive. During any medical treatment there is a risk of hemorrhage. Horses that are dysphagic may require enteral support via nasogastric intubation or esophagostomy.

Surgical removal of the diphtheritic membrane is not recommended because it can precipitate fatal hemorrhage or severe cranial nerve deficits. If surgical occlusion of the affected artery is performed, spontaneous remission of the mycotic lesion is likely, and debulking the plaque is unnecessary. Surgical treatment aims to occlude the artery over which the mycotic plaque is situated. Prior endoscopic examination is generally adequate to identify which artery or arteries are affected. If the lesion is extensive and overlies both the internal and external carotid arteries, both arteries can be occluded simultaneously. Anomalies of the arterial anatomy sometimes occur, and these can result in failure of the surgery due to failure to prevent back-bleeding from the circle of Willis. Angiography may be helpful to identify anomalies of the arteries if this is suspected.

The major blood supply to the brain of a horse is the basilar artery. Thus, occlusion of both internal carotid arteries or of the common carotid artery can be undertaken without risk of cerebral ischemia. Retrograde blood flow from the contralateral internal carotid artery and from the basilar artery means that occlusion of the common carotid artery does not significantly affect blood pressure in the internal carotid artery. Thus, emergency ligation of the common carotid artery would not prevent hemorrhage from guttural pouch mycosis.

The internal carotid artery can be ligated immediately distal to its origin from the common carotid artery, outside the guttural pouch. The surgical approach is similar to that used in the hyovertebrotomy approach to the guttural pouch, but is placed more ventrally. The internal carotid artery usually originates on the cardiac side of the occipital artery and travels deep to that vessel in a more rostral direction. In some horses it can be difficult to distinguish between the internal carotid artery and the occipital artery, and both arteries may originate from a single trunk; in these cases, both arteries can be safely ligated together.

The internal carotid is not an end-artery and therefore the placement of a simple ligature on the cardiac side of the lesion will not always be successful, because retrograde hemorrhage (from the cerebral arterial circle of Willis) may occur. The placement of a single ligature does not reduce the blood pressure in the vessel distal to the ligature. However, in many cases, thrombosis of the vessel occurs following ligation, and this prevents serious hemorrhage. In order to prevent retrograde flow in the internal carotid artery distal to the site of ligature placement, a balloon-tipped silicone rubber catheter (4–8-French gauge), detachable latex balloon, or a 6-French gauge venous thrombectomy catheter can be placed into the internal carotid artery. The catheter is advanced about 13 cm to occlude the artery distal to the mycotic lesion; the catheter tip usually impacts at this distance, being the site of the second flexure of the sigmoid at the roof of the guttural pouch. The catheter is inflated with sterile saline and secured by ligation. The redundant part of the catheter is folded over and buried in the deeper tissues prior to wound closure.

The external carotid artery can be ligated at the same time as ligation of the internal carotid artery via the same incision. However, numerous collateral vessels are present that can result in retrograde flow to the lesion. The most likely of these is the major palatine artery. A balloon-tipped catheter or 6-F venous thrombectomy catheter can be inserted into the major palatine artery via an incision 3 cm caudal to the corner incisor tooth. The catheter is advanced in retrograde fashion 40–44 cm until its tip can be inflated in the maxillary artery immediately caudal to the caudal alar foramen. The mucosal incision is closed and the redundant portion of the catheter is brought out between the commissures of the lips, and tied inside a stockinette hood fashioned around the horse's head. The catheter is removed after 10 days.

If the internal carotid artery is not being occluded at the same time as the external carotid artery, a second balloon-tipped catheter needs to be placed. The catheter or venous thrombectomy catheter is inserted 12 cm into the transverse facial artery and directed in a retrograde fashion into the external carotid artery. The balloon is partly inflated, and the catheter withdrawn until resistance is met, at which point the balloon will be impacted against the origin of the superficial temporal artery. The balloon is deflated and advanced 2–3 cm in retrograde fashion into the external carotid artery, and then fully inflated. The wound is closed and the redundant portion of catheter fixed to the hood as above. The major potential complication of external carotid artery occlusion is blindness, especially when it is combined with internal carotid artery occlusion.

The use of long balloon-tipped catheters has been associated with a high complication rate due to incisional infection and catheter breakage. If wound infection occurs, the catheter can be removed by a simple cut-down procedure, performed under local anesthesia. These potential complications can be avoided if a detachable balloon is used for distal arterial occlusion. Embolization microcoils can also be used to produce arterial occlusion, but the procedure requires fluoroscopy, specialized equipment, and expertise.

## Prognosis

The prognosis for cases of guttural pouch mycosis not showing neurological deficits is generally good following arterial occlusion surgery. Although a small proportion of horses showing pharyngeal paralysis recover normal swallowing function, destruction on humane grounds is a more likely outcome and is indicated as soon as the patient shows signs of dehydration or aspiration pneumonia. Modest improvement of pharyngeal function can continue for more than a year after resolution of the infection. Laryngeal hemiplegia resulting from guttural pouch mycosis can be managed as for the idiopathic form recurrent laryngeal neuropathy.

Serious neurological complications, including cerebral abscessation, can occur several days following apparent successful arterial occlusion in a small percentage of horses. The flow of septic emboli or fungi to the brain may have been induced by the surgical manipulation of the artery in these cases.

## OTHER DISORDERS OF THE GUTTURAL POUCHES

Other disorders of the guttural pouches include rupture of the longus capitis and rectus capitis ventralis muscles, and avulsion fractures of the basioccipital and basisphenoid bones. The longus capitis and rectus capitis ventralis muscles insert onto the basisphenoid and occipital bones. Fractures at the junction of the basisphenoid and occipital bones may occur as an avulsion injury in horses that have reared over backwards. Affected horses usually present with epistaxis and variable degrees of neurological damage of the brainstem; signs of vestibular disease (including head tilt, nystagmus, and ataxia) are common. Endoscopic examination can be used to confirm that the origin of the epistaxis lies in the guttural pouches. There may be pharyngeal collapse, and blood is seen draining from the guttural pouch drainage ostium. Hemorrhage, blood clots, and submucosal hematoma formation may be seen in the rostral part of the pouch, compressing the pouch medially. This endoscopic appearance differentiates the condition from guttural pouch mycosis. The submucosal hematoma may be seen in the median septum in both guttural pouches, but it tends to be larger on one side. Radiographic examination identifies free fluid in the floor of the guttural pouches, avulsed bony fragments ventral to the basisphenoid bone, and a step in the base of the skull indicative of a fracture of the basisphenoid and basioccipital bones (Fig. 8.9). There is no effective treatment apart from symptomatic therapies, and the prognosis depends on the degree of neurological damage. The hematoma usually resolves spontaneously; antibiotic treatment is indicated to prevent abscess formation.

### Foreign bodies

Wire foreign bodies can penetrate into the retropharyngeal tissues and guttural pouch, where they may damage the neurovascular structures. The clinical signs include epistaxis, nasal discharge, dyspnea, dysphagia, and pain in the upper neck with restricted movement. The diagnosis is determined by radiographic examination. Although the radiographic identification of metallic material in the caudal wall of the guttural pouch is easy, projections in two planes are required for an accurate stereotactic location of the object.

### Neoplasia

Neoplasia of the guttural pouches is rare. Ectopic melanosis (see Fig. 8.1) is a common feature of the mucosa of the guttural pouches of grey horses, and primary melanomas can arise here. All regions of the horse richly endowed with lymphoreticular tissue are potential sites for development of lymphoma, and this tumor can arise in the tissues abutting onto the guttural pouches. Other reported tumors at this site include squamous cell carcinoma, fibrosarcoma,

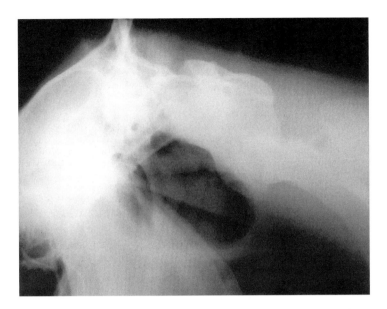

**Fig. 8.9.** Lateral radiographic projection of a horse with vestibular dysfunction after a traumatic head injury (flipped over backward). Note the evidence of hemorrhage (soft tissue opacity) dorsal to the guttural pouch and the presence of bony fragments from avulsion of bone by the *longus capitus mm.*

hemangioma, and hemangiosarcoma. Clinical signs can include parotid swelling, epistaxis, cranial nerve dysfunction, dyspnea, and dysphagia.

## FURTHER READING

Baptiste, K. 1997. Functional anatomy observations of the pharyngeal orifice of the equine guttural pouch (auditory tube diverticulum). *Vet J* 153:311–319.

Bayly, W.M., and Robertson, J.T. 1982. Epistaxis caused by foreign body penetration of a guttural pouch. *J Am Vet Med Assoc* 180:1232–1234.

Caron, J.P., Bailey, J.V., Barber, S.M., and Hurtig, M.B. 1987. Balloon-tipped catheter arterial occlusion for prevention of hemorrhage caused by guttural pouch mycosis: 13 cases (1982–1985). *J Am Vet Med Assoc* 191:345–349.

Cheramie, H.S., Pleasant, R.S., Robertson, J.L., Moll, H.D., Carrig, C.B., Freeman, D.E., and Jensen, M.E. 1999. Evaluation of a technique to occlude the internal carotid artery of horses. *Vet Surg* 28:83–90.

Colles, C.M., and Cook, W.R. 1983. Carotid and cerebral angiography in the horse. *Vet Rec* 113:483–489.

Cook, W.R. 1968. The clinical features of guttural pouch mycosis in the horse. *Vet Rec* 83:336–345.

Freeman, D.E. 1991. Guttural pouches. In *Equine Respiratory Disorders*. J. Beech, ed. Philadelphia: Lea & Febiger, pp 305–330.

Freeman, D.E., and Donawick, W.J. 1980. Occlusion of internal carotid artery in the horse by means of a balloon-tipped catheter: Evaluation of a method designed to prevent epistaxis caused by guttural pouch mycosis. *J Am Vet Med Assoc* 176:232–235.

Freeman, D.E., and Donawick, W.J. 1980. Occlusion of internal carotid artery in the horse by means of a balloon-tipped catheter: Clinical use of a method to prevent epistaxis caused by guttural pouch mycosis. *J Am Vet Med Assoc* 176:236–240.

Greene, H.J., and O'Connor, J.P. 1986. Haemangioma of the guttural pouch of a 16-year-old thoroughbred mare: Clinical and pathological findings. *Vet Rec* 118: 445–446.

Hardy, J., and Leveille, R. 2003. Diseases of the guttural pouch. *Vet Clinics N Am Equine Pract* 19:123–158.

Judy, C.E., Chaffin, M.K., and Cohen, N.D. 1999. Empyema of the guttural pouch (auditory tube diverticulum) in horses: 91 cases (1977–1997). *J Am Vet Med Assoc* 215:1666–1670.

Lane, J.G. 1998. Disorders of the ear, nose and throat. In *Equine Medicine, Surgery and Reproduction*. T. Mair, S. Love, J. Schumacher, and E. Watson, eds. London: W.B. Saunders, pp 81–117.

Leveille, R., Hardy, J., Robertson, J.T., Willis, A.M., Beard, W.L., Weisbrode, S.E., and Lepage, O.M. 2000. Transarterial coil embolization of the internal and external carotid arteries for prevention of hemorrhage from guttural pouch mycosis in horses. *Vet Surg* 29:389–397.

Matsuda, Y., Nakanishi, Y., and Mizuno, Y. 1998. Occlusion of the internal carotid artery by means of microcoils for preventing epistaxis caused by guttural pouch mycosis in horses. *J Vet Med Sci* 61:221–225.

Ragle, C.A. 2003. Guttural pouch disease. In *Current Therapy in Equine Medicine*, 5th ed. N.E. Robinson, ed. Philadelphia: W.B.Saunders, pp 386–390.

Seahorn, T.L., and Schumacher, J. 1991. Nonsurgical removal of chondroid masses from the guttural pouches of two horses. *J Am Vet Med Assoc* 199:368–369.

Stick, J.A., Wilson, T., and Kunze, D. 1980. Basilar skull fractures in three horses. *J Am Vet Med Assoc* 176:228–231.

Sweeney, C.R., Freeman, D.E., Sweeney, R.W., Rubin, J.L., and Maxson, A.D. 1993. Hemorrhage into the guttural pouch (auditory tube diverticulum) associated with rupture of the longus capitis muscle in three horses. *J Am Vet Med Assoc* 202: 1129–1131.

Tate, L.P., Blikslager, A.T., and Little, E.D.E. 1995. Transendoscopic laser treatment of guttural pouch tympanites in eight foals. *Vet Surg* 24:367–372.

Tetens, J., Tulleners, E.P., Ross, M.W., Orsini, P.G., and Martin, B.B. 1994. Transendoscopic contact neodymium:yttrium aluminium garnet laser treatment of tympany of the auditory tube diverticulum in two foals. *J Am Vet Med Assoc* 204:1927–1929.

# The Pharynx

## ANATOMY

The pharynx is a funnel-shaped musculomembranous sac that represents both a part of the digestive tract and a part of the respiratory tract. The tube connects the nasal cavity to the larynx. It is wider and larger rostrally than caudally. Its long axis is directed obliquely ventrad and caudad. The pharynx is attached by its muscles to the palatine, pterygoid, and hyoid bones, and to the cricoid and thyroid cartilages.

The cavity of the pharynx has seven openings: the two choanae (posterior nares), two pharyngeal openings of the auditory tubes (Eustachian tubes), the oral opening (isthmus faucium), the laryngeal opening (aditus laryngis) and the esophageal opening (aditus esophagi). Caudal to the openings of the auditory tubes, there is a median cul-de-sac (the pharyngeal recess). The dorsal part of the pharynx (nasopharynx) is lined by ciliated epithelium, and the submucosa contains numerous lymphoid aggregates, especially around the pharyngeal recess. The ventral part (oropharynx) is lined by stratified squamous epithelium. The two parts of the pharynx are separated by the soft palate.

The soft palate extends caudally from the hard palate to the base of the larynx. The soft palate has an oral mucous membrane on its ventral surface, and a respiratory mucosa on its dorsal surface. Within the substance of the soft palate are located the palatine glands, the palatine aponeurosis, and the palatinus and palatopharyngeus muscles.

Several different muscles alter and control the size and configuration of the nasopharynx, including muscles that control the position of the tongue, muscles that control the position of the hyoid apparatus, a constrictor group of muscles in the dorsal pharynx, and muscles that control the position of the soft palate.

The position of the soft palate is determined by the activity of different groups of antagonistic muscles, including the levator veli palatini, tensor veli palatini, palatinus, and palatopharyngeus muscles. The levator veli palatini muscle elevates the soft palate during swallowing and vocalization. The tensor veli palatini muscle expands the nasopharynx during inspiration by tensing the palatine aponeurosis, depressing the rostral part of the soft palate toward the tongue. The palatinus and palatopharyngeus muscles control the position of the caudal half of the soft palate. Contraction of the palatinus and palatopharyngeus muscles shortens the soft palate and depresses the caudal part toward the tongue. The innervation of the soft palate is through the pharyngeal branch of the vagus nerve, mandibular branch of the trigeminal nerve, and the glossopharyngeal nerve. The caudal free margin of the soft palate continues dorsally on either side of the larynx to form the palatopharyngeal arch.

## DORSAL DISPLACEMENT OF THE SOFT PALATE

Dorsal displacement of the soft palate (Fig. 9.1) can be intermittent or persistent:

- Intermittent dorsal displacement of the soft palate occurs during exercise, and is a cause of severe exercise intolerance, usually associated with an abnormal respiratory noise.
- The caudal border of the soft palate dislocates from its normal subepiglottic position to obstruct the airway.
- The condition commonly arises secondary to other diseases of the respiratory tract, including inflammatory diseases affecting the pharynx, or diseases that promote fatigue.
- Intermittent dorsal displacement of the soft palate generally occurs when a horse reaches the point of maximum exertion.
- The diagnosis is based on the history, clinical signs, and endoscopic examination.
- Endoscopy during exercise on a high-speed treadmill may be necessary to confirm the diagnosis.
- Conservative treatments include tack modifications, rest, and treatment of underlying pharyngeal inflammation.
- Surgical treatments include staphylectomy, strap (sternothyrohyoid) muscle resection, the Llewellyn procedure, epiglottic augmentation, tension palatoplasty, and laryngeal tie-forward.

The function of the palatopharyngeal arch is to provide an airtight seal that locks the larynx into the caudal wall of the nasopharynx. There is no communication between the nasopharynx and oropharynx. Thus, the larynx can be thought of as being like a "collar stud" that fits through a "buttonhole" in the soft palate. This mechanism renders the horse at exercise an obligatory nose-breather. The intranarial siting of the larynx provides streamlining of the air-

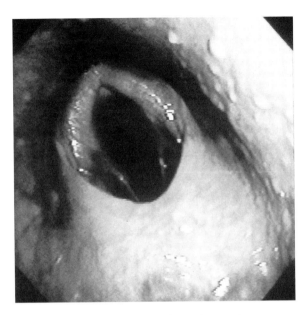

**Fig. 9.1.** Dorsal displacement of the soft palate. The epiglottis is not visible, and the soft palate is billowing dorsally during exhalation.

way. The larynx is suspended and held in place by the hyoid apparatus. Rostrally the palatal arch passes ventral to the epiglottis; laterally, it passes lateral to the aryepiglottic folds; and posteriorly, it runs caudal to the corniculate processes of the arytenoid cartilages. Thus, the free border of the palate is not visible by endoscopy when the larynx occupies its normal intranarial position. The conformation and position of the hyoid apparatus not only affects the position of the larynx, but also may influence the size and configuration of the pharynx.

The nasopharynx must withstand large changes in intraluminal pressure, from 30–60 cm $H_2O$ during inspiration and expiration, without cartilage or bony support. In addition, the nasopharynx is exposed to turbulent airflow at peak velocities of 90–100 liters/second, which causes vibration of the soft tissues within the nasopharynx that tend to lift the soft palate during expiration. The stability of the nasopharynx during these large changes in intraluminal pressure, and airflow is achieved by the contraction of skeletal muscles. Two mechanisms may help resist the collapsing inspiratory pressure and the uplifting expiratory pressure: extrinsic factors, including the muscles affecting hyoid and laryngeal positioning and the resulting geometry and tension on the nasopharynx; and intrinsic factors, such as dynamic nasopharyngeal muscle activity.

## Extrinsic factors

Historically, the epiglottis has been considered to play an important role in stabilizing the soft palate, and a relationship between epiglottic hypoplasia and dorsal displacement of the soft palate has been recognized. A theory was proposed that the epiglottis functions to hold the soft palate down, thereby preventing dorsal displacement. However, this theory seems unlikely, because horses with epiglottic retroversion and horses that have had the epiglottis surgically removed do not demonstrate dorsal displacement of the soft palate.

In addition to the muscles that are part of the nasopharyngeal walls, the hyoid apparatus, larynx, and muscles that affect the interrelationship between the larynx and the hyoid apparatus may tense the soft palate and nasopharynx. The muscles thought to play an important role in the position of the hyoid apparatus include the geniohyoid, genioglossus, omohyoid, and sternohyoid. Dysfunction of one or more of these muscles could result in an unstable nasopharynx.

## Intrinsic factors
The coordinated function of four muscles determines the soft palate position:

- Tensor veli palatini muscle (innervated by the mandibular branch of the trigeminal nerve)
- Levator veli palatini muscle (innervated by the pharyngeal branch of the vagus nerve)
- Palatinus muscle (innervated by the pharyngeal branch of the vagus nerve)
- Palatopharyngeus muscle (innervated by the pharyngeal branch of the vagus nerve)

Dorsal displacement of the soft palate can be persistent or, more commonly, intermittent. Horses with persistent dorsal displacement of the soft palate present with severe exercise intolerance and abnormal respiratory noise; there may also be dysphagia and coughing. Persistent dorsal displacement of the soft palate may be associated with concurrent epiglottal entrapment or with neurological deficits.

Intermittent dorsal displacement of the soft palate arises as an acute respiratory obstruction that occurs during fast exercise. The free border of the palatal arch becomes dislodged from its normal subepiglottic position (i.e., the collar stud disengages from the buttonhole), and the unsupported soft tissue is inhaled into the rima glottidis. The condition can occur secondary to underlying conditions, and may be a symptom rather than a disease in its own right. The underlying causes which have been proposed include

- Conditions causing fatigue—e.g., unfitness; primary cardiovascular disorders; primary pulmonary diseases, particularly small airway inflammation; and other concurrent obstructions of the conducting airways, such as recurrent laryngeal neuropathy
- Disorders of the palate itself or which compromise its function—e.g., congenital and iatrogenic defects, ulceration of the free border, intrapalatal cysts, and pharyngeal paralysis

- Disorders of the epiglottis—e.g., hypoplasia, deformity, entrapment, sub-epiglottic cysts, and epiglottitis
- Conditions causing mouth breathing—e.g., neglected dental enamel points; retained temporary premolar caps; bits which are too harsh for the patient's mouth; and excessive flexion of the neck when being ridden, typically seen in dressage and show horses
- Conditions provoking pharyngeal discomfort—e.g., pharyngeal lymphoid hyperplasia, pharyngitis, pharyngeal cysts, current upper respiratory tract infections, the presence of excessive discharges including mucopus or blood, and neoplasia
- Neuromuscular dysfunction involving the extrinsic and/or intrinsic muscles

Studies of the condition using high-speed treadmill endoscopy suggest that different forms of intermittent dorsal displacement of the soft palate can occur, and some are associated with other dynamic respiratory abnormalities.

## Clinical signs

Intermittent dorsal displacement of the soft palate affects horses during exercise. The abrupt respiratory obstruction that accompanies intermittent dorsal displacement of the soft palate not only causes a loud vibrant noise ("gurgling") but precipitates a serious interference with the progress of the horse ("choking up," "choking down"). In most cases, the horse completely loses its stride rhythm as it makes gulping attempts to restore the larynx into the intranarial position. Occasionally a horse will continue running noisily but with the severe handicap produced by partial asphyxiation. As soon as the normal anatomical configuration is restored, the horse is able to resume galloping and will not appear distressed thereafter.

Intermittent dorsal displacement of the soft palate generally occurs when a horse reaches the point of maximum exertion, typically in the later stages of a race or during a competitive gallop in training. Racehorses (including trotters and pacers) are mostly affected, but the dysfunction can occur in other occupations, such as eventing.

The noise is due to vibration of the caudal edge of the soft palate during exhalation. In some affected horses (up to 30%) no noise will be heard. Billowing of the cheeks may also be observed because of airflow diverted into the oral cavity.

## Diagnosis

The diagnosis is based on the history, clinical signs, and endoscopic examination. If there is any doubt, endoscopic examination during exercise on a high-speed treadmill may be necessary. Although a ridden exercise test should be included for cases of suspected intermittent dorsal displacement of the soft palate, it is unusual for a choking up episode to occur without the exertion of a race or competitive gallop.

Intermittent dorsal displacement of the soft palate during resting endoscopy is frequently observed in normal horses and should not be regarded as an indication of potential dynamic dysfunction during exercise. However, endoscopic confirmation of displacement of the soft palate dorsal to the epiglottis despite multiple (two or more) swallows during an examination immediately after exercise is suggestive of the diagnosis. Persistent dorsal displacement of the soft palate should always be regarded as significant, and is an indication for further investigation, such as radiography or endoscopy per os. Endoscopic findings at rest are poorly correlated with those during exercise on a high-speed treadmill. Endoscopy during exercise is currently the most effective way of diagnosing intermittent dorsal displacement of the soft palate. If endoscopy during exercise is performed, displacement of the palate may be observed at different stages during the exercise protocol, as well as at different phases of the respiratory cycle (i.e., inspiration, expiration, or swallowing). Displacement of the palate that persists for 8 seconds or longer is considered significant. Horses that are prone to dorsal displacement of the soft palate may demonstrate displacement during a standing endoscopic examination when the external nares are occluded; this procedure creates a negative pressure in the pharynx that is comparable to that occurring during exercise (see Fig. 9.1).

Ulceration of the free border of the soft palate is a not uncommon observation during standing endoscopy. In the past it had been assumed that such ulceration occurs as a result of repeated displacement and replacement of the soft palate, but a recent study suggests that there is no significant correlation between ulceration and displacement of the palate during high-speed treadmill exercise. The significance of ulceration is, therefore, uncertain, and it should not be assumed to be indirect evidence of intermittent dorsal displacement of the soft palate.

In addition to diagnosing dorsal displacement of the soft palate, attempts must be made to identify any predisposing factor(s). Even when a physical evaluation is combined with endoscopy, radiography, bronchoalveolar lavage and detailed clinical pathology, there are frequent cases where a specific cause is not found.

## Treatment

Every attempt should be made to eliminate the predisposing factors, including unfitness, or, alternatively, to provide additional time or medication for recovery from respiratory tract infections.

### Conservative measures and medical treatments

Routine dental attention should be directed to the removal of enamel points from the cheek teeth and to displace loose temporary premolar caps. Noninfectious inflammatory airway disease should be treated.

Devices aimed to prevent the horse from retracting the tongue and opening the mouth during exercise can be helpful. These include the tongue-tie or tongue-strap, and the figure-eight or Australian noseband. Other tack modifications to decrease head flexion may also be tried.

The pharyngeal branch of the vagus nerve is known to control the action of three of the four intrinsic soft palate muscles. This nerve traverses the medial wall of the guttural pouch and may, conceivably, be affected by inflammatory lesions affecting the mucosa at this site. The high prevalence of pharyngeal lymphoid hyperplasia, which also usually involves the walls of the guttural pouches, in young horses may explain why intermittent dorsal displacement of the soft palate is common in this age group. Owners of affected 2-year-olds may consider waiting until the following year before considering surgical treatments since the pharyngitis may resolve during the intervening time period.

### Surgical treatments

Various surgical treatments are available. These include staphylectomy, strap (sternothyrohyoid) muscle resection, the Llewellyn procedure, epiglottic augmentation, tension palatoplasty and laryngeal tie-forward. In cases of persistent dorsal displacement of the soft palate associated with epiglottal entrapment, surgical treatment of the epiglottal entrapment should be undertaken.

#### Staphylectomy

Historically, it was believed that intermittent dorsal displacement of the soft palate was due to elongation of the soft palate. Treatments were therefore devised to reduce the length or "tighten" the free border of the palate. Attempts to stiffen or thicken the free border of the palatal arch have included chemical and physical cautery. However, the most frequent technique comprises resection of the edge of the palate, staphylectomy. This technique appears to be illogical inasmuch as the effect of the surgery is to increase the size of the intrapharyngeal ostium so that the intranarial configuration of the larynx would be expected to be less stable. However, there is agreement that a proportion of horses are improved by staphylectomy—59% in one survey—and it has been suggested that the improvement arises through a reduction in the bulk of the tissues available to obstruct the rima glottidis.

Staphylectomy is performed under general anesthesia and through a conventional laryngotomy incision at the cricothyroid membrane. The caudal free edge of the soft palate is identified, and a crescent-shaped section of the soft palate (0.75 cm at the midline, tapering to each side) is resected. The laryngotomy wound can be partially or completely closed, or left open to heal by secondary intention. Dysphagia is a major complication of staphylectomy and occurs if too much tissue is resected, resulting in loss of the seal between the oropharynx and nasopharynx. Nd:YAG or diode laser augmentation of the free border of the soft palate has also been used to induce scar tissue formation and to discourage palatal displacement.

#### Strap muscle resection

Inhibition of the laryngeal retraction that precedes dorsal displacement of the soft palate may be achieved by section of the strap muscles—sternothyrohyoideus myectomy. The procedure can be performed on the standing horse under local analgesia, but is more safely and more accurately carried out under general anesthesia.

In the standing sedated horse, the head is elevated in cross-ties, and local anesthetic solution is infiltrated at the junction of the mid and proximal cervical area. A 10 cm ventral midline incision is made, and curved forceps are used to undermine each sternohyoid muscle. Following transection of the muscles proximally, the distal segment of muscle is grasped and pulled cranially prior to transection distally so that a 15 cm segment is removed. The smaller sternothyroid muscles are then exposed on the ventral surface of the trachea, and a section of each of these muscles is similarly resected. The skin is apposed in an appropriate manner.

The same procedure can be performed with the horse placed under general anesthesia. The omohyoid muscle can also be resected. Careful ligation of all vessels should be undertaken prior to subcutaneous and skin closure with placement of Penrose drains.

The complications of strap muscle resection are usually minor. Seroma or abscess formation is sometimes seen, usually after omohyoid resection. The overall success rate is reported to be around 60%, and is similar to that achieved by staphylectomy. On the basis that myectomy and staphylectomy performed independently produce approximately 60% success, some surgeons hold that the two techniques performed together increase the possibility of inhibiting dorsal displacement of the soft palate.

### Llewellyn procedure—Sternothyroid muscle resection and staphylectomy

The horse is placed under general anesthesia in dorsal recumbency. A 10 cm ventral midline incision is made centred on the cricothyroid membrane. The paired sternohyoid muscles are bluntly separated on the midline, and the tendon of insertion of the sternothyroid muscle on the thyroid cartilage is exposed. Removal of a section of the muscle and its tendon is then performed bilaterally. A laryngotomy and staphylectomy are then performed. Some surgeons also perform a sternohyoid myectomy (removing a 5 cm portion) or epiglottic augmentation at the same time.

### Epiglottic augmentation

With the horse in dorsal recumbency, a laryngotomy is performed and the epiglottis inverted into the lumen of the larynx by grasping the aryepiglottic fold on one side. Polytetrafluoroethylene (Teflon) is injected submucosally along the ventral surface of the epiglottis. Three injections are usually made, one along each side and one in the midline. A total of 3–7 ml is used. Alternatively, one midline injection of 3 ml can be made, followed by digital redistribution on the ventral surface of the epiglottis. The Teflon results in thickening of the epiglottis by 30–50% due to sterile granuloma formation and fibrosis.

### Tension palatoplasty

The oral palato-pharyngoplasty (Ahern procedure) is performed with the horse under general anesthesia and placed in dorsal or lateral recumbency. Through an oral approach with long-handled scissors, an elliptical incision is made in the oral palatine mucosa starting 1–2 cm caudal to the hard palate and extending caudally 1 cm past the palatopharyngeal arch. The palatine mucosa and submucosa down to the aponeurosis of the soft palate is resected. Care must be taken not to invade the aponeurosis; otherwise, a palatal fistula may result. The palatine mucosa is reapposed with simple interrupted sutures of absorbable material. This procedure reduces flaccidity of the soft palate at the point where the prodromal billowing arises. Excision of a section of glossoepiglottic tissue is often performed via a ventral laryngotomy incsion concurrently with the palatopharyngoplasty.

An alternative procedure involves cautery of the same area of the oral surface of the palate. Similar success rates have been reported. Cautery of the nasal surface of the soft palate can also be undertaken using transendoscopic laser surgery in standing horses.

### Laryngeal tie-forward
This is an experimental treatment that is currently being investigated. With the horse under general anesthesia, sutures are used to displace the thyroid cartilage rostrally by 3–4 cm.

## Prognosis
A cautious prognosis must be given for all horses in which intermittent displacement of the soft palate is diagnosed. The results of the surgical treatments outlined above are, at best, unpredictable.

## PHARYNGEAL LYMPHOID HYPERPLASIA

Pharyngeal lymphoid hyperplasia, also known as follicular pharyngitis, is a common and normal condition in young horses, especially those less than 2 years old (Fig. 9.2):

- Resolution of hyperplasia occurs as the horse ages, and it is unusual in horses older than 5 years of age.
- Extensive pharyngeal lymphoid hyperplasia could affect performance and cause an abnormal respiratory noise.
- Diagnosis is achieved by endoscopic examination.
- Most cases do not require specific treatment.

Pharyngeal lymphoid hyperplasia is probably the result of exposure to novel antigens, including bacteria, viruses, organic dusts, and other allergens. It affects virtually all young horses, and as such is considered a normal maturation process. Resolution of the hyperplasia occurs as the horse ages and the immune system matures. It is unusual in horses older than 5 years of age. The

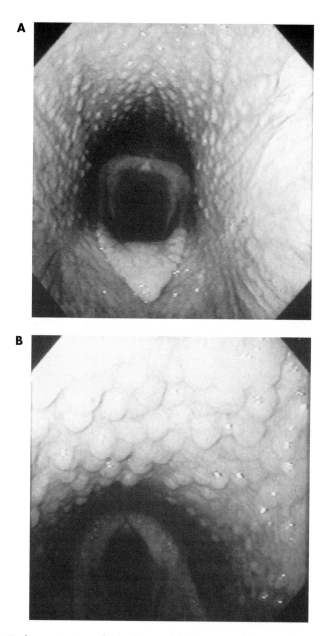

**Fig. 9.2.** Endoscopic view of the pharynx of two young horses with Grade II (A) and Grade III (B) lymphoid pharyngeal hyperplasia. *(See also color section.)*

condition is characterized by extensive follicles of lymphoid hyperplasia on the walls of the nasopharynx and pharyngeal recess.

## Clinical signs

In most cases, there appears to be little interference with the performance of young horses with pharyngeal lymphoid hyperplasia. However, some clinicians believe that extensive pharyngeal lymphoid hyperplasia might affect performance because of a disturbance of normal laminar airflow and a reduction of pharyngeal diameter. An abnormal respiratory noise may be heard in such cases. In addition, inflammation of the pharynx and discomfort associated with engorged follicles has been proposed to lead to dynamic collapse and dorsal displacement of the soft palate.

## Diagnosis

Diagnosis is determined by endoscopic examination. The degree of pharyngeal lymphoid hyperplasia can be classified using the following grading system:

- Grade 1: A few small inactive whitish follicles over the dorsal wall (normal)
- Grade 2: Numerous small inactive follicles, with occasional hyperemic follicles, extending downward over the lateral pharyngeal walls (see Fig. 9.2A)
- Grade 3: More active follicles located close together, covering the entire dorsal and lateral walls of the pharynx (see Fig. 9.2B)
- Grade 4: Large edematous follicles, frequently coalesced into broad-based and polypoid structures

Grade 1 and 2 lesions are not associated with clinical signs. Grade 3 and 4 lesions might be associated with an abnormal respiratory noise, and possibly with exercise intolerance. However, the precise relationship between pharyngeal lymphoid hyperplasia and exercise intolerance is difficult to establish.

## Treatment

A variety of different treatments have been used for pharyngeal lymphoid hyperplasia. However, since this reaction is believed to be a normal maturation process, most cases do not require specific treatment. Treatment should be confined to the rare cases where a significant clinical problem exists.

Medical treatments have included intensive vaccination against equine influenza and equine herpesviruses 1 and 4. Pharyngeal sprays containing antimicrobial and anti-inflammatory agents can also be applied to the affected region once or twice a day for 7–14 days. Rest may also be necessary in severe cases.

Grade 4 pharyngeal lymphoid hyperplasia, which is refractory to medical management, has been treated surgically with 50% trichloracetic acid, electrocautery, and cryotherapy. Topical treatment with trichloracetic acid and cryotherapy can be performed under endoscopic control in standing horses. Electrocautery is performed via a laryngotomy incision with the horse in dorsal recumbency. Laser photovaporization could also be used.

In addition to generalized lymphoid hyperplasia, large discrete polypoid aggregates can arise. These are more likely to be clinically significant by virtue of their size. These masses may be resected via a laryngotomy incision, or excised transendoscopically with an Nd:YAG laser.

Surgical treatments are rarely necessary for pharyngeal lymphoid hyperplasia and should be undertaken cautiously. A possible untoward sequela might be the development of a pharyngeal cicatrix.

## NASOPHARYNGEAL CICATRICES

A nasopharyngeal cicatrix is a transverse stricturing web of fibrous tissue in the nasopharynx:

- Nasopharyngeal cicatrices occur most commonly in horses older than 5 years of age.
- Most cases present with signs of exercise intolerance, abnormal respiratory noise, or dyspnea.
- The diagnosis is achieved by endoscopy.
- Surgical treatments have been described for severe lesions.

Nasopharyngeal cicatrices have been reported most commonly in Texas, and appear to be rare elsewhere. The cicatrix is frequently associated with laryngeal abnormalities.

### Clinical signs
Nasopharyngeal cicatrices occur most commonly in horses older than 5 years of age. Females are reported to be affected more commonly than males. No breed predeliction has been reported. Most cases present with signs of exercise intolerance, abnormal respiratory noise, or dyspnea, although some cases have been identified as an incidental finding during routine endoscopic examination in asymptomatic horses.

### Diagnosis
The diagnosis is achieved by endoscopic examination. A constriction is present in the nasopharynx, involving only the soft palate or involving the whole circumference of the pharynx (i.e., soft palate, walls, and roof of the pharynx). Other abnormalities are commonly present, including arytenoid chondropathy, epiglottic deformity, and deformity of the pharyngeal ostia of the guttural pouches.

### Treatment
Treatment may not be required if there is no respiratory impairment. Successful treatment of cicatrices has been described in three horses; the cicatrix was cut in one or more places in all three horses, and in one horse a cuffed orotracheal tube was passed nasally to dilate the stricture. The nasopharynx appeared to regain about 75% of its normal diameter in all three horses. Other proposed treatments include laser ablation or bougie dilation. Treatment of any associated lesion, such as arytenoid chondropathy, may be required.

## CLEFT PALATE (PALATOSCHISIS)

Cleft palate is an uncommon congenital deformity of unknown etiology:

- Most defects affect the caudal aspect of the soft palate (Fig. 9.3A).
- Acquired cleft palates can occur as a complication of dental or upper airway surgery (Fig. 9.3B).

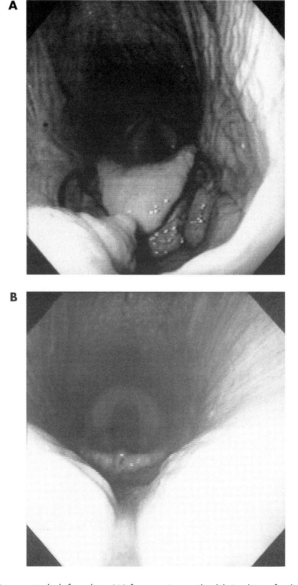

**Fig. 9.3.** Congenital cleft palate (A) from a 6-month-old Arabian foal with dysphagia since birth. The lateral aspect of the soft palate is absent and the oral mucosa is visible from the nasopharynx. Also shown, an iatrogenic cleft palate (B), which occurred during surgical correction of an epiglottic entrapment using an oral hook.

- Most affected animals present within the first few weeks of life with signs of the appearance of milk at the nostrils, coughing after nursing and un-thriftiness.
- Aspiration pneumonia is a common and serious complication.
- Diagnosis is confirmed by digital and visual examination of the oral cavity, and endoscopy.
- Surgical treatment via a mandibular symphysiotomy and/or transhyoid pharyngotomy can be attempted.

Defects of the hard and soft palates may be congenital or iatrogenic (see Fig. 9.3). The hard palate is formed by the fusion of the palatine processes of the incisive and maxillae bones and the horizontal plates of the palatine bone. These palatine processes normally fuse during embryological life in a rostral to caudal plane around day 47 of gestation. Cleft palate is an uncommon con-genital deformity. Most defects preferentially affect the caudal aspect of the soft palate, but can rarely extend to the hard palate. Midline clefts are more common than lateral defects. Hard palate cleft results from a failure of the lat-eral palatine processes of these bones to fuse during embryonic development. The etiology of soft palate congenital cleft is unknown, but the condition is heritable in other species.

Acquired cleft palates are a complication of dental or upper airway surgery (see Fig 9.3B). Hard palate clefts (oronasal fistulae) result from inadvertent fracture of the palate by a tooth punch during repulsion of upper cheek teeth. Soft palate clefts can result from using a hook knife through a nasal approach for treatment of epiglottal entrapment.

The hard palate has a static role in separating the respiratory and digestive tracts, and the soft palate dynamically closes the choanae during swallowing. Failure of this separation between airway and digestive tract leads to contam-ination of the nasal cavity and tracheal aspiration of feed material. The degree of nasal and airway contamination is dependent on the size and location of the cleft. A cleft rostral to the levator veli palatini muscle on the soft palate results in nasal or nasopharyngeal contamination. Clefts caudal to levator veli pala-tini muscles cause less consistent airway contamination.

A cleft soft palate leads to dorsal displacement of the soft palate during ex-ercise and, therefore, an increase in expiratory impedance. This expiratory re-sistive load appears to be due to the soft palate's inability to form a proper laryngopalatal seal around the epiglottis and arytenoid cartilages. During ex-halation, this results in airflow being directed to the oropharynx, thus lifting the soft palate into the nasopharynx and partially occluding its lumen, caus-ing an expiratory obstruction.

## Clinical signs

There is no breed or gender predisposition for congenital cleft palate. Most af-fected animals present within the first few weeks of life with signs of the ap-pearance of milk at the nostrils, coughing after nursing, unthriftiness, stunted growth, purulent nasal discharge, fever, depression, and signs of aspiration pneumonia. Some horses with more caudal and shorter clefts go unnoticed for many months and are presented with a history of recurrent lower airway infection, stunted growth, and an occasional observation of feed material at the nostrils. Cleft palate can also occur in association with wry nose and other congenital abnormalities.

Acquired cleft palate usually presents clinical signs shortly after a surgical procedure for treatment of upper airway disease or, more rarely, after treatment of dental disease.

## Diagnosis

A presumptive diagnosis of congenital cleft palate can be made on the basis of the typical clinical signs. The definitive diagnosis is made by a combination of an oral examination and endoscopic evaluation of the nasal cavity and nasopharynx. In young foals, digital palpation can assess the integrity of the hard palate. The endoscopic diagnosis of cleft palate is made through observation of a lack of palate continuity or by observation of oral structures, including the pale oropharynx mucosa with its numerous folds and rounded elevations containing the tonsils and the glossoepiglottic fold at the base of the epiglottis. Congenital hard palate cleft is always on the midline, and soft palate cleft may be on the midline (axial) or to one side (abaxial).

## Treatment

The treatment of choice for cleft palate is one-stage surgical correction of the defect, but the high complication rates (dehiscence of the repair site, chronic nasal discharge, and high mortality rates) and frequent need for revisions have limited the number of horses receiving surgical treatment. The status of the lower airway influences the anesthetic risk to the patient. Delay in repair increases the chance of lower airway infection and poor growth, but the size of the oral cavity and nasopharynx in young foals limits exposure for surgical manipulation.

Mandibular symphysiotomy and/or transhyoid pharyngotomy are the most widely described surgical approaches. Both approaches allow acceptable access with long instruments so primary repair of the cleft palate is possible. A mucosa-periosteal sliding flap is used to close the hard palate. If adequate soft palate tissue is available for repair with minimal tension on the incision site, the standard method for closure of the soft palate in horses involves a three-layer closure of the defect, using a combination of vertical and horizontal mattress patterns. However, if significant soft palate tissue is missing so that palate repair without tension is impossible, buccal mucosal flaps can be used. This technique can be done only via a mandibular symphysiotomy.

## Prognosis

The rate of successful healing of a repaired cleft palate may be as high as 70% after one or more surgeries. It is not uncommon for one or two revisions to be needed to obtain sufficient healing to resolve clinical signs.

Reported complications associated with mandibular symphysiotomy include dehiscence of the lip, osteomyelitis of the mandibular pin tracts, and submandibular abscesses. In addition, tongue paralysis can result from damage to the hypoglossal or lingual nerves during surgery. One potential long-term complication following transhyoid pharyngotomy is epiglottic retroversion at exercise, because this approach has the potential to cause trauma to the hyoepiglotticus muscle and/or its innervation.

## SUBEPIGLOTTIC, PHARYNGEAL, AND PALATAL CYSTS

Developmental cysts are occasionally recognized in the pharynx as a cause of dyspnea and/or dysphagia:

- Pharyngeal cysts may occur in the subepiglottic position (most common), dorsal pharynx, or soft palate.
- Subepiglottic cysts (Fig. 9.4) are thought to be derived from the embryological remnants of the thyroglossal duct.
- Large subepiglottic cysts can cause dysphagia and respiratory obstruction in foals.
- In older horses, pharyngeal cysts present with signs of nasal discharge, dysphagia, poor performance, and abnormal respiratory sounds at exercise.

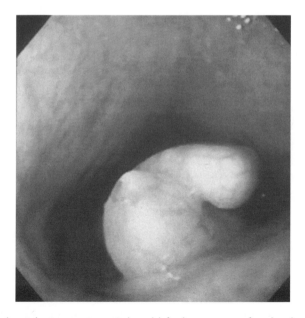

**Fig. 9.4.** Subepiglottic cyst in a 5-day-old foal presenting for dysphagia. The cyst was intermittently visible in the nasopharynx (as seen in this picture), and was primarily hidden under the soft palate in the oropharynx. *(See also color section.)*

- Diagnosis is made by endoscopic and/or radiographic examination.
- Surgical treatment is recommended.

As mentioned, the most frequently encountered of these lesions is the subepiglottic cyst which is thought to be derived from the embryological remnants of the thyroglossal duct, a structure which runs from the level of the epiglottis to the anterior mediastinum. Trauma or inflammation has also been proposed as a potential cause of subepiglottic cysts. Less commonly, cysts may occur in the dorsal pharynx, the walls of the pharynx and in the soft palate. Cysts in the dorsal pharynx may represent remnants of the craniopharyngeal duct or Rathke's pouch, and palatal cysts may be of salivary origin.

Although cysts have been recognized in all breeds, they are most commonly reported in Thoroughbreds and Standardbreds. It is believed that most subepiglottic cysts are present from birth, but they may not be discovered until the horse is mature and commences training.

Subepiglottic cysts consist of smooth-walled, sometimes multilobular, structures filled with straw-colored slightly tenacious fluid. They arise from within the loose glossoepiglottic mucosa lying between the base of the tongue and the epiglottis. They are covered by stratified squamous, pseudostratified, or cuboidal epithelium. It is very rare for a subepiglottic cyst to be found that is not located within an epiglottal entrapment.

## Clinical signs
The age and manner by which the cysts cause clinical signs are dependent on their size. Large cysts can cause dysphagia and respiratory obstruction in foals. Such foals may present within a few days of birth with reflux of milk from the nares. These cases require endoscopic examination for differentiation from foals with palatal clefts or laryngeal dysfunction. They may also show clinical signs of coughing, bilateral mucopurulent nasal discharge, and aspiration pneumonia.

In older horses, pharyngeal cysts may present with a variety of signs, including nasal discharge, dysphagia, poor performance, and abnormal respiratory sounds at exercise. The nature and severity of the clinical signs varies with the size of the cysts. Unlike foals, aspiration pneumonia is rare in older horses. Horses with small subepiglottic cysts may present with a history of choking up at exercise and will require differentiation from dorsal displacement of the soft palate.

## Diagnosis
The diagnosis of pharyngeal cysts is easily established by endoscopic examination, provided that the cystic lesions are available to be seen. Subepiglottic cysts vary in size from 1–5 cm in diameter. They appear as smooth-walled cystic masses situated under or slightly lateral to the epiglottis and above the caudal margin of the soft palate. In some cases the cyst may be hidden from view by the caudal edge of the soft palate; in such cases the area should be

observed for several minutes and the horse made to swallow, which should allow the cyst to become visible (often in association with an epiglottal entrapment).

Occasionally horses with subepiglottic cysts have concurrent persistent dorsal displacement of the soft palate; in these cases, the cyst will not be visible by nasal endoscopy and the horse will fail to return the soft palate to a subepiglottic position despite numerous swallowing attempts. Other diagnostic procedures, such as plain and contrast radiography, can help to identify a soft tissue mass in the subepiglottic position in these cases. Alternatively, the cyst may be visualised by endoscopy performed through the mouth with the horse placed under general anesthesia. Soft palate cysts may also not be easily identified by nasal endoscopy, and contrast radiography of the oropharynx can be helpful to outline them.

## Treatment

Surgical resection of subepiglottic cysts can be performed in several ways. A snare of stainless steel or obstetrical wire, or an ecraseur can be passed through the mouth of the horse placed under general anesthesia. The cyst is placed into the loop of the snare with one hand, and then the snare is pulled tight to amputate the cyst. Care is needed to ensure that only the cyst and its mucosal lining are incorporated in the snare. Healing is usually rapid, and the horse can be returned to work in 1–2 weeks.

Surgical resection can also be performed through a standard laryngotomy incision with the horse in dorsal recumbency. The epiglottis is everted into the larynx, and the cyst brought into view by applying traction to the aryepiglottic folds and the subepiglottic tissues, using Alice tissue forceps. The cyst is dissected away from the surrounding tissues and excised through its stalk at the base of the epiglottis. The mucosal defect can be sutured or left to heal by secondary intention. Treatment for concurrent epiglottal entrapment, if present, should be performed at the same time. In foals, where the cyst may have an inflammatory etiology, the aryepiglottic and glossoepiglottic mucosa around the cyst should be excised to prevent recurrence. Rest for 4–6 weeks is recommended following surgical resection.

If available, an Nd:YAG laser passed through an endoscope inserted via the mouth can also be used to dissect the cyst free. Access for surgical dissection of other pharyngeal and soft palate cysts is difficult but ventral laryngotomy offers the best option. Iatrogenic fenestration of the soft palate is a likely surgical complication when excision of palatal cysts is attempted. Non-contact laser ablation can also be used.

## Prognosis

Subepiglottic cystic lesions can often be excised intact and a favorable prognosis can be given. Recurrence is unlikely. Prognosis for other pharyngeal cysts depends on their size and accessibility for surgical resection. The prognosis for horses with soft palate cysts is generally poor.

## PHARYNGEAL PARALYSIS

Pharyngeal paralysis causes dysphagia, with food and water exiting via the nostrils. Although dynamic collapse of the pharyngeal walls and intractable dorsal displacement of the soft palate would lead to partial asphyxiation during exercise, this is most unlikely to be a major presenting sign. Paralysis may result from a brain-stem lesion involving the pharyngeal nuclear regions of the glossopharyngeal (IX) and vagus (X) nerves, or a lesion affecting the peripheral parts of these nerves. Guttural pouch mycosis is the most common cause of pharyngeal paralysis (hemiplegia). Other causes of pharyngeal paralysis include heavy metal poisoning (such as lead) and botulism.

## PHARYNGEAL NEOPLASIA

Neoplasia of the nasopharynx is rare. However, all tissues that are rich in lymphoreticular elements are susceptible to lymphoma development, and this tumor occasionally arises in the nasopharynx. Squamous cell carcinoma (Fig. 9.5) may invade the nasopharynx from the nasal cavity, or it may metastasize to the retropharyngeal lymph nodes from a primary site in the oral cavity. Other tumors at this location are very rare.

Signs relate to the size and location of the tumor masses. Dyspnea due to airway obstruction, dysphagia, nasal discharge, and enlargement of submandibular lymph nodes are likely. Neoplastic destruction of the palate may lead to the formation of an oronasal fistula and ingesta-stained nasal discharge.

Diagnosis is achieved by endoscopic, radiographic, and histopathologic examination. Computed tomographic scanning provides information regarding the size and extent of the tumor. Treatment is rarely possible. Radiotherapy can be used to treat some tumors in this area. Alternatively, treatment by intralesional chemotherapy or laser excision might be considered in appropriate cases.

## PHARYNGEAL TRAUMA

Iatrogenic injury to the pharynx may occur as a result of nasogastric intubation and as a result of surgical treatments of other upper airway diseases. The use of an indwelling nasogastric tube in horses with gastric reflux has rarely been associated with pressure necrosis and rupture of the pharyngeal wall. Retropharyngeal emphysema and cellulitis, and descending sepsis along the fascial planes of the neck can result.

Iatrogenic palatal defects can arise through overenthusiastic resection surgery or laser surgery for dorsal displacement of the soft palate, and damage from treatment of epiglottal entrapment. Excessive resection surgery of the caudal border of the soft palate often leads to chronic palatal instability lead-

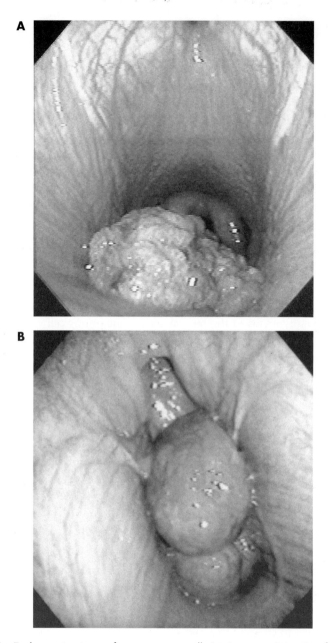

**Fig. 9.5.** Endoscopic views of a squamous cell carcinoma originating from the oral cavity partially obstructing the nasopharynx (A) and a giant cell tumor originating from the dorsal pharyngeal recess completely obstructing the nasopharynx (B). The giant cell tumor is viewed via retrograde examination through the tracheotomy incision. The slits on either side of the mass are the guttural pouch openings. *(See also color section.)*

ing to more severe signs of dorsal displacement of the soft palate. Horses with an iatrogenically induced palatal defect may be subjected to treatment via a mandibular symphysiotomy or an oral approach, depending on the size and location of the defect.

## PHARYNGEAL AND RETROPHARYNGEAL FOREIGN BODIES

Foreign bodies, including metal objects, twigs and thorns can occasionally cause penetrating wounds to the pharynx and initiate infection in the retropharyngeal tissues and/or guttural pouch:

- Foreign bodies in the pharynx or retropharyngeal area are a rare cause of dysphagia and dyspnea.
- Swelling of the parotid region may be present.
- Diagnosis is made by endoscopic and radiographic examination.
- Endoscopic or surgical removal may be possible.

### Clinical signs
Affected horses usually present with a combination of dysphagia, dyspnea, swelling in the parotid region, purulent or bloody nasal discharge, and pain in the throat region with reluctance to flex the poll.

### Diagnosis
The diagnosis is confirmed and the location of the foreign body established by a combination of endoscopy, radiography, and ultrasonography. Computed tomographic scanning provides precise information regarding the extent and location of the foreign body and damage to tissues.

### Treatment
Treatment involves removal of the foreign body and elimination of infection. The approach to removal of the foreign body is dependent on the location of the object. Perioperatively, antibiotics and nonsteroidal anti-inflammatory drugs should be administered. A temporary tracheotomy may be required if there is severe dyspnea.

## RETROPHARYNGEAL ABSCESS

A retropharyngeal abscess may develop as a result of septic lymphadenopathy (e.g., *Streptococcus equi* infection) or following trauma to the pharynx:

- *Streptococcus equi* is the most common reason for retropharyngeal abscess formation.
- Parotid swelling is accompanied by signs of dysphagia and dyspnea.
- Swelling/impingement of the medial compartment of the guttural pouch may be seen via endoscopic examination.
- Diagnostic ultrasonography and percutaneous centesis are valuable diagnostic procedures.

• Treatment options include prolonged antibiotic therapy, surgical drainage, and percutaneous needle drainage.

## Clinical signs

A unilateral retropharyngeal swelling develops, which causes lateral and dorsal compression of the nasopharynx, ventral compression of the guttural pouch, compression of the larynx and esophagus, and lateral swelling of the parotid region (Fig. 9.6). Dyspnea, inspiratory stertor, dysphagia, fever, increased salivation, nasal discharge, and coughing may be noted.

## Diagnosis

Diagnosis is determined by a combination of the physical examination, endoscopy, radiography, ultrasonography, and hematology. External palpation over the parotid region of the affected side frequently produces a pain response. Hematology reveals leukocytosis and hyperfibrinogenemia. On endoscopic examination per nasum, the nasopharynx appears constricted on the affected side. The swelling may also cause distortion of the larynx, with medial displacement of the corniculate process on the affected side. Endoscopic examination of the guttural pouch often shows compression of the medial compartment, often with a mass projecting from a caudoventral direction. In some cases, purulent exudate may be observed draining into the guttural pouch. Occasionally, an abscess may rupture into the nasopharynx, in which case exudate will be seen draining from this site.

Lateral radiographic projection identifies a soft tissue mass that impinges on the caudoventral aspect of the guttural pouch and causes a ventral depression of the roof of the pharynx. The roof of the pharynx appears thickened. Transcutaneous ultrasonography can be used to identify the abscess in some

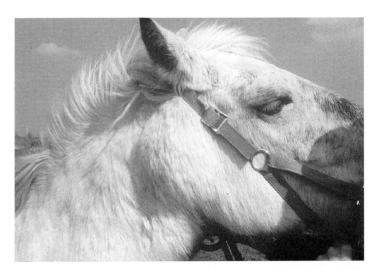

**Fig. 9.6.** Parotid swelling due to a large retropharyngeal abscess.

cases. Percutaneous needle aspiration is challenging due to the depth of the abscess and the presence of vital structures. Ultrasonographic guidance may allow the clinican to obtain an adequate sample for bacterial culture and sensitivity.

## Treatment

Treatment options include medical therapy with broad spectrum antibiotics and nonsteroidal anti-inflammatory drugs, surgical drainage of the abscess, or percutaneous needle aspiration and instillation of antibiotics directly into the abscess cavity. The latter technique is performed under ultrasound guidance. In some cases a tracheotomy may be necessary, and nasogastric tube feeding may be required in cases affected by severe dysphagia. Surgical drainage can be achieved via an approach similar to the modified Whitehouse approach for guttural pouch surgery or via Viborg's triangle. Drainage via Viborg's triangle can be undertaken in the standing horse using regional infiltration with local anesthetic solution. An 18-gauge needle can be inserted in the middle of Viborg's triangle and directed dorsally and cranially at an angle of about 45°. When pus can be aspirated, a scalpel is advanced along the line of the needle until the abscess cavity is opened.

## Prognosis

The prognosis is usually good. Surgical treatment provides rapid resolution of the problem, whereas medical treatment alone may take many weeks.

## FURTHER READING

Adams, R., Calderwood-Mays, M.B., and Peyton, L.C. 1988. Malignant lymphoma in three horses with ulcerative pharyngitis. *J Am Vet Med Assoc* 193:674–676.

Ahern, T.J. 1993. Oral palatopharyngoplasty: A survey of one hundred post-operative raced horses. *Equine Vet Sci* 13:670–672.

Anderson, J., Tulleners, E.P., Johnston, J.J. 1995. Sternothyrohyoideus myectomy or staphylectomy for treatment of intermittent dorsal displacement of the soft palate in racehorses: 209 cases (1986–1991) *J Am Vet Med Assoc* 206:1909–1912.

Burrows, G.E. 1982. Lead poisoning in the horse. *Equine Pract* 4:30–36.

Ducharme, N.G. 2002. DDSP: Anatomy, diagnosis and surgical options. *Proc 12th Ann Vet Symp Am Coll Vet Surg*, pp 205–208.

Ducharme, N.G., Hackett, R.P., Woodie, J.B., Dykes, N., Erb, H.N., Mitchell, L.M., and Soderholm, L.V. 2003. Investigations into the role of the thyrohyoid muscles in the pathogenesis of dorsal displacement of the soft palate in horses. *Equine Vet J* 35:258–263.

Gaughan, E.M., and DeBowes, R.M. 1993. Congenital diseases of the equine head. *Vet Clinics N Am Equine Pract* 9:93–110.

Hahn, C.N., Mayhew, I.G., and Mackay, R.J. 1999. Botulism. In *Equine Medicine and Surgery*, 5th ed. P.T. Colahan, A.M. Merritt, J.N. Moore, and I.G. Mayhew, eds. St. Louis: Mosby, pp 981–983.

Hamilton, D.P. 1973. Pharyngeal rupture in a horse. *J Am Vet Med Assoc* 162:466.

Hardy, J., and Leveille, R. 2003. Diseases of the guttural pouch. *Vet Clinics N Am Equine Pract* 19:123–158.

Hardy, J., Stewart, R.H., Beard, W.L., and Yvorchuk-St-Jean, K. 1992. Complications of nasogastric intubation in horses: Nine cases (1987–1989). *J Am Vet Med Assoc* 201:483–486.

Harrison, I., and Raker, C. 1988. Sternothyrohyoideus myectomy in horses: 17 cases (1984–1985). *J Am Vet Med Assoc* 193:1299–1300.

Haynes, P. 1983. Dorsal displacement of the soft palate and epiglottic entrapment: Diagnosis, management, and interrelationship. *Comp Cont Ed Pract Vet* 5:S379–389.

Haynes, P.F., Beadle, R.E., McClure, S.R., and Roberts, E.D. 1990. Soft palate cysts as a cause of pharyngeal dysfunction in two horses. *Equine Vet J* 22:369–371.

Holcombe, S.J., Beard, W.L., Hinchcliff, K.W., and Robertson, J.T. 1994. Effect of sternothyrohyoid myectomy on upper airway mechanics in exercising horses. *J Applied Physiol* 77:2812–2816.

Holcombe, S.J., Derksen, F.J., and Stick, J.A. 1999. Pathophysiology of dorsal displacement of the soft palate in horses. *Equine Vet J Suppl* 30:45–48.

Holcombe, S.J., Robertson, J.T., and Richardson, L. 1994. Surgical repair of iatrogenic soft palate defects in two horses. *J Am Vet Med Assoc* 205:1315–1317.

Jones, D. 1994. Squamous cell carcinoma of the larynx and pharynx in horses. *Cornell Vet* 84:15–24.

Kiper, M.L., Wrigley, R., Traub-Dargatz, J., and Bennett, D. 1992. Metallic foreign bodies in the mouth or pharynx of horses: Seven cases (1983–1989). *J Am Vet Med Assoc* 200:91–93.

Koch, D.B., and Tate, L.P. 1978. Pharyngeal cysts in horses. *J Am Vet Med Assoc* 173:860–862.

Lane, J.G. 1985. Palatine lymphosarcoma in two horses. *Equine Vet J* 17:465–467.

Lane, J.G. 1998. Disorders of the ear, nose and throat. In *Equine Medicine, Surgery and Reproduction*. T. Mair, S. Love, J. Schumacher, and E. Watson, eds. London: W.B.Saunders, pp 81–117.

McClure, S.R., Robertson, J.T., and Snyder, J.R. 1994. Transnasal incision of restrictive nasopharyngeal cicatrix in three horses. *J Am Vet Med Assoc* 205:461–463.

Nelson, A.W., Curley, B.M., and Kainer, R.A. 1971. Mandibular symphysiotomy to provide adequate exposure for intraoral surgery in the horse. *J Am Vet Med Assoc* 159:1025–1031.

Parente, E.J., and Martin, B.B. 1995. Correlation between standing endoscopic examinations and those made during high speed exercise in horses: 150 cases. *Proc 41st Ann Conv Am Assoc Equine Pract*, p 170.

Parente, E.J., Martin, B.B., and Tulleners, E.P. 2002. Dorsal displacement of the soft palate in 92 horses during high-speed treadmill examination (1993–1998). *Vet Surg* 31:507–512.

Raker, C.W., and Boles, C.R. 1978. Pharyngeal lymphoid hyperplasia in the horse. *J Equine Med Surg* 2:202–207.

Robertson, J.T. 1991. Pharynx and larynx. In *Equine Respiratory Disorders*. J. Beech, ed. Philadelphia: Lea and Febiger, pp 331–387.

Schuh, J.C.L. 1986. Squamous cell carcinoma of the oral, pharyngeal and nasal mucosa in the horse. *Vet Pathol* 23:205.

Schumacher, J., and Hanselka, D.V. 1987. Nasopharyngeal cicatrices in horses: 47 cases (1972–1985) *J Am Vet Med Assoc* 191:239–242.

Semevolos, S.A., and Ducharme, N.G. 2002. Cleft palate. In *Manual of Equine Gastroenterology*. T. Mair, T. Divers, and N. Ducharme eds. London: W.B. Saunders Co, pp 79–87.

Stick, J.A. 1993. Current therapy of epiglottic and palate abnormalities. *Equine Pract* 5:34–36.

Stick, J.A., and Boles, C. 1980. Subepiglottic cyst in three foals. *J Am Vet Med Assoc* 177:62–64.

Sullivan, E.K., and Parente, E.J. 2003. Disorders of the pharynx. *Vet Clinics N Am Equine Pract* 19:159–167.

Sweeney, C.R., Sweeney, R.W., Raker, C.W., and Freeman, D.E. 1985. Upper respiratory tract obstruction caused by a pharyngeal abscess in a filly. *J Am Vet Med Assoc* 187:268–270.

Todhunter, R.J., Brown, C.M., and Stickle, R. 1987. Retropharyngeal infections in five horses. *J Am Vet Med Assoc* 187:600–604.

Tulleners, E.P., Schumacher, J., Johnston, J., and Richardson, D.W. 1992. Pharynx. In *Equine Surgery*. J.A. Auer, ed. Philadelphia: W.B.Saunders Co, pp 446–459.

Walker, M.A., Schumacher, J., Schmitz, D.G., McMullen, W.C., Ruoff, W.W., Crabill, M.R., Hawkins, J.F., Hogan, P.M., McClure, S.R., Vacek, J.R., Edwards, J.F., Helman, R.G., and Frelier, P.F. 1998. Cobalt 60 radiotherapy for treatment of squamous cell carcinoma of the nasal cavity and paranasal sinuses in 3 horses. *J Am Vet Med Assoc* 212:848–851.

# The Larynx

The larynx is a short tubular structure that connects the pharynx to the trachea. It functions as a valve, regulating airflow and preventing aspiration of food, and is the major organ of the voice.

## ANATOMY AND FUNCTION

The larynx, trachea, and lungs develop embryologically from the ventral wall of the foregut, as a respiratory diverticulum. The epithelium and glandular structures are derived from endoderm, but the cartilages and muscles originate from mesenchyme of the fourth and sixth branchial arches.

The larynx is related dorsally to the pharynx and the proximal esophagus. Ventrally, it is covered by the sternohyoid and omohyoid muscles, fascia, and skin. Laterally it is related to the parotid and mandibular glands, the medial pterygoid, digastricus, stylohyoid, and pharyngeal constrictor muscles. It is attached to the basihyoid and thyrohyoid, and to the first tracheal ring by the cricotracheal ligament.

The skeleton of the larynx consists of a framework of cartilages, that are connected by joints (diarthrodial) and ligaments, and moved by extrinsic and intrinsic muscles. There are three single cartilages—the cricoid, thyroid, and epiglottis—and one paired cartilage—the arytenoids. The thyroid, cricoid, and most of the arytenoids are composed of hyaline cartilage. The epiglottis and parts of the arytenoids are composed of elastic cartilage. The thyroid and cricoid cartilages frequently become mineralized with age.

The joints of the larynx include the cricothyroid, cricoarytenoid, and thyrohyoid joints. Ligaments include the cricothyroid, thyrohyoid, hyoepiglottic, thyroepiglottic, and vocal ligaments. The extrinsic muscles consist of the sternothyrohyoideus, thyrohyoideus, and hyoepiglotticus muscles. The intrinsic muscles include the cricothyroideus, cricoarytenoideus dorsalis and lateralis, arytenoideus transversus, thyroarytenoideus (including vocalis and vestibularis), thyroarytenoideus accessorius, and tensor ventriculi lateralis.

The cricothyroid muscles, which tense the vocal ligaments and folds, and thereby adduct the vocal folds, are supplied by branches of the cranial laryngeal nerves. The other intrinsic muscles receive their motor innervation from the recurrent laryngeal nerve. Abduction of the arytenoids is produced by contraction of the cricoarytenoideus dorsalis, and adduction is produced by the thyroarytenoideus, arytenoideus transversus, and cricoarytenoideus lateralis muscles.

The epithelial lining of the larynx changes at the level of the vocal folds from stratified squamous rostrally to pseudostratified columnar ciliated caudally. The mucous membrane is gathered into discrete folds where it passes between the arytenoids and the epiglottis; here it forms the aryepiglottic folds. It forms the vocal folds (or "true vocal cords") where it covers the vocal ligaments and muscles, and it forms the vestibular folds (or "false vocal cords") where it covers the vestibular ligaments and muscles. Between the vocal and vestibular folds is a shallow depression, the lateral ventricle, which opens into the laryngeal saccule. The laryngeal saccule is a blind-ending mucosal sac, 2.5–3 cm long, that extends dorsocaudally between the medial surface of the thyroid and the lateral surface of the arytenoid.

The aditus laryngis, or pharyngeal aperture of the larynx, is a large oval opening bounded by the epiglottis, the aryepiglottic folds, and the corniculate processes of the arytenoids. Between the aditus laryngis and the vocal folds is the vestibule of the larynx, which has the vestibular folds and laryngeal ventricles as its lateral walls. The middle, narrow part of the cavity of the larynx is called the glottis or rima glottidis. It is bounded by the vocal cords and medial surface of the arytenoids. The posterior compartment of the laryngeal cavity continues with the trachea. It is enclosed by the cricoid cartilage and cricothyroid membrane, and has a transverse diameter of about 4–5 cm.

The blood supply to the larynx comes from the caudal laryngeal artery and branches of the ascending pharyngeal artery.

During swallowing, the airway is closed off by adduction of the arytenoid cartilages and caudal movement of the epiglottis. The caudal movement of the epiglottis occurs passively as a result of rostral movement of the larynx. Solid food passes over the epiglottis, and liquid material is diverted laterally around the aryepiglottic folds.

## IDIOPATHIC LARYNGEAL HEMIPLEGIA/RECURRENT LARYNGEAL NEUROPATHY

Laryngeal hemiplegia due to recurrent laryngeal neuropathy is the most common cause of abnormal respiratory noise in the exercising horse:

- The left side of the larynx is almost invariably involved.
- Recurrent laryngeal neuropathy leads to dysfunction and atrophy of the intrinsic laryngeal muscles, particularly the cricoarytenoideus dorsalis, which leads to a failure of abductory function of the left arytenoid cartilage.
- Exercise intolerance occurs as a result of reduced cross-sectional area of the rima glottidis, decreased inspiratory flow, hypercapnia, and hypoxemia.
- Diagnosis is based on the history, palpation of the larynx, endoscopic examination, and exercise tests.
- Endoscopic evaluation during exercise on a high-speed treadmill may be required to determine the significance of hemiparesis.
- Treatment is not always required in performance or pleasure horses.
- Exercise intolerance is most likely in racehorses.
- Surgical treatments include ventriculocordectomy, prosthetic laryngoplasty, and arytenoidectomy.
- Improvement in exercise tolerance is easier to achieve with surgery than abolition of abnormal noise.

Idiopathic laryngeal hemiplegia (recurrent laryngeal neuropathy) is caused by damage to the recurrent laryngeal branch of the vagus nerve. It results in a permanent dysfunction of the intrinsic muscles of the larynx. This causes partial obstruction of the airway during exercise (Fig. 10.1) and compromised athletic performance due to hypoxia. The condition almost invariably involves the left side of the larynx, but very rarely right-sided or bilateral cases are encountered. The disease manifests itself as a failure to achieve or to maintain full symmetrical arytenoid abduction under conditions of greatest respiratory demand. The resistance to normal airflow causes turbulence in the airstream that is the source of the characteristic abnormal inspiratory sounds—"whistling" or "roaring." Recurrent laryngeal neuropathy is the most common cause of abnormal respiratory noise in the exercising horse.

Although the condition is commonly referred to as *laryngeal hemiplegia,* in fact there is a wide variation of disease severity from mild hemiparesis to marked hemiparesis to hemiplegia. As a result, the clinical signs and clinical significance are variable. Pathological changes can be found in the left recurrent laryngeal nerve and the muscles it supplies in some normal horses, indicating subclinical disease can occur.

The underlying neurological disease, recurrent laryngeal neuropathy, consists of a distal axonopathy whereby the larger myelinated nerve fibres degenerate from the motor end-plate proximally toward the cell body of the neurone. The effect is atrophy of those muscles predominantly supplied by the large myelinated fibers (Fig. 10.2), and for this reason the major adductor, the cricoarytenoideus lateralis is afflicted before the major dilator of the rima glottidis, the cricoarytenoideus dorsalis. However, defects of adduction rarely provide overt clinical signs.

The structural changes in the nerves are believed to arise through an underlying defect of axonal transport. The condition may be related to the absolute

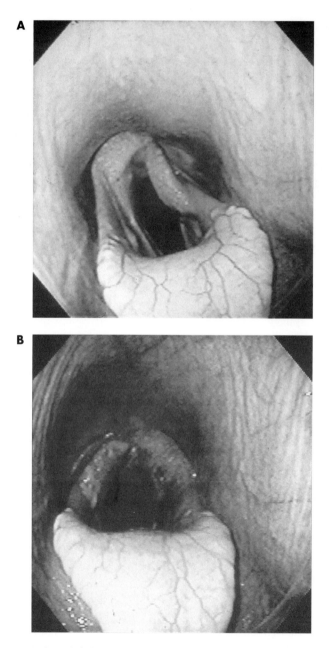

**Fig. 10.1.** Grade 4 left laryngeal hemiplegia prior to surgical correction (A) and after prosthetic laryngoplasty (B). Note the position of the left arytenoid at rest after surgical intervention. *(See also color section.)*

length of the recurrent laryngeal nerve fibers, which are the longest lower motor neurones in the horse. The left nerve is significantly longer than the right. Although the disease is most severe in the left recurrent laryngeal nerve, milder lesions can also be found in the right recurrent nerve and in some long peripheral nerves of the distal hindlimb. It is possible that the distal axonopa-

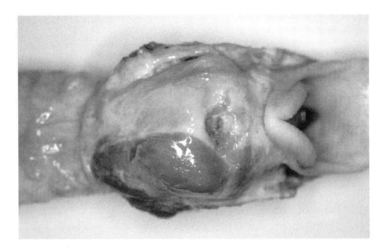

**Fig. 10.2.** Post-mortem appearance of the larynx of a horse affected by Grade 4 left laryngeal hemiplegia showing atrophy of the intrinsic laryngeal musculature on the left side.

thy of recurrent laryngeal neuropathy has an inherited basis; however, the precise mode of inheritance is unknown. Other, less common causes of recurrent laryngeal neuropathy include trauma to the recurrent nerve by perivascular injection of irritant drugs; damage to the vagal trunk by guttural pouch mycosis or strangles abscessation; toxicity by heavy metals, such as lead, or organophosphates; and nutritional deficiencies, such as thiamine.

Clinical signs of recurrent laryngeal neuropathy, including exercise intolerance and stridor at exercise, are caused by failure of the principal abductor of the larynx, the cricoarytenoideus dorsalis muscle. The degree of neurogenic myopathy correlates with the severity of the nerve lesion. During exercise, the arytenoid cartilages are normally held in full symmetrical abduction, which is sustained throughout all stages of the respiratory cycle. Prolonged and constant dilatation is necessary to prevent dynamic collapse of the larynx in the face of increased negative inspiratory pressures. Failure of the neuromuscular unit results in partial obstruction of the airway. As the cross-sectional area of the rima glottidis is reduced, the pressure differentials within the larynx increase to maintain the airflow necessary to sustain exercise. The collapsing forces rise and the paralyzed cord is drawn even further across the airway (Venturi effect). When the demands for inspiratory flow reach their peak, affected horses show flow limitation, increased inspiratory resistance, inability to maintain normal coupling between respiration and stride, and depression of arterial oxygen tension. The abnormal inspiratory noise produced with exercise is the result of air turbulence created by the asymmetric larynx.

## Prevalence

Recurrent laryngeal neuropathy has been identified in foals and fetuses. Clinically, horses of any age from birth onward may be affected. However, it is not clear whether the disorder is invariably present from birth or whether it is progressive.

Horses over 16 hands tall are most susceptible, and the condition is rare in ponies. It is estimated that about 50% of horses more than 17 hands tall are clinically affected. Stallions and geldings appear to be at increased risk compared to mares.

The prevalence of idiopathic laryngeal hemiplegia in the Thoroughbred is not known and there are widely varying estimates (0.96–95%) in the literature. The frequency of true hemiplegia—i.e., where there are no active abductory or adductory movements by the left arytenoid cartilage and vocal fold, is in the order of 2%. The clinical signs of laryngeal hemiplegia in racehorses usually appear before the horse is 6 years old. However, in the performance horse, the signs may not appear until later.

## Clinical signs

Affected horses usually produce consistent inspiratory sounds that can be heard throughout the period of exertion at the canter and gallop. The sounds range from a low-grade musical whistle to a harsh roaring noise. The sound usually gets louder the longer and harder the horse works. Disappearance of the noise usually occurs within a short time of pulling up, and a resting respiratory rate is attained in a normal time period.

Some horses with laryngeal hemiplegia produce adventitious respiratory noises only under extreme exertion, and examination by endoscopy during high-speed treadmill exercise may be necessary to determine whether the noise stems from abrupt dynamic collapse of the paralyzed arytenoid cartilage or from secondary dorsal displacement of the soft palate.

Exercise intolerance or poor performance in addition to an abnormal noise is common in racehorses. Event and steeplechase horses can also experience exercise intolerance because they compete at high exertional levels over significant distances. The effect on exercise tolerance in horses performing less strenuous exercise can be very difficult to estimate. In many competition horses, hunters, and pleasure horses, the disease manifests simply as an adventitious noise with little or no effect on performance or exercise tolerance. However, head and neck position can influence the performance-limiting effects of laryngeal hemiplegia. Head and neck flexion alone can cause upper airway obstruction by decreasing the cross-sectional area of the respiratory tract; this increase in respiratory impedance can compound the effects of laryngeal dysfunction.

## Diagnosis

Diagnosis is determined by a combination of physical examination, endoscopy, and exercise tests. In some cases, endoscopic examination during high-speed treadmill exercise may be necessary to determine the clinical significance of the lesion.

Palpation of the larynx is performed to identify atrophy of the intrinsic laryngeal musculature, evidenced by prominence of the muscular process, especially on the left side. The muscular process is palpated as a distinct "knuckle" cranial to the dorsal border of the thyroid cartilage on the affected side. Palpation should seek evidence of a cicatrix from previous surgery. Both jugular veins are examined for evidence of thrombosis. In addition, an assessment of the strength of the slap response is performed, which is more accurately judged by palpation than endoscopic examination. The horse is slapped over the saddle area to induce a thoracolaryngeal reflex, which results in an adductory flicker of the contralateral arytenoid. The test is performed with the horse breathing quietly and during the expiratory phase of respiration. The response to slapping over both sides of the thorax is compared.

The arytenoid depression test is performed immediately after exercise. The right side of the larynx is forced to adduct by digital pressure on the right arytenoid muscular process. If the horse has left laryngeal hemiplegia, the additional obstruction caused by forced adduction of the right side results in a notable increase in stridor.

The Grunt-to-the-Stick test depends upon startling the horse by threatening with a stick. Laryngeal fixation in an incompletely closed position together with a rapid rise in pressure within the airway produces a low-pitched grunt. This is a test of the competence of laryngeal adduction, but the results are inconsistent.

Endoscopic examination at rest is the standard method of assessing laryngeal function. A rhythmic bilaterally symmetrical abductory movement of the arytenoids occurring during inspiration is observed in the resting horse. Asymmetry of the rima glottidis in cases of true left laryngeal hemiplegia is usually obvious (see Fig. 10.1), but in cases of hemiparesis the asymmetry may be more subtle and difficult to assess. Distortion of the image that arises from the eccentric position of the endoscope in the nasopharynx must be taken into account. Thus, when the endoscope is introduced through the right nostril, false negative diagnoses are possible, but from the left side the left arytenoid cartilage may give the false impression of inadequate abduction. Whenever doubt exists, the endoscopy should be performed through each nostril in turn.

Nasal occlusion and induced swallowing (such as instilling water through the endoscope) are used to induce abduction of the arytenoids so that dynamic evaluation of arytenoid function is improved. A rapid abduction of the arytenoids occurs immediately after swallowing. A comparison should be made between the left and right sides.

Difficulties in interpreting the results of endoscopy are made worse by the fact that many "normal" horses demonstrate some degree of asynchronous abduction of the arytenoids at rest. A grading system with reproducible parameters is very helpful to eliminate the subjectivity of assessing laryngeal function. Several different grading systems exist. A commonly used grading system is summarized by the following:

- Grade 1: Normal. All movements, both adductory and abductory are synchronized at rest and after exercise. Complete synchronous arytenoid abduction is present.

- Grade 2: Asynchronous movement, such as hesitation, flutters, adductor weakness of the left arytenoid during inspiration or expiration, or both, but full abduction is induced by swallowing or nasal occlusion.
- Grade 3: Asynchronous movement of the left arytenoid is present during inspiration or expiration, or both. The left arytenoid is no longer capable of full abduction, and during adduction compensation by the right arytenoid crossing the midline may be evident.
- Grade 4: Marked asymmetry of the larynx at rest, and there is lack of substantial movement of the left arytenoid.

Grades 1 and 2 are considered to be within the acceptable limits of clinical normality; Grade 4 is considered abnormal, and affected horses would be expected to produce abnormal inspiratory noises during the exercise test. Grade 3 comprises equivocal dysfunction; some horses show no untoward inspiratory sounds at exercise, and others produce a characteristic whistle.

Endoscopic examination during high-speed treadmill exercise is necessary to provide a complete assessment of laryngeal function, because the interpretation at rest may be misleading. Treadmill testing is particularly helpful to clarify the significance of Grade 3 motility. If possible, treadmill endoscopy is performed with the horse wearing its usual tack, and with its head carriage simulating the usual position during competition.

## Treatment

Treatment is not required in all cases. Many competition horses and pleasure horses perform adequately with the disease. Allowing horses to work with less head and neck flexion can sometimes resolve problems associated with exercise intolerance in performance horses without necessitating surgical intervention.

A number of different surgical procedures have been used to treat the obstructive effects of recurrent laryngeal neuropathy. These include various ventriculectomy and cordectomy procedures, prosthetic laryngoplasty, temporary and permanent tracheostomy, subtotal arytenoidectomy, and laryngeal reinnervation (nerve/muscle pedicle grafting).

### Ventriculectomy and cordectomy

Ventriculectomy (also known as sacculectomy, or Hobday or Williams procedure) involves removal of the mucous membrane lining from the laryngeal ventricle and saccule. The procedure is often combined with excision of the vocal fold (i.e., cordectomy). The benefits of the ventriculocordectomy procedures are at best slight. It was originally believed that the ventriculectomy would abduct and stabilize the arytenoid and vocal cord, and prevent dynamic collapse of these structures during exercise. However, recent studies suggest that the procedure has little effect on airflow. Despite these findings, the laryngeal saccule is known to be a resonator and is a major source of the abnormal noise associated with laryngeal hemiplegia. Removal of the saccule, therefore, will remove a source of turbulent airflow and may improve exercise tolerance in a small number of cases. Concurrent removal of the vocal cord provides a larger airway and appears to be more effective at decreasing respiratory noise.

Despite the limitations, ventriculectomy or ventriculocordectomy is still commonly performed. It is often done concurrently with laryngeal prosthesis surgery. Some clinicians favor the use of ventriculocordectomy alone in mild cases of recurrent laryngeal neuropathy. Unlike the laryngeal prosthesis surgery, complications from the ventriculocordectomy are very rare. The procedure is also indicated in those horses which, on the treadmill, are obstructed by the dynamic collapse of the vocal fold rather than by the arytenoid cartilage.

In draft horses used for pulling, a ventriculectomy without a cordectomy can be used, since it is believed that the ability to close the glottis is important in enabling the horse to develop an abdominal press. However, the ventriculectomy will not greatly improve the abnormal inspiratory noise, so draft horses used for showing may need another procedure performed if noise reduction is required.

A number of different surgical techniques are available for performing the ventriculectomy and ventriculocordectomy. The horse is placed in dorsal recumbency under general anesthesia. Surgery is performed through a laryngotomy incision. The mucosal lining of the saccule is everted, usually using a toothed burr, and then excised. If a cordectomy is to be performed at the same time, the vocal cord is grasped with Alice tissue forceps, and a 5 mm margin is excised from the vocal process to the floor of the larynx. The excised margins of the ventricle may be apposed with sutures or left unsutured. The laryngotomy can be left open to heal by secondary intention, or it can be closed to allow primary healing. The advantage of leaving the wound open is that it provides an alternative airway should laryngeal edema occur; however, the healing time is prolonged and a significant amount of wound discharge is expected. The advantage of primary healing is more rapid recovery and absence of the normal wound discharge. Closure of the wound requires meticulous closure of the cricothyroid membrane (to prevent subcutaneous emphysema), and thorough wound lavage prior to suturing the different tissue layers. Infection of the wound is a possible complication. An alternative is to close only the cricothyroid membrane, and to leave the other layers to heal by secondary intention.

Ventriculocordectomies can be performed in the standing horse by transendoscopic laser surgery, or by sharp surgery through a laryngotomy incision. An oral approach in the anesthetized horse has been described.

## Prosthetic laryngoplasty

Prosthetic laryngoplasty (abductor prosthesis operation; tie-back operation) is considered to be the treatment of choice for recurrent laryngeal neuropathy in most countries. The surgery involves the extralaryngeal placement of a suture or a pair of sutures between the cricoid cartilage and the muscular process of the arytenoid. The objective is that the suture will mimic the action of the cricoarytenoideus dorsalis muscle as if it were in a semicontracted state. However, the procedure should be regarded as a gross physiological disturbance because when the rima glottidis is fixed in an abducted position, the ability of the larynx to protect the lower airways during deglutition is compromised. A degree of dysphagia is inevitable. Nevertheless, most horses show relief of laryngeal obstruction and are only subclinically dysphagic. Physiological studies have confirmed that prosthetic laryngoplasty is effective in the restoration of normal respiratory function and in the prevention of dynamic collapse of the paralyzed arytenoid in cases of recurrent laryngeal neuropathy. The prosthetic laryngoplasty is usually combined with a ventriculocordectomy, since it improves the cross-sectional area of the rima glottidis and it results in less postoperative noise.

The horse is placed in right lateral recumbency (for treatment of left laryngeal hemiplegia). The head is extended and the neck elevated with padding to improve surgical access. A 5–8 cm skin incision is made ventral and parallel to the linguofacial vein, extending rostrally to the level of the cricotracheal space. Following incision of the subcutaneous tissues, blunt dissection continues between the linguofacial vein and the omohyoid muscle, down to the caudal border of the cricoid cartilage and the lateral surface of the larynx. The cricopharyngeal and thyropharyngeal muscles are separated with scissors to allow access to the muscular process. The choice of prosthesis material and needle varies between surgeons, but a heavy nonabsorbable material is generally used. The needle is inserted by carefully sliding it under the caudal edge of the cricoid and pushed through the cricoid such that it is placed approximately 1 cm from the dorsal midline and at least 1.5 cm rostral to the caudal border. Care must be taken to avoid penetration of the underlying mucosa and penetration of the airway. The needle is guarded as it is pushed through the cricoid to avoid damage to the esophagus or common carotid artery. A second suture can be passed in a more axial position at this time. The ends of the sutures are then passed under the cricopharyngeus muscle, ensuring that they do not get entangled. The first suture is then passed through the muscular process in an axial-to-abaxial direction approximately 0.3 cm from the apex. Room is left to allow the second suture to be placed dorsal to the first. The first suture is then tied; this can be done at the same time as endoscopic examination of the larynx to judge the degree of abduction. The second suture is then tied. Subcutaneous tissues and skin are then closed routinely. A ventriculocordectomy is then performed via a laryngotomy or using a laser transendoscopically *per nasum*. Following surgery, horses are confined to a stable for 4–6 weeks with handwalking exercise only. If coughing associated with eating occurs, dampening dry food with water is helpful.

Published success rates for laryngoplasty range from 48%–95%, depending on the criteria used to assess success. The success rate appears to be lower in Thoroughbred racehorses compared with horses performing less demanding activities. The objective of this surgery is to achieve abduction of the affected arytenoid in a position midway between the resting position and full abduction (see Fig. 10.1B). Excessive abduction may result in aspiration of food and possible inhalation pneumonia. Inadequate abduction fails to improve the airway calibre. It should be recognized that a reduction in the degree of arytenoid abduction is likely to occur post-surgery.

There are many potential complications that can arise with this surgery, including coughing, chondritis, fistula formation, dysphagia, inhalation pneumonia, wound sepsis, and dehiscence, and failure of the sutures to maintain arytenoid abduction. Coughing and nasal discharge of food and water are the most common complications. Fortunately, in most horses these complications resolve with time. Coughing is usually associated with eating and relates to the aspiration of food particles into the airway. Regurgitation of food and water is less common, and probably results from interference with neuromuscular control of deglutition. However, horses that show severe or persistent dysphagia following surgery may need to have the suture removed.

A major complication of the laryngoplasty, reported to affect around 20% of cases, is failure to maintain abduction. If a prosthetic laryngoplasty fails because the suture pulls through the cartilage, the suture breaks, or the muscular process fractures, a repeat prosthetic laryngoplasty may be attempted. Careful dissection is required because of the previous surgery. In addition, the arytenoid and muscular process must be freed from the thyroid (using curved, sharp scissors).

## Temporary tracheotomy tubing

The purpose of the tracheotomy tube is to provide an alternative airway and to bypass the site of airway obstruction. It may be used when other surgical techniques for laryngeal hemiplegia have failed, but their major virtue is that intubation is performed under local analgesia and disruption of the training program is minimal. Tracheotomy tubing provides a short-term expedient to racehorses that would otherwise be sidelined by alternative surgery. When the tracheotomy tube is eventually removed, the defect heals quickly by second intention and the option to perform a ventriculectomy or laryngoplasty operation will not have been compromised.

## Permanent tracheostomy

Permanent tracheostomy involves the creation of a fistula between the tracheal lumen and the skin surface of the ventral neck. Unfortunately, the results are generally not aesthetically acceptable. There is a regular requirement for nursing care to remove exudation from the skin adjacent to the stoma and to maintain local hygiene.

## Arytenoidectomy

Total, partial, and subtotal arytenoidectomies aim to remove the intralaryngeal structures that are causing obstruction. Thus, the usual indications for arytenoidectomy are the removal of infected cartilage in cases of chronic chondropathy and the removal of the left arytenoid cartilage when other techniques to treat laryngeal hemiplegia have failed. These surgeries are considered salvage operations, because the normal upper airway mechanics cannot be reestablished and a partial airway obstruction will persist. A partial arytenoidectomy is the procedure of choice for performance animals. This involves removal of the entire arytenoid cartilage apart from the muscular process.

### Laryngeal reinnervation

Nerve/muscle pedicle grafting aims to transplant cubes of muscle taken from the omohyoideus, together with their motor supply, through the first and second cervical nerves into the atrophied cricoarytenoideus dorsalis muscle to restore abductory function to the larynx. Following surgery, the grafts grow in response to mechanical stimulation so that at least a year must be allowed to achieve optimum results. Abduction of the arytenoid cartilage occurs only during exercise because the omohyoid is an accessory muscle of respiration. The technique has the advantage over prosthetic laryngoplasty because no complications can arise from aspiration through a permanently abducted rima glottidis.

A similar surgical approach to the laryngoplasty is used. The ventral branch of the first cervical nerve is identified as it travels over the lateral surface of the larynx, and a branch of the nerve with a 5 mm section of omohyoideus muscle is excised and transposed to a recipient incision made in the cricoarytenoideus dorsalis. The muscle pedicle is secured with sutures. From three to five such nerve-muscle pedicles should be transposed.

## Prognosis

Prosthetic laryngoplasty appears to be the best practicable option currently available for treatment of recurrent laryngeal neuropathy. Although it is recognized that this surgery can produce complications in the forms of coughing, nasal reflux of ingesta, or recurrence of dyspnea, the risks are justifiable in horses that cannot otherwise be effective athletes. Nerve/muscle pedicle grafting is a promising alternative, which is most likely to be applicable to horses where recurrent laryngeal neuropathy is confirmed at an early stage, and when the prolonged convalescent period is likely to be less restrictive. Reinnervation techniques may also be developed in the future.

## RIGHT LARYNGEAL HEMIPLEGIA

Right laryngeal hemiplegia is uncommon. Although rare cases of idiopathic right or bilateral laryngeal hemiplegia have been described, other causes of damage to the recurrent laryngeal nerve should be sought.

Identification of right laryngeal hemiplegia should prompt careful palpation of the larynx to identify any malformations that may be associated with a fourth branchial arch defect. Other potential causes of right laryngeal hemiplegia include perivascular injections around the jugular vein, strangles abscessation and tumors of the head and neck, guttural pouch mycosis, and trauma.

Treatment of right laryngeal hemiplegia involves identification and treatment of the underlying cause, if appropriate. Surgical treatment by laryngoplasty can also be undertaken.

## EPIGLOTTAL ENTRAPMENT

Epiglottal entrapment occurs when the cartilage of the epiglottis becomes enveloped by a fold of glossoepiglottic mucosa and aryepiglottic folds (Fig. 10.3):

- Horses with a congenitally hypoplastic epiglottis are predisposed to epiglottal entrapment.
- Clinical signs include exercise intolerance, inspiratory and/or expiratory noises at exercise, intermittent gurgling from secondary dorsal displacement of the soft palate, and coughing after eating.
- Diagnosis is determined by endoscopic examination.
- Occasionally there may be an associated persistent dorsal displacement of the soft palate, which obscures the epiglottis during endoscopy.
- Treatment involves surgical division of the entrapping membrane or resection.

The aryepiglottic folds are thick bands of mucous membrane that attach to the ventral surface of the epiglottis along its lateral free borders and extend

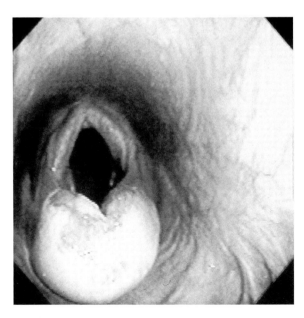

**Fig. 10.3.** Epiglottic entrapment by the aryepiglottic fold. The outline of the epiglottis is visible, but has lost its normal scalloped cartilage border, and superficial blood vessels are obscured by the entrapping mucosa. *(See also color section.)*

caudodorsally along the lateral aspects of the arytenoid cartilages to blend dorsally with the mucous membrane that covers the corniculate processes. These aryepiglottic folds are continuous with the redundant mucosa of the glossoepiglottic fold on the lingual surface of the epiglottis. The subepiglottic epithelium is loose and redundant, which allows for epiglottic elevation during swallowing. Tissue comprising both the aryepiglottic folds and the glossoepiglottic mucosa becomes entrapped over the epiglottis in this disorder.

The etiology of epiglottal entrapment is often not known. The condition can be reproduced on most equine laryngeal post-mortem specimens by pulling the glossoepiglottic mucosa over the tip of the epiglottis, but it is not clear why some horses develop the condition in life and others do not. Inflammation and swelling of the aryepiglottic and subepiglottic tissue might be a predisposing factor.

Not surprisingly, horses with a congenitally hypoplastic epiglottis are predisposed to epiglottal entrapment because it is easier for the aryepiglottic tissue to envelop a small epiglottis. Likewise, horses with subepiglottic cysts are predisposed to epiglottal entrapment. Both of these possibilities are evaluated via endoscopic and/or radiographic examination prior to surgical correction of epiglottal entrapment. Epiglottal entrapment has been observed in foals in association with cleft palate.

Reports of the prevalence of epiglottal entrapment in endoscopic surveys of athletic horses at rest suggest an incidence in the range of 0.75–3.3%.

## Clinical signs

The entrapped mucosa acts as an obstruction to airflow and results in turbulent airflow both during inspiration and during expiration. The degree of airway obstruction depends on the amount of tissue that has become entrapped, degree of inflammation and swelling, and presence of secondary dorsal displacement of the soft palate. The clinical signs associated with epiglottal entrapment are highly variable and include exercise intolerance, inspiratory and/or expiratory noises at exercise, intermittent gurgling from secondary dorsal displacement of the soft palate, coughing after eating, and headshaking. Some horses with epiglottal entrapment may be asymptomatic.

## Diagnosis

Diagnosis of epiglottal entrapment is determined via endoscopic examination. The epiglottis will be visible in outline (assuming that it is not obscured by a displaced soft palate) but will have lost its normal scalloped cartilage border, and superficial blood vessels are obscured by the entrapping mucosa (see Figure 10.3). The entrapment may form a small rim of tissue that covers only the apex and lateral borders of the epiglottis, or it may cover most of the laryngeal surface of the epiglottis. Sometimes it will appear incomplete and cover only the apex and one lateral border of the epiglottis. The caudal margin of the entrapping mucosa is generally visible. The mucosa overlying the epiglottis may become ulcerated, especially in long-standing entrapments. Occasionally, an ulcer will erode completely through the entrapped mucosa to allow the tip of the epiglottis to protrude through the entrapment.

When persistent dorsal displacement of the soft palate is present, the epiglottis cannot be visualized, in which case a lateral radiograph of the pharynx is indicated to determine whether entrapment is present. Metallic markers of known length can be placed on each side of the mandible to calculate the amount of magnification on the radiograph. On this projection, the epiglottis should measure at least 7.0 cm from tip to the hyoid articulation; an epiglottis with a length less than 5.5 cm is indicative of hypoplasia and surgery would be contraindicated.

Epiglottal entrapment may be intermittent, and it is important, as a routine part of the endoscopic procedure, to stimulate a series of deglutition sequences in an attempt to provoke the condition. However, epiglottal entrapment may be present only during vigorous exercise, so high-speed treadmill endoscopy provides the ideal opportunity to establish a diagnosis of intermittent entrapment.

## Treatment

The treatment options for epiglottal entrapment include resection via a ventral laryngotomy, axial division per os using a hooked bistoury, axial division per nasum using a hooked bistoury, transendoscopic laser division, and transendoscopic electrosurgical axial division. Axial division per nasum and transendoscopic laser division can be performed in the standing horse, but the other techniques require general anesthesia. If the entrapment is intermittent, axial division per os or resection via a laryngotomy should be used. Persistent entrapments can be treated by any of the techniques.

Resection via laryngotomy involves retraction of the epiglottis back toward the larynx, followed by grasping the aryepiglottic fold on one side. The entrapping membrane is identified and grasped with Alice tissue forceps on either side of the midline. The membrane is then incised along its midline down to the tip of the epiglottis and the incision continued along the edges of the epiglottis for approximately one-third of the length of the epiglottis, at which point the folds are amputated. The laryngotomy incision is left to heal by secondary intention.

Axial division per nasum using a hooked bistoury is not recommended because of the risk of iatrogenic damage to the soft palate. The aryepiglottic mucosa is quite tough, and care is required to prevent a palatal injury when the hook suddenly cuts free from the entrapment. If the horse moves or swallows while the entrapped membrane is being cut, the knife may inadvertently damage the soft palate and create a cleft (see Chapter 9, Fig. 9.3B). Alternatively, if the horse swallows on the bistoury, it may lodge within the proximal esophagus where it can cause iatrogenic damage. Axial division using a hooked bistoury can be safely performed per os with the horse under general anesthesia. The palate is manually displaced dorsally, and the hook knife placed around the entrapping mucosa by palpation or under endoscopic visualization.

Transnasal laser incision is performed under sedation with topical application of local anesthetic solution to the epiglottis and membranes. The membranes are incised along the midline by dragging the fiber from caudal to rostral. As the incision is made through the entrapping membrane, the tissues will retract laterally. Care must be taken not to damage the epiglottis itself.

**Prognosis**

The possibility of recurrence of entrapment is greatest with the axial section techniques, but even this is uncommon. Iatrogenic trauma to the epiglottal cartilage can provoke granulomas or distortion, which may compromise the relationship between the epiglottis and the soft palate. Chronic coughing associated with low-grade dysphagia is a rare but recognized complication of resection of the glosso-epiglottal mucosa.

## ARYTENOID CHONDROPATHY (ARYTENOID CHONDRITIS; ARYTENOID CHONDROSIS)

Arytenoid chondritis consists of the development of suppuration within the matrix of one or both arytenoid cartilages:

- Arytenoid chondritis causes inflammation, thickening, granulation protuberance and deformation of the arytenoid cartilage either uni- or bilaterally.
- Exercise intolerance and abnormal respiratory noise are the main presenting clinical signs.
- Mild cases affecting the left arytenoid require careful differentiation from laryngeal hemiplegia due to recurrent laryngeal neuropathy.
- The definitive diagnosis is determined via endoscopic examination.
- Radiographic examination detects the extent/mineralization of an associated granulomatous mass.
- Medical treatment or laser excision of granulation tissue may be effective in mild cases if arytenoid mobility is still present.
- Partial arytenoidectomy is the preferred surgical treatment for advanced cases.

Arytenoid chondritis is progressive, and is characterized by distortion, dystrophic mineralization, protruberances of cartilage or granulation tissue, and central necrosis associated with fistulation. Mucopurulent material may drain from the sinus tracts in the cartilage. Loss of abductory function of the affected arytenoid results from a combination of thickening of the cartilage, inflammation of the musculature surrounding the arytenoid, and involvement of the cricoarytenoid articulation. The cause is unknown, but might result from trauma to the affected arytenoid cartilage or infection/inflammation of the corniculate process and arytenoid cartilage from mucosal damage. The condition is more common unilaterally and is seen in all breeds and ages, but presents most frequently in young male Thoroughbreds. The condition appears to be more prevalent in the U.S. than in Europe.

## Clinical signs

The clinical signs associated with arytenoid chondritis arise through a combination of airway obstruction and compromised glottic protection. The severity of clinical signs varies with the severity of laryngeal obstruction. The onset of signs can be sudden and severe, or insidious and progressive. Stridorous inspiratory noise during exertion and exercise intolerance are the most common signs. If there is bilateral disease, signs may be present at rest. Coughing may be evident at any stage.

## Diagnosis

The diagnosis of arytenoid chondritis is primarily made by endoscopic examination to identify distortion of the affected cartilage (Fig. 10.4). As the microabscesses develop, the cartilage thickens and axially displaces toward the midline with reduced mobility. In the early stages, particularly when the left side is involved, cursory endoscopic examination may suggest a diagnosis of laryngeal hemiplegia. As the condition advances, the distortion of the cartilage becomes more obvious, and granulomatous eruptions appear on the medial face of the corniculate process. Contact lesions ("kissing" lesions) may develop on the contralateral arytenoid cartilage, and sometimes a larger amount of granulation tissue may be present on the opposing normal arytenoid cartilage than the affected cartilage. The palatopharyngeal arch may appear more prominent on the affected side. If both arytenoids are affected, the rima glottidis may be reduced to a narrow slit.

Digital pressure placed over the affected arytenoid frequently causes airway

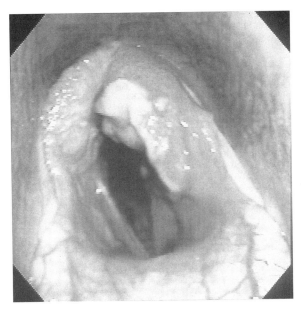

**Fig. 10.4.** Chondritis of the left arytenoid cartilage. Note the granulomatous, exudative, thickened appearance of the affected arytenoid cartilage. (See also color section.)

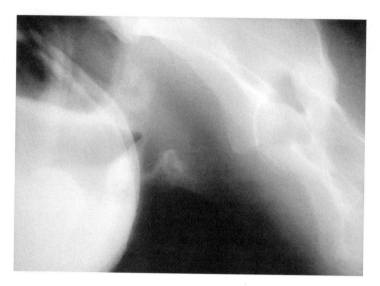

**Fig. 10.5.** Lateral radiographic projection of a horse with arytenoid chondritis. Note the calcification of the granulomatous mass caudal and dorsal to the arytenoid cartilages.

obstruction, dyspnea, and a stridorous noise. Lateral radiographs of the larynx usually show focal mineralization even in early cases (Fig. 10.5). The lateral ventricle may be obliterated, and the affected corniculate process may appear enlarged.

## Treatment

The progress of arytenoid chondritis may be arrested in the early stages by the prolonged (i.e., 6 weeks) use of potentiated sulphonamide and nonsteroidal anti-inflammatory medication, but once the chronic stage has been reached, the only effective treatment option is likely to be arytenoidectomy. In cases where there is only a projection of granulation tissue but arytenoid motility remains good, laser excision of the granulation tissue followed by medical treatment might be effective.

There are three types of arytenoidectomy depending on the extent of cartilage removal:

- Total arytenoidectomy involves removal of the entire arytenoid cartilage, including the corniculate process and muscular process.
- Partial arytenoidectomy involves removing all of the arytenoid apart from the muscular process.
- Subtotal arytenoidectomy involves retention of the corniculate process and muscular process, and occasionally the articular facet.

Total arytenoidectomy frequently results in significant dysphagia, and is therefore rarely performed apart from cases of laryngeal neoplasia. Partial and subtotal arytenoidectomies are safer, and can be used in cases of arytenoid chondropathy and failed prosthetic laryngoplasty. Partial arytenoidectomy is

most commonly performed in cases of arytenoid chondropathy. If both arytenoids are affected by chondropathy, bilateral arytenoidectomy can be performed, but the prognosis for an athletic horse is poor. Even unilateral partial
arytenoidectomy is associated with continued upper airway obstruction, so the
surgery is mainly used as a salvage procedure.

Partial arytenoidectomy is performed with the horse in dorsal recumbency
and intubated via a tracheotomy. A routine laryngotomy is performed, and if
additional exposure is required, the thyroid and cricoid cartilages can be incised. The thyroid is incised on the midline, taking care not to damage the base
of the epiglottis. The cricoid is also incised on the ventral midline. The vocal
cord and ventricle are removed first. This leaves an opening at the ventral aspect of the arytenoidectomy site to permit drainage of submucosal hemorrhage. There are various different techniques of arytenoidectomy, but most
aim to preserve the mucosa. In one technique, the mucosa dissection is begun
with two vertical incisions from dorsal midline to ventral at the caudal border
of the arytenoid and at the rostral border, just caudal to the corniculate
process. These incisions are connected by a horizontal incision along the ventral border of the arytenoid. A periosteal elevator or spatula is used to elevate
the mucosa from the underlying cartilage, leaving the dorsal attacments. If the
mucosa cannot be separated without damage due to disease, it can be resected
en bloc. The abaxial border of the arytenoid is freed by blunt dissection. The
muscular process is isolated and transected. The arytenoid is then elevated and
freed by cutting the remaining corniculate mucosa rostrally. Any remaining
dorsal attachments are also cut, and the cricoarytenoid joint capsule is cut caudally. The cartilage is removed. The mucosa is trimmed and sutured with synthetic absorbable material in a simple interrupted pattern. The ventral end of
the incision may be left open to drain. Any "kissing" lesions on the contralateral arytenoid can be debrided as necessary. The larygotomy incision can be
left open to heal by secondary intention, or the cricothyroid membrane may
be sutured.

Postoperatively, a tracheotomy tube is left in place until there is endoscopic
evidence of a satisfactory airway (usually 5–7 days). The tracheotomy tube
and the laryngotomy wound are cleaned twice a day. Antibiotic and anti-
inflammatory medications are continued for 5–7 days. The horse should be
kept stabled for 4 weeks and then given 4–8 weeks of paddock rest. All feeding should be from the ground to minimize the risk of aspiration. The diameter of the laryngeal airway is believed to increase for 3–4 months after surgery.
If the mucosa was removed during surgery, the area is left to granulate and
healing will be prolonged. Granulation tissue and excessive mucosa evident 1
month after surgery can be removed by laser excision.

## Prognosis

Partial arytenoidectomy offers the best compromise to salvage a horse afflicted
with laryngeal chondritis for breeding or for quiet exercise, but full athletic
capacity cannot be restored by any surgery. An intermittent or persistent
cough occurs in about 10% of horses following surgery, and appears likely fol-

lowing bilateral arytenoidectomy. Aspiration pneumonia is a potential complication, and postoperative respiratory noise due to vibration of the residual arytenoid mucosa can be observed. Collapse of the aryepiglottic fold can also occur due to absence of support by the missing arytenoid. Evaluation of the horse on a high-speed treadmill may be needed to diagnose the precise cause of any long-term respiratory noise or exercise intolerance.

## LARYNGEAL NEOPLASIA

Neoplasia of the larynx is rare. However, neoplastic masses and infiltrates must be considered as a differential diagnosis of arytenoid chondropathy. Arytenoid chondroma has been identified and can be successfully treated by arytenoidectomy. Squamous cell carcinoma and lymphosarcoma can also arise at this site (Fig. 10.6).

## FOURTH BRANCHIAL ARCH DEFECTS

Fourth branchial arch defects is a syndrome of irreparable congenital defects resulting from a failure of development of some or all of the derivatives of the fourth branchial arch:

• Fourth branchial arch defects is an unusual and untreatable condition of the larynx.

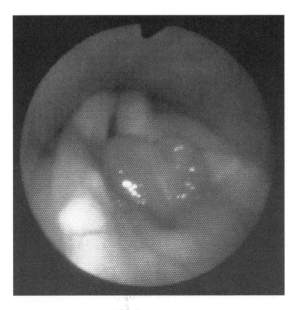

**Fig. 10.6.** Laryngeal lymphosarcoma. A neoplastic mass is obscuring the view of the aditus laryngis. *(See also color section.)*

- The prevalence of fourth branchial arch defects in Thoroughbred horses is around 0.2%.
- Clinical signs can include abnormal respiratory sounds at exercise, eructation, nasal discharge, coughing, and recurrent colic.
- The involuntary aerophagia can be confused with the noises produced by "wind-suckers."
- A tentative diagnosis can be made based on the results of palpation, endoscopy, and radiography.
- Rostral displacement of the palatal arch is often identified by endoscopy, but sometimes it occurs only at exercise.
- Defective arytenoid motility can be confused with recurrent laryngeal neuropathy.
- There is no effective treatment.

The structures that are derived from the fourth branchial arch—and which may be defective—include the wings of the thyroid cartilage, the cricothyroid articulation, the cricothyroideus muscles and the upper esophageal sphincter muscles (crico- and thyropharyngeus muscles). Any permutation of aplasia or hypoplasia of these structures may arise uni- or bilaterally.

The absence of a firm bond between the wing of the thyroid and the cricoid cartilages deprives the larynx of a stable skeleton to facilitate the function of its intrinsic musculature. In the face of such defects, the action of the cricoarytenoideus dorsalis muscle will be ineffective and the ability of the arytenoid to abduct is reduced. This may be mistaken as laryngeal hemiplegia due to recurrent laryngeal neuropathy on initial examination.

The absence of the cricopharyngeus muscles has two effects. The inability to close the upper esophageal sphincter can result in involuntary aerophagia. The absence of a means to anchor the palatal pillars into a position caudal to the apices of the corniculate cartilages may result in rostral displacement of the palatal arch (RDPA). (Fig. 10.7).

The prevalence of fourth branchial arch defects in Thoroughbred horses is not less than 0.2%, and the condition has been identified in other breeds, including the Hanovarian, warmbloods, and the Haflinger. There is no current evidence that the syndrome is genetically transmitted.

## Clinical signs

The presenting signs of horses with fourth branchial arch defects are variable and reflect the severity of the defect in the individual horse. Signs include abnormal respiratory sounds at exercise, eructation, nasal discharge, coughing, and recurrent colic. The involuntary aerophagia and eructation may be confused with the noises produced by "wind-suckers."

## Diagnosis

A complete evaluation of the extent of fourth branchial arch defects can only be made at exploratory surgery or post-mortem, but the combined findings of

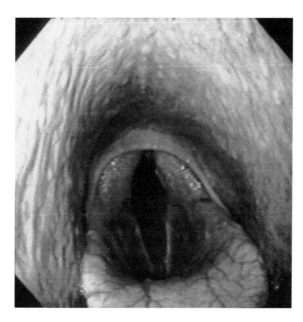

**Fig. 10.7.** Rostral displacement of the palatopharyngeal arch associated with fourth branchial arch defect. The caudal pillars of the soft palate form a hood that partly obscures the corniculate processes dorsally. *(See also color section.)*

palpation, endoscopy, and radiography are generally sufficient to make a diagnosis. An abnormally wide gap can be palpated between the caudal margin of the thyroid and the rostral edge of the cricoid; in the normal larynx the two structures overlap.

The two typical endoscopic features of fourth branchial arch defects are RDPA, in which the caudal pillars of the soft palate form a hood that partly obscures the corniculate processes dorsally (see Fig. 10.7) and may even leave the upper esophagus open, and defective arytenoid motility. A small number of cases of fourth branchial arch defects can be detected only as dynamic RDPA during treadmill exercise.

Radiographic examination provides additional information to establish the diagnosis. When the upper esophageal sphincter is absent, lateral radiographs reveal a continuous column of air extending from the pharynx into the esophagus. The RDPA is seen as a "dewdrop" intruding into this air column from the dorsal wall.

**Treatment**

There are no effective means to reconstruct the absent structures. Laser treatment of the rostrally displaced palatopharyngeal arch has been described.

**Prognosis**

Affected horses are generally ineffective athletes, but they may be useful in less arduous occupations as pleasure horses. Repeated aerophagia leaves those animals without an upper esophageal sphincter susceptible to recurrent episodes of colic.

## EPIGLOTTIC FLACCIDITY

Epiglottic flaccidity is an abnormality of epiglottic rigidity:

- The clinical signs of epiglottic flacidity are caused by the secondary effects of dorsal displacement of the soft palate or retroversion of the epiglottis.
- Diagnosis is determined by endoscopic examination.
- Epiglottal augmentation with Teflon can be successful as a treatment in some cases.

The cause of epiglottic flaccidity is uncertain. Experimental blocking of the hypoglossal innervation of the geniohyoideus muscle will cause epiglottal flaccidity, so it is possible that a neuropathy affecting this nerve may be the cause in some horses. A flaccid epiglottis is believed to be unable to resist the dynamic collapse of the soft palate, resulting in dorsal displacement of the soft palate.

There is some confusion as to the terms *epiglottic flaccidity* and *epiglottic hypoplasia,* and some authors have used the term *epiglottic hypoplasia* to describe both conditions. In the current text, the term *epiglottic hypoplasia* is used to describe an abnormally short epiglottis, and the term *epiglottic flaccidity* is used to describe an abnormality of epiglottic rigidity. The two conditions may sometimes present simultaneously.

### Clinical signs
The clinical signs of epiglottic flaccidity are caused by the secondary effects of dorsal displacement of the soft palate or retroversion of the epiglottis, or both. Exercise intolerance and an abnormal respiratory noise are expected. Some non-racehorses may have evidence of epiglottic flaccidity, but it is unlikely to be clinically significant in these cases.

### Diagnosis
Diagnosis is achieved by endoscopic examination. Sedation may make the epiglottis appear flaccid, so the examination should be performed in the unsedated horse. The epiglottis appears flaccid and lies directly on the soft palate throughout its length. It conforms to the contours of the palate rather than maintaining its own shape. The lateral edges of the epiglottis may curl upward, and the normal serrated margin may not be observed. Nasal occlusion results in the soft palate billowing upward, with air leaking through the laryngopalatal junction and easy inducement of dorsal displacement of the soft palate. The flaccid epiglottis distorts with the soft palate rather than remaining stationary and allowing the palate to distort around it.

In some horses, the epiglottis may appear normal at rest, but flaccidity is noted prior to dorsal displacement of the soft palate when the horse is endoscopically evaluated during exercise on a high-speed treadmill. Conversely, some horses may have a flaccid-appearing epiglottis at rest that assumes a normal appearance during exercise.

## Treatment

The mechanical rigidity of the epiglottis may be increased by the injection of polytetrafluoroethylene (Teflon). The procedure may reduce the incidence of secondary dorsal displacement of the soft palate. Teflon is injected submucosally along the ventral surface of the epiglottis via a laryngotomy incision. Three injections are usually made, one along each side and one in the midline. A total of 3–7 ml is used. Alternatively, one midline injection of 3 ml can be made, followed by digital redistribution on the ventral surface of the epiglottis. The Teflon results in thickening of the epiglottis by 30–50% due to sterile granuloma formation and fibrosis.

## Prognosis

Some horses respond favorably to this treatment, but others continue to demonstrate dorsal displacement of the soft palate. Excessive granulation and abscess formation has been reported as an untoward sequela in a few cases.

## EPIGLOTTIC HYPOPLASIA

Epiglottic hypoplasia describes an abnormally short epiglottis, which predisposes to dorsal displacement of the soft palate and epiglottal entrapment. There is no specific treatment.

The normal epiglottis of adult Thoroughbreds measures 8–9 cm in length. An epiglottis that measures less than 5.5 cm is considered to be hypoplastic. The cause of epiglottal hypoplasia is unknown.

## Clinical signs

Horses with epiglottal hypoplasia are predisposed to epiglottal entrapment and/or dorsal displacement of the soft palate. Clinical signs relate to the presence of these secondary problems.

## Diagnosis

The diagnosis of epiglottal hypoplasia is based on measurement of the length of the epiglottis (measured from the basihyoid to the tip of the epiglottis) on a lateral radiograph. Metallic markers of known length are placed on each mandible so that the magnification factor for the radiograph can be determined. An abnormally short epiglottis is observed by endoscopy.

## Treatment

There is no specific treatment for epiglottal hypoplasia. Treatment of associated epiglottal entrapment or dorsal displacement of the soft palate can be undertaken, but there is a high risk of recurrence. Epiglottic augmentation by injection of polytetrafluoroethylene (Teflon) will not increase epiglottic length and is unlikely to successfully resolve the problem.

## Prognosis

The long-term prognosis for athletic activity is poor, especially if the condition is associated with dorsal displacement of the soft palate.

## EPIGLOTTITIS

Epiglottitis describes inflammation of the epiglottis, and clinical signs can include coughing, dysphagia, and dyspnea. The condition usually responds to antibiotic therapy.

Inflammation of the epiglottis can cause airway obstruction and interfere with deglutition. Causes include inhaled irritants, respiratory tract infection, traumatic injury, and ingestion of poor quality roughage. The condition has been observed in association with intermittent dorsal displacement of the soft palate and epiglottal entrapment.

## Clinical signs

Clinical signs include exercise intolerance, increased respiratory noise, coughing, dysphagia, and airway obstruction.

## Diagnosis

The diagnosis is determined via endoscopic examination. The mucosa of the epiglottis and aryepiglottic folds appears inflamed and swollen. There may be ulceration or granulation on the epiglottis, which may also appear dorsally elevated (Fig. 10.8). The degree of swelling and inflammation may make it difficult to differentiate from epiglottal entrapment or dorsal displacement of the soft palate. Chondritis of the epiglottis can develop, and this may result in epiglottic deformity.

## Treatment

A temporary tracheotomy may be necessary if there is severe dyspnea. Broad-spectrum antibiotic and nonsteroidal anti-inflammatory medications are indicated, and topical application of anti-inflammatory drugs can be beneficial (glycerin throat spray).

## Prognosis

The prognosis is generally good, but complications including epiglottic deformity, intermittent or persistent dorsal displacement of the soft palate, and epiglottal entrapment have been reported.

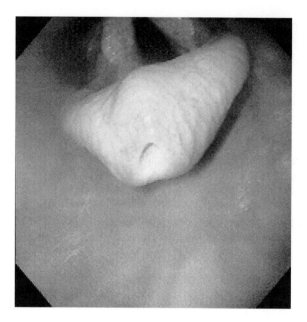

**Fig. 10.8.** Epiglottitis in an 8-year-old horse. The mucosa of the epiglottis appears inflamed and swollen, and there is ulceration of the tip and swelling of the dorsal surface of the epiglottis.

## DORSAL EPIGLOTTIC ABSCESS

Dorsal epiglottic abscess is probably caused by secondary infection of the tissues following mucosal damage. Affected horses show exercise intolerance, an abnormal respiratory noise, and cough while eating. The diagnosis is made by endoscopy; a smooth mass is present on the dorsal surface of the epiglottis. Aspiration via the endoscope confirms that the mass is an abscess. Treatment includes lancing of the abscess and lavage of the cavity followed by antibiotic treatment. The abscess can be lanced with the horse under general anesthesia using either a transoral approach or a ventral laryngotomy. Alternatively, the abscess can be ablated using an Nd:YAG laser.

## PERSISTENT FRENULUM OF THE EPIGLOTTIS

Persistent frenulum is a rare congenital abnormality that causes dysphagia in foals. Persistent dorsal displacement of the soft palate is identified by endoscopic examination per nasum. Endoscopy per os, performed under general anesthesia, reveals a ventrally displaced tip of epiglottis, with a ridge of tissue on the ventral aspect of the epiglottis attaching to the soft tissues caudal to the base of the tongue. Treatment involves surgical transecton of the tissue.

## LARYNGEAL WEB

Laryngeal web is a rare congenital abnormality due to failure of the larynx to completely recanalize during development. Affected foals present with respiratory stertor, distress, and dysphagia. The diagnosis is achieved by endoscopic examination; a web of tissue is seen on the ventral aspect of the rima glottidis with fusion of the vocal cords. Resection of the web or laser excision could be considered, but the affected foal should be assessed for other congenital abnormalities. An acquired form of laryngeal web, associated with ventral glottic stenosis, has been recorded rarely in adult horses following surgical treatments of the larynx.

## PERILARYNGEAL ACCESSORY BRONCHIAL CYST

There is one report in the veterinary literature of a perilaryngeal accessory bronchial cyst. This is a developmental congenital defect. In the reported case, the abnormality resulted in laryngeal hemiplegia associated with malformation of the cricoid and thyroid, or damage to the recurrent laryngeal nerve. Clinical signs include abnormal respiratory noise and exercise intolerance. Laryngeal hemiplagia is evident on endoscopic examination, and a fluctuant swelling is palpable in the laryngeal region. Surgical resection of the cyst may be possible.

## FURTHER READING

Baxter, G.M. 1992. Paralaryngeal accessory bronchial cyst as a cause of laryngeal hemiplegia in a horse. *Equine Vet J* 24:67–69.

Blikslager, A., Tate, L., and Tudor, R. 1999. Transendoscopic laser treatment of rostral displacement of the palatopharyngeal arch in four horses. *J Clin Laser Med Surg* 17:49–52.

Davenport-Goodall, C.L.M., and Parente, E.J. 2003. Disorders of the larynx. *Vet Clinics N Am Equine Pract* 19:169–187.

Dixon, P.M., McGorum, B.C., Railton, D.I., Hawe, C., Tremaine, W.H., Pickles, K., and McCann, J. 2001. Laryngeal paralysis: a study of 375 cases in a mixed breed population of horses. *Equine Vet J* 33:452–458.

Dixon, P.M., McGorum, B.C., Railton, D.I., Hawe, C., Tremaine, W.H., Pickles, K., and McCann, J. 2002. Clinical and endoscopic evidence of progression in 152 cases of equine recurrent laryngeal neuropathy (RLN). *Equine Vet J* 34:29–34.

Dixon, P.M., Railton, D.I., and McGorum, B.C. 1994. Ventral glottic stenosis in 3 horses. *Equine Vet J* 26:166–170.

Duncan, I.D., Amundson, J., Cuddon, R., Sufit, R., Jackson, K.F., and Lindsay, W.A. 1991. Preferential denervation of the adductor muscles of the equine larynx I: Muscle pathology. *Equine Vet J* 23:94–98.

Duncan, I.D., Reifenrath, P., Jackson, K.F., and Clayton, M. 1991. Preferential dener-
    vation of the adductor muscles of the equine larynx II: Nerve pathology. *Equine Vet
    J* 23:99–103.
Edwards, R.B. 1999. Diseases of the larynx. In *Equine Medicine and Surgery,* 5th ed.
    P.T. Colahan, I.G. Mayhew, A.M. Merritt and J.N. Moore, eds. St. Louis: Mosby,
    pp 512–522.
Fulton, I.C., Stick, J.A., and Derksen, F.J. 2003. Laryngeal reinnervation in the horse.
    *Vet Clinics N Am Equine Pract* 19:189–208.
Goulden, B., Anderson, L., and Davies, A. 1976. Rostral displacement of the
    palatopharyngeal arch: A case report. *Equine Vet J* 8:95–98.
Hammer, E.J., Tulleners, E.P., Parente, E.J., and Martin, B.B. 1998. Videoendoscopic
    assessment of dynamic laryngeal function during exercise in horses with grade III
    left laryngeal hemiparesis at rest: 26 cases (1992–1995). *J Am Vet Med Assoc*
    212:399–403.
Hawkins, J.F., and Tulleners, E.P. 1994. Epiglottitis in horses: 20 cases (1988–1993) *J
    Am Vet Med Assoc* 205:1577–1580.
Hawkins, J.F., Tulleners, E.P., Ross, M.W., Evans, L.H., and Raker, C.W. 1997.
    Laryngoplasty with or without ventriculocordectomy for treatment of left laryngeal
    hemiplegia in 230 racehorses. *Vet Surg* 26:484–491.
Hay, W.P. 1996. Diagnosis and treatment of arytenoid chondritis in horses. *Comp Cont
    Ed Pract Vet* 18:812–817.
Honnas, C.M., and Wheat, J.D. 1988. A transnasal surgical approach to divide the
    aryepiglottic fold axially in the standing horse. *Vet Surg* 17:246–251.
Jones, D. 1994. Squamous cell carcinoma of the larynx and pharynx in horses. *Cornell
    Vet* 84:15–24.
Klein, H., Deegen, E., and Stockhofe, N. 1989. Rostral displacement of the palatopha-
    ryngeal arch in a seven-month-old Hanoverian colt. *Equine Vet J* 21:382–383.
Kraus, B.M., and Parente, E.J. 2003. Laryngeal hemiplegia in non-racehorses. In
    *Current Therapy in Equine Medicine,* 5th ed. N.E. Robinson, ed. Philadelphia: W.B.
    Saunders, pp 383–386.
Lane, J.G. 1998. Disorders of the ear, nose and throat. In *Equine Medicine, Surgery
    and Reproduction.* T. Mair, S. Love, J. Schumacher, and E. Watson, eds. London:
    W.B. Saunders, pp 81–117.
Lees, M.J., Barber, S.M., and Farrow, C.S. 1987. A congenital laryngeal web defect in
    a Quarter Horse. *Equine Vet J* 19:561–563.
Lumsden, J.M., Derksen, F.J., Stick, J.A., Robinson, N.E., and Nickels, F.A. 1994.
    Evaluation of partial arytenoidectomy as a treatment for equine laryngeal hemiple-
    gia. *Equine Vet J* 26:125–129.
Mair, T.S., and Lane, J.G. 1996. The differential diagnosis of sudden onset respiratory
    distress. *Equine Vet Educ* 8:131–136.
Marks, D., Mackay-Smith, M.P., Cushing, L.S., and Leslie, J.A. 1970. Prosthetic device
    for surgical correction of laryngeal hemiplegia in horses. *J Am Vet Med Assoc*
    157:157–163.
Parente, E.J. 2003. Arytenoid chondrosis. In *Current Therapy in Equine Medicine,* 5th
    ed. N.E. Robinson, ed. Philadelphia: W.B. Saunders, pp 381–383.
Peloso, J.G., Stick, J.A., Nickels, F.A., Lumsden, J.M., and Derksen, F.J. 1992. Epiglot-
    tic augmentation by use of polytetrafluoroethylene to correct dorsal displacement of
    the soft palate in a Standardbred horse. *J Am Vet Med Assoc* 201:1393–1395.

Robertson, J.T. 1991. Pharynx and larynx. In *Equine Respiratory Disorders*. J. Beech, ed. Philadelphia: Lea and Febiger, pp 331–387.

Russell, A.P., and Slone, D.E. 1994. Performance analysis after prosthetic laryngoplasty and bilateral ventriculectomy for laryngeal hemiplegia in horses: 70 cases (1986–1991). *J Am Vet Med Assoc* 204:1235–1241.

Specht, T.E., Peyton, L.C., Nixon, A.J. 1989. Spontaneous recovery from idiopathic right laryngeal hemiplegia in a horse. *Can Vet J* 30:593–594.

Speirs, V.C., Tulleners, E.P., Ducharme, N.G., and Hackett, R.P. 1992. Larynx. In *Equine Surgery*. J.A. Auer, ed. Philadelphia: W.B. Saunders, pp 460–488.

Tetens, J., Derksen, F.J., Stick, J.A., Lloyd, J.W., and Robinson, N.E. 1996. Efficacy of prosthetic laryngoplasty with and without bilateral ventriculocordectomy as treatments for laryngeal hemiplegia in horses. *Am J Vet Res* 57:1668–1673.

Trotter, G.W., Aanes, W.A., and Snyder, S.P. 1981. Laryngeal chondroma in a horse. *J Am Vet Med Assoc* 178:829.

Tulleners, E.P. 1990. Transendoscopic contact neodymium:yttrium aluminium garnet laser correction of epiglottic entrapment in standing horses. *J Am Vet Med Assoc* 196:1971–1980.

Tulleners, E.P. 1991. Correlation of performance with endoscopic and radiographic assessment of epiglottic hypoplasia in racehorses with epiglottic entrapment corrected by use of contact neodydium:yttrium aluminium garnet laser. *J Am Vet Med Assoc* 198:621–626.

Tulleners, E.P. 1991. Use of transendoscopic contact neodymium:yttrium aluminium garnet laser to drain dorsal epiglottic abscesses in two horses. *J Am Vet Med Assoc* 198:1765–1769.

Tulleners, E.P. 1994. Arytenoidectomy. In *Current Practice of Equine Surgery*. N.A. White and J. Moore, eds. Philadelphia: J.B. Lippincott, pp 255–261.

Tulleners, E.P., and Hamir, A. 1991. Evaluation of epiglottic augmentation by use of polytetrafluoroethylene paste in the horse. *Am J Vet Res* 52:1908–1916.

Tulleners, E.P., Harrison, I.W., and Raker, C.W. 1988. Management of arytenoid chondropathy and failed laryngoplasty in horses: 75 cases (1979–1985) *J Am Vet Med Assoc* 192:670–675.

Tulleners, E.P., Ross, M.W., and Hawkins, J. 1996. Management of right laryngeal hemiplegia in horses: 28 cases (1987–1996). In *Proceedings Am Coll Vet Surg*, p 21.

White, N.A., and Blackwell, R.B. 1980. Partial arytenoidectomy in the horse. *Vet Surg* 9:5–12.

Yarborough, T.B., Voss, E., Herrgesell, E.J. 1999. Persistent frenulum of the epiglottis in four foals. *Vet Surg* 28:287–291.

# Dynamic Airway Collapse During Exercise

**11**

The dynamics of airflow change dramatically between the resting and exercising horse. The equine athlete under maximum exertion, increases airflow by almost twentyfold relative to the resting animal, and creates negative pressures within the airway ninefold greater than the resting animal. During inspiration, in particular, the tissues abutting onto the extrathoracic airway must resist these marked forces of collapse, especially in the face of muscular fatigue. In this regard, the soft structures of the external nares and the pharynx and larynx are most vulnerable.

It is unlikely that dynamic collapse can be seen endoscopically during quiet breathing, unless by partial asphyxiation by forced nostril closure. It has been only since the advent of high-speed treadmills and the equipment to perform endoscopic examination during peak exertion that the dynamic causes of airway collapse have been confirmed.

The method of the treadmill exercise test is important in obtaining accurate results. Head and neck position should mimic the natural clinical position as far as possible. Certain disorders have been observed only when the horse is under tack.

## PHARYNGEAL COLLAPSE

It is normal for the walls of the pharynx to collapse slightly during exercise and for the soft palate, which makes up the floor of the nasopharynx, to billow slightly upward during inspiration. However, collapse due to excessive negative pressure in the pharynx or to dysfunction of the supporting musculature causes a severe obstruction with associated signs of exercise intolerance and abnormal respiratory noise. Increased negative pressure in the nasopharynx might occur as a result of an obstruction rostral to the pharynx, such as space-occupying masses, nasal deformity, and Horner's syndrome resulting in engorgement of the vasculature in the nasal cavity. Myopathies causing muscular weakness, such as hyperkalemic periodic paralysis (Fig. 11.1), or neuropathies could also cause pharyngeal collapse. A hind brain lesion was found to be the cause of nasopharyngeal roof collapse in one reported case. Other adjacent dynamic abnormalities, such as mild guttural pouch tympany, could also potentially result in pharyngeal collapse. Diagnosis of dynamic pharyngeal collapse has been recorded in 3–8% of horses undergoing treadmill evaluation for poor performance.

The diagnosis is determined via endoscopic examination during exercise on a high-speed treadmill, or endoscopy at rest with nasal occlusion. The lateral walls or roof of the nasopharynx are seen to collapse, causing a significant narrowing in axial-abaxial and dorsoventral planes of the pharyngeal airway. Treatment depends on identifying and treating any underlying cause. The prognosis for horses without an identifiable primary cause is poor.

## DYNAMIC DORSAL DISPLACEMENT OF THE SOFT PALATE

Dorsal displacement of the soft palate is a dynamic event that occurs only under conditions of extreme exertion. Treadmill endoscopy provides the means to observe the events that lead to the spontaneous displacement of the

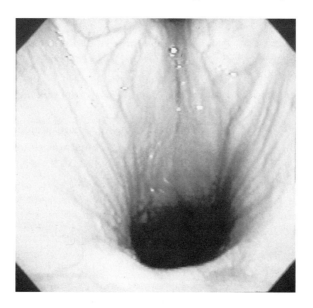

**Fig. 11.1.** Pharyngeal collapse in 2-year-old Quarter Horse gelding homozygous for hyperkalemic periodic paralysis. Homozygous individuals often demonstrate mild to moderate inspiratory noise at rest, and complete pharyngeal collapse is observed during endoscopic examination.

palatal arch above the epiglottis and to differentiate idiopathic dorsal displacement of the soft palate from other forms.

## INTERMITTENT EPIGLOTTAL ENTRAPMENT

Frequently, epiglottal entrapment is not a stable anatomical arrangement but may consist of the intermittent gathering of the glossoepiglottic mucosa over the apex of the epiglottis. Although most cases of intermittent epiglottal entrapment can be provoked by the repeated stimulation of deglutition sequences, a small number are not confirmed by endoscopy until treadmill exercise is used. In one study, intermittent epiglottal entrapment was diagnosed in 2 of 348 horses undergoing endoscopy during exercise on a high-speed treadmill for the evaluation of poor performance.

## ARYEPIGLOTTIC FOLD COLLAPSE (AXIAL DEVIATION OF THE ARYEPIGLOTTIC FOLDS)

Aryepiglottic fold collapse is a cause of dynamic airway obstruction during exercise:

- Affected horses present with a history of exercise intolerance and an abnormal respiratory noise during exercise.
- Diagnosis is determined via endoscopic examination during exercise on a high-speed treadmill.
- In young horses, especially those with other concurrent upper airway abnormalities, conservative treatment and prolonged rest may be beneficial.
- Treatment by resection of the affected aryepiglottic fold(s) can be performed using transendoscopic laser surgery in the standing horse.

The aryepiglottal mucosal folds extend from the lateral margins of the epiglottis to the corniculate processes of the arytenoid cartilages. Dynamic collapse of one or both of these folds toward the midline is a relatively common observation during treadmill endoscopy of horses with a history of exercise intolerance. The inversion of soft tissue structures causes a major obstruction of the rima glottidis but the etiology is unknown. Immaturity is a possible predisposing factor in young horses, especially if other concurrent dynamic upper airway abnormalities are present.

### Clinical signs
Affected horses have exercise intolerance with or without a consistent harsh inspiratory noise. There is no known breed or gender predisposition. All ages can be affected, but there might be a higher prevalence in young horses (2- and 3-year-olds).

## Diagnosis

Diagnosis of aryepiglottic fold collapse can be made only by endoscopic examination during exercise on a high-speed treadmill. No abnormalities are identified on resting endoscopy, and nostril occlusion fails to induce aryepiglottic fold collapse. During exercise, the aryepiglottic folds collapse axially over the lateral margins of the larynx on inspiration. The problem may be unilateral (usually right-sided) or bilateral. The collapse tends to worsen as the exercise period proceeds. The severity of the axial deviation of the aryepiglottic fold varies. In mild cases, the fold remains abaxial to the vocal fold. In moderate cases, the fold deviates across the vocal fold, but less than halfway between the vocal fold and the midline. In severe cases, the fold reaches or crosses the midline of the glottis. In severe bilateral cases, the folds may contact each other in the midline causing a complete obstruction of the larynx. There may or may not be other observable upper airway abnormalities, but the condition has no obvious association with any other disease.

## Treatment

Several treatments have been proposed, but there is little information regarding efficacy. Horses with moderate or severe aryepiglottic fold collapse, and horses with mild aryepiglottic fold collapse associated with exercise intolerance, but with no other identifiable problems, are candidates for surgical treatment.

Attempts to stiffen and induce fibrosis in the aryepiglottic folds may be made using an Nd:YAG laser through the endoscope. The folds are blanched on their rostral margins using a contact technique. A similar effect may be produced using electrocautery applied through a laryngotomy incision.

Resection of the aryepiglottic folds can be achieved standing using topical anesthesia or with the horse under general anesthesia. In the standing procedure, the aryepiglottic fold is grasped with bronchoesophagoscopic forceps passed via the contralateral nasal passage. The fold is elevated caudodorsally. The endoscope and Nd:YAG or diode laser fiber are passed up the ipsilateral nasal passage. A 2 cm right-angled triangle of tissue is excised using the laser in contact mode. If the resection is performed with the horse under general anesthesia, the approach is made orally, and a nasotracheal tube is used rather than an orotracheal tube. Postoperative treatment with antibiotics and nonsteroidal anti-inflammatories is continued for 7 days. Topical antimicrobial/anti-inflammatory spray may also be administered.

If the horse is affected by concurrent intermittent dorsal displacement of the soft palate, cauterization or resection of the aryepiglottic fold can be combined with caudal palatoplasty (staphylectomy) performed via a ventral laryngotomy.

In young horses and those with multiple upper airway abnormalities, a conservative approach with a prolonged period of rest may be beneficial.

## Prognosis

The outcome has been favorable in the small number of cases treated by surgical resection of the folds, and to date, no untoward effects of the treatment have been recorded.

## EPIGLOTTIC RETROVERSION

Epiglottic retroversion is a rare cause of upper respiratory tract noise during exercise. The cause is unknown, but may involve loss of motor function of the hyoepiglotticus muscle (innervated by the hypoglossal nerve). Alternatively, contraction of the geniohyoideus muscle, which pulls the hyoid arch rostral and increases tension on the hyoepiglottic ligament, may be involved. Typically, an inspiratory gurgling noise is produced. Endoscopically, the epiglottis elevates and retroverts into the glottis during inspiration. Attempted treatments have included epiglottic augmentation with polytetrafluoroethylene and stabilization of the epiglottis with a suture between the epiglottis and the thyroid cartilage.

## DYNAMIC ROSTRAL DISPLACEMENT OF THE PALATOPHARYNGEAL ARCH

The fourth branchial arch defect syndrome has been described previously. Even with careful palpation, radiography, and endoscopy, a definitive diagnosis may not be achieved at rest, particularly when the defects are minor. The only evidence of this lesser expression of fourth branchial arch defect may be dynamic rostral displacement of the palatal arch (see Chapter 10, Fig. 10.7.) observed during treadmill endoscopy.

## DYNAMIC LARYNGEAL COLLAPSE

During quiet breathing, the reliability of endoscopic examination as a means to interpret laryngeal function is far from satisfactory. In the absence of the collapsing forces at inspiration, resting horses with recurrent laryngeal neuropathy may recruit sufficient motility to appear relatively normal. However, exercise may lead to fatigue of the residual abductor musculature so that treadmill endoscopy reveals dynamic collapse of the affected arytenoid cartilage.

Axial collapse of the ipsilateral vocal cord and ventricle during exercise is also recognized in some horses affected by laryngeal hemiplegia. This can occur even if the laryngeal hemiplegia has been effectively treated by prosthetic laryngoplasty. For this reason, performing a ventriculocordectomy at the same time as laryngoplasty is recommended by many clinicians.

## FURTHER READING

Blikslager, A.T., and Tate, L.P. 2000. History, instrumentation, and techniques of flexible endoscopic laser surgery in horses. *Vet Clinics N Am Equine Pract* 16:251–268.
Davenport-Goodall, C.L.M., and Parente, E.J. 2003. Disorders of the larynx. *Vet Clinics N Am Equine Pract* 19:169–187.

Edwards, R.B. 1999. Diseases of the larynx. In *Equine Medicine and Surgery*, 5th ed. P.T. Colahan, I.G. Mayhew, A.M. Merritt, and J.N. Moore, eds. St. Louis: Mosby, pp 512–522.

Kannegieter, N., and Dore, M. 1995. Endoscopy of the upper respiratory tract during treadmill exercise: A clinical study of 100 horses. *Aust Vet J* 72:101–107.

King, D.S. 2003. Axial deviation of the aryepiglottic folds. In *Current Therapy in Equine Medicine*, 5th ed. N.E. Robinson, ed. Philadelphia: W.B. Saunders, pp 378–380.

King, D.S., Tulleners, E.P., Martin, B.B., Parente, E.J, and Boston, R. 2001. Clinical experiences with axial deviation of the aryepiglottic folds in 52 racehorses. *Vet Surg* 30:151–160.

Mair, T.S., and Pearson, G.R. 1990. Melanotic hamartoma of the hind brain in a riding horse. *J Comp Pathol* 102:240–243.

Martin, B., Reef, V., and Parente, E. 2000. Causes of poor performance of horses during training, racing, or showing: 348 cases (1992–1996). *J Am Vet Med Assoc* 216:554–558.

Parente, E.J., Martin, B.B., and Tulleners, E.P. 1998. Epiglottic retroversion as a cause of upper airway obstruction in two horses. *Equine Vet J* 30:270–272.

Smith, C.M., Taylor, R.J., and Dixon, P.M. 1994. Unilateral ventral displacement of the roof of the nasopharynx as a cause of stridor in a pony. *Vet Rec* 134:140–141.

Strand, E., and Staempfli, H.R. 1993. Dynamic collapse of the roof of the nasopharynx as a cause of poor performance in a Standardbred colt. *Equine Vet J* 25:252–254.

Tulleners, E.P. 1996. Instrumentation and technique in transendoscopic upper respiratory tract laser surgery. *Vet Clinics N Am Equine Pract* 12:373–395.

# Postanesthetic Upper Respiratory Tract Obstruction

Postanesthetic upper respiratory tract obstruction can arise for different reasons. Mild obstruction due to nasal edema is the most common. Bilateral laryngeal paralysis is rare, but can cause serious life-threatening airway obstruction.

## NASAL EDEMA

Nasal edema or congestion is usually the result of passive venous congestion that occurs after prolonged general anesthesia, especially in horses maintained in dorsal recumbency. Trauma to the nasopharynx associated with endotracheal intubation may also contribute to the problem.

A loud inspiratory snoring noise is heard immediately after extubation. This problem usually resolves spontaneously without treatment. A nasopharyngeal tube can be placed through one nostril to provide a clear airway. In severe cases, nasotracheal intubation is required. Phenylephrine nasal spray (5–10 mg in 10 ml water) or furosemide (1 mg/kg IV) is administered to reduce the degree of edema.

## BILATERAL LARYNGEAL PARALYSIS

The precise cause of bilateral laryngeal paralysis following general anesthesia is unknown. Potential causes include compression of the recurrent laryngeal nerve between the endotracheal tube and noncompliant neck structures, damage to the recurrent laryngeal nerve from hypoxia or hypotension, and overextension of the neck when the horse is positioned in dorsal recumbency. Impaired laryngeal function may occur as a result of $\alpha_2$-adrenergic agonist use, and preexisting laryngeal disease might predispose to the problem.

Severe upper airway obstruction becomes evident when the horse stands after extubation. A loud, high-pitched inspiratory stridor develops with marked dyspnea. The horse rapidly becomes hypoxic and may develop cardiovascular collapse. The horse may be uncontrollable, complicating emergency treatment. Once the horse collapses, emergency tracheotomy can be performed, but it is often too late. Affected horses die from irreversible shock, pulmonary edema, and hypoxia.

Attempted treatments involve urgent establishment of a patent airway. This may be achieved by placing a nasotracheal tube or performing a tracheotomy. The horse may need to be re-anesthetized to permit these procedures. Alternatively a paralytic agent such as succinylcholine may be used. As soon as an airway is established, oxygen insufflation is instituted.

## FURTHER READING

Dixon, P.M., Railton, D.I., and McGorum, B.C. 1993. Temporary bilateral laryngeal paralysis in a horse associated with general anaesthesia and post anaesthetic myositis. *Vet Rec* 132:29–32.

Flaherty, D., Nolan, A., and Reid, J. 1996. Complications during recovery from anaesthesia in the equine patient. *Equine Vet Educ* 8:17–22.

Kollias-Baker, C.A., Pipers, F.S., Heard, D., and Seeherman, H. 1993. Pulmonary edema associated with transient airway obstruction in three horses. *J Am Vet Med Assoc* 202:1116–1118.

Lukasik, V.M., Gleed, R.D., Scarlett, J.M., Ludders, J.W., Moon, P.F., Ballenstedt, J.L., and Sturmor, A.T. 1997. Intranasal phenylephrine reduces post anesthetic upper airway obstruction in horses. *Equine Vet J* 29:236–238.

Southwood, L.L., and Gaynor, J.S. 2003. Postanesthetic upper respiratory tract obstruction. In *Current Therapy in Equine Medicine*. N.E. Robinson, ed. Philadelphia: W.B. Saunders, pp 391–393.

# The Trachea

## ANATOMY

The trachea extends from the larynx to the hilus of the lungs, where it divides into the left and right principal bronchi. Its average length is 75–80 cm, and its average calibre is 5–6 cm. The trachea is a tube comprised of 50–60 hyaline cartilage rings that maintain its structure. The cartilage rings are incomplete dorsally. A fibroelastic membrane encloses and connects adjacent rings; in the spaces between the rings, this membrane is known as the tracheal annular ligament. Smooth muscle is attached dorsally to the inner surface of the cartilaginous plates, and combines with the mucosa and adventitia to form the dorsal tracheal membrane. The trachea is normally cylindrical, but in the cervical part, the dorsal surface is flattened due to contact with the longus colli muscle. The sternothyroideus and sternohyoideus muscles lie on the ventral aspect of the cervical trachea, and the esophagus lies dorsal to it at its origin. In the distal neck, the esophagus lies to the left side.

The trachea is lined by pseudostratified columnar ciliated epithelium with numerous goblet cells. The epithelial surface is covered by a layer of mucus that is constantly being propelled proximally the pharynx. The mucocilary escalator is an important part of the nonspecific pulmonary defense system that protects the lower airway from inhaled dust particles and other foreign material.

## TRACHEAL EXAMINATION

Examination of the trachea includes palpation, auscultation, endoscopy, and radiography. "Tracheal rattle" is the term used to describe the sound generated by the oscillation of accumulated mucus within the tracheal lumen during respiration. Deep palpation of the proximal trachea is performed to assess inducibility of cough to indicate the degree of tracheal irritation. Horses have a high threshold for inducible cough and will not normally respond to deep tracheal/laryngeal palpation.

## SURGERY OF THE TRACHEA

Surgery of the trachea can include intubation, permanent tracheostomy, tracheal resection and anastomosis, the application of external prostheses, and laser surgery.

### Tracheotomy intubation

Tracheotomy intubation involves implantation of a tube directly into the trachea to provide an alternative airway when the upper respiratory tract is completely or partly obstructed or when it may become obstructed—for example, after laryngeal surgery. Tracheotomy can be used as the primary means to manage pharyngeal or laryngeal obstructions or when other methods to treat recurrent laryngeal neuropathy or arytenoid chondritis have failed.

The surgery is performed through a ventral midline incision on the standing horse under local anesthesia. In most cases, the surgery is performed at the junction of the upper and middle thirds of the trachea; the trachea is superficial and easily palpable at this site. A 6–8 cm incision is made through the skin and cutaneous colli muscle. The septum between the paired sternothyrohyoideus muscles is divided to expose the ventral surface of the trachea. After clearing the overlying fascia, a transverse incision is made into the tracheal lumen without transection of a complete tracheal cartilage ring. The incision should involve about 120° of the tracheal circumference. If necessary, semicircles of cartilage are removed from adjacent tracheal rings, leaving a narrow bridge of cartilage on either side of the hole by which to maintain the structural stability of the trachea.

A self-retaining metallic tube is placed for racing purposes. A similar technique may be used for anesthetic maintenance when the presence of an endotracheal tube passed per os is an encumbrance to the surgeon.

The wound and tracheotomy tube should be cleaned at least once daily. Obstruction of the tube by secretions can occur unless careful cleaning and aftercare are performed. When the tube is removed permanently, the wound is left open to heal by secondary intention. The wound normally granulates quickly, and healing is usually complete in about 1 month.

Complications of tracheotomy intubation are unusual. Local infection and cellulitis can occur, but are generally responsive to antibiotic therapy. Subcutaneous emphysema occasionally develops around the site, but this usually resolves within 1–2 weeks. Tracking of emphysema along the fascial planes of the neck to the thorax, resulting in pneumomediastinum and possibly pneumothorax, is a rare event. Stenosis of the trachea can occur if the tracheal cartilage rings are traumatized. The risk of stenosis may be higher in foals because they have soft, pliable cartilage rings. Traumatic dissection or placement of the tracheotomy tube, use of a large, tight-fitting tube, or prolonged intubation may increase the risk of subsequent stenosis.

## Permanent tracheostomy

Permanent tracheostomy is indicated in horses with severe upper airway obstructive diseases that are not amenable to other forms of treatment, or where other forms of treatment have failed. Examples might include some cases of nasopharyngeal cicatrix, arytenoid chondritis, neoplasia of the upper airway, and severe nasal cavity obstruction.

Permanent tracheostomy can be performed with the horse standing or under general anesthesia. The standing procedure has advantages because the surgical structures are maintained in a more normal anatomical orientation and less tension is placed on the wound. The horse is sedated and restrained in stocks with cross-ties with the head extended. Local anesthetic solution is infiltrated in an inverted U pattern, dorsal and lateral to the 2nd–6th tracheal rings. A 3 cm wide x 6 cm long rectangular piece of skin is excised, starting 3 cm distal to the cricoid cartilage. The paired sternothyrohyoideus muscles are separated, and dissection is continued laterally around the abaxial borders of the muscles. Following isolation of the muscle bellies, they are clamped at the proximal and distal ends of the wound and then transected. A section of the omohyoid can be removed in a similar fashion. A ventral midline incision, and two paramedian incisions, approximately 15 mm on either side of the midline, are made through the tracheal rings without penetrating the mucosa. The cartilage segments are dissected free and removed, leaving the tracheal mucosa intact. Four or preferably five tracheal rings are removed. Subcutaneous tissue is sutured to the tracheal fascia prior to incision of the tracheal mucosa in a "double Y" pattern. The tracheal mucosa and submucosa are sutured to the skin with simple interrupted sutures of absorbable material.

Antibiotics are administered for 5–7 days. The stoma is cleaned twice a day until sutures are removed at 14 days. Thereafter daily cleaning is required for about a month, but subsequently cleaning is usually only needed once or twice a week. Post-operative swelling and partial dehiscence are the most common complications. Most incisions will heal satisfactorily by second intention if partial dehiscence occurs.

Long-term complications are rare. The procedure has been used in broodmares with no apparent effect on foaling. Although the defense mechanisms of air warming/humidifying of the upper respiratory tract are bypassed, this does not appear to cause significant problems. Development of a cough at exercise is seen in a proportion of cases; maintenance of dust-free conditions is recommended if this occurs.

## Tracheal resection and anastomosis

Resection and anastomosis of the trachea is rarely performed. Surgical success requires restricted head movement and maintenance of neck flexion to prevent disruptive tension on the tracheal anastomosis during healing. Maintaining neck flexion reduces the suture line tension by about 50%. No more than 5 tracheal rings can be removed. Resection of 3 rings can be performed relatively easily, but the force required to appose the ends is increased by 100% when 5 rings are removed.

Indications for tracheal resection include acquired tracheal stenosis following temporary tracheotomy. Other indications might include intraluminal webbing, mucosa fibrosis, cut cartilage rings, and telescoping of cut edges of cartilages over each other.

The procedure is performed with the horse in dorsal recumbency. A ventral midline incision from the cricoid cartilage to the thoracic inlet is required so that the entire cervical trachea can be mobilized. This reduces the tension of the resected ends of the trachea. The trachea can tolerate extensive mobilization in this way, and has a good collateral blood suppply. The trachea is freed from the surrounding fascia, and the diseased trachea is resected. A circumferential mucosal flap is created on the free ends of the remaining trachea. An endotracheal tube is passed through the distal end of the transected trachea to continue gaseous anesthesia. The mucosal cuffs are then turned back over the normal tracheal cartilages and sutured to the adventia with fine, absorbable suture material. This directly apposes the mucosa and provides an airtight seal at the anastomosis site. The endotracheal tube is removed from the distal trachea and replaced by an orotracheal tube that is passed down into the distal tracheal segment. The head is then flexed to 90° and the anastomosis performed with 25 g stainless steel wire in a simple interrupted pattern. Sutures are placed 0.5–1.0 cm apart and through half the width of each tracheal ring without entering the tracheal lumen. Tension sutures encompassing tracheal rings proximal and distal to those removed may be placed if required to relieve tension on the anastomotic site. Following removal of the endotracheal tube, the surgical field is flooded with saline to check for air leaks. A suction drain is placed next to the trachea prior to wound closure.

A martingale harness with a line running from the girth to the halter is fitted for anesthetic recovery, and kept in place for 3 weeks after surgery. This is effective at reducing tension on the anastomosis site. Slings or assisted recovery from anesthesia may be used as indicated. Postoperative antibiotics are administered for 10 days.

Buds of granulation tissue frequently develop at the mucosa postoperatively, but following complete healing, restoration of 90% of the tracheal diameter can be achieved. Failure of the anastomosis will result in subcutaneous emphysema and eventual stenosis. Complete dehiscence is potentially disastrous. Malalignment of the cartilage rings may result if long tension sutures are placed.

Use of a tracheal prosthesis following surgical resection of a segment of diseased trachea has been described. A 45 cm reinforced polyvinyl chloride hose prosthesis was used. The horse developed complications that necessitated euthanasia after 9 months.

## External prosthesis to stent collapsed tracheal cartilages

Collapsed, deformed tracheal rings can be reshaped and supported by external stents. The technique has limited application in the horse because many cartilage deformities are too severe to allow effective reconstruction.

A stent fashioned from a 60 ml polypropylene syringe case can be used. The case is cut longitudinally in half, and numerous small holes are drilled into it. Alternatively, a wire spring covered with polyethylene tubing that is spiraled onto the affected segment of trachea can be used. The support is applied through a ventral midline incision with the horse placed under general anesthesia. Chondrotomies consisting of one or more partial or full-thickness incisions across the width of each affected cartilage ring may be necessary to permit reshaping. Fine monofilament sutures are preplaced as necessary around the affected segments of tracheal rings to elevate them into a normal position. The support is then applied (placing it under the recurrent laryngeal nerve), and the preplaced sutures are tied to it. A continuous closed suction drain is placed adjacent to the trachea prior to wound closure.

Postoperative antibiotics are given for 7–10 days. The suction drain is removed after 3 days. Potential complications include infection and damage to adjacent nerves. The implant may need to be removed in young growing horses to allow tracheal growth.

## Laser surgery

Intraluminal tracheal masses, such as granulation tissue or inflammatory granulomas, can be excised using contact laser surgery, usually with an Nd:YAG or diode laser. Granulation tissue usually results from traumatic tracheal perforation or tracheal surgery. Rarely, it may follow transtracheal aspiration. Transendoscopic laser excision can be performed in the standing sedated patient following the topical application or local anesthetic solution to the larynx and trachea. When dissection of the mass is nearly complete, the laser fiber is removed and replaced by grasping forceps, which are used to hold the mass and complete its removal by gentle traction. Alternatively, the mass can be grasped by bronchoesophagostomy forceps prior to dissection with the laser fiber.

## CONGENITAL TRACHEAL COLLAPSE (COLLAPSED TRACHEA)

Congenital tracheal collapse is seen in Shetland ponies and miniature horses:

- Dorsoventral flattening of the trachea occurs.
- Clinical signs include inspiratory stridor and coughing.
- Treatment is rarely possible.

Congenital narrowing of the trachea through flattening of the cartilage rings is uncommon in horses. However, it is sometimes encountered in Shetland ponies and miniature horses. This disease usually results in dorsoventral flattening, and is also known as "scabbard trachea." In most cases, the tracheal rings are deformed and take the shape of shallow arcs; the dorsal tracheal membrane is stretched and the tracheal lumen is elliptical rather than circular.

## Clinical signs

The abnormality may be subclinical in some animals, especially those that lead a sedentary lifestyle. Others are presented with persistent coughing and adventitious respiratory sounds at exercise. Clinical signs are most commonly seen in ponies over 10 years of age. It is possible that aging changes, such as calcification and inflammation, exacerbate the obstruction and are the reason why clinical signs develop later in life. Once clinical signs develop, they are often persistent. Inspiratory stridor and a "honking" noise are typical, and are exacerbated by exercise. Many affected animals develop a chronic paroxysmal cough.

## Diagnosis

A palpable vibration is often present over the cervical trachea. In some cases, a deformity of the tracheal cartilage rings is palpable. Confirmation of the abnormality is established by endoscopic examination, which identifies dorsoventral flattening in most cases (Fig. 13.1). Radiographic examination demonstrates severe dorsoventral flattening of the tracheal lumen.

## Treatment

In most cases, there is no effective means to correct this deformity. The entire trachea is often involved. Surgery (external prosthesis) might be possible if the defect is confined to a short segment of trachea, but this is very unusual.

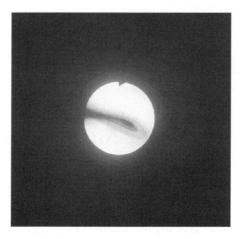

**Fig. 13.1.** Endoscopic view of dorsoventral tracheal collapse in a Shetland pony. *(See also color section.)*

Affected ponies may be managed conservatively by retirement and use of cough suppressors, such as butorphanol tartrate.

## TRACHEAL STENOSIS

Tracheal stenosis is a narrowing or stricture of the tracheal lumen:

- It may arise as a congenital deformity or secondary to trauma.
- It can occur as a complication of tracheotomy.
- Inspiratory noise and dyspnea may be present.
- Tracheal resection and anastomosis may be performed if the affected segment is short.

Congenital defects of the tracheal cartilage rings (other than tracheal collapse) are rare (Fig. 13.2). Clinical signs may not become apparent until the horse starts work. Acquired tracheal stenosis is more common than congenital defects of the cartilagenous rings. The most common cause of acquired tracheal stenosis is technical errors following tracheotomy tube placement. If a complete tracheal ring is cut longitudinally (rather than transversely incising between tracheal rings or removing a crescent-shaped segment of a ring), the dorsal tips of the cartilage will override, due to loss of ventral support. The trachea collapses laterally, and the cut mucosal edges heal with a web across the lumen. Tracheal stenosis can also occur as a result of transection through the tracheal annular ligament for more than 180° of its circumference. The tracheal cartilage rings are also vulnerable to fracture by kicks from other horses or by running against paddock rails. Prolonged or traumatic tracheal intubation causes mucosal damage and hemorrhage. This damage usually heals without complication, but could potentially lead to tracheal stenosis, as has been reported in some other species.

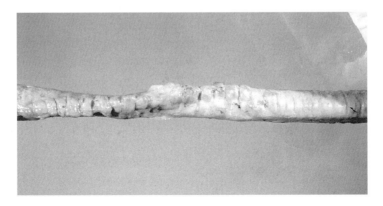

**Fig. 13.2.** Congenital tracheal deformity and stenosis. *(See also color section.)*

## Clinical signs

Mild tracheal stenosis may produce no overt clinical signs, but inspiratory dyspnea and an adventitious respiratory noise may be produced with more severe lesions, especially at exercise.

## Diagnosis

The level of stenosis may be detected by palpation and auscultation. Confirmation of the luminal distortion is achieved by endoscopy (see Fig. 13.1) and radiography.

## Treatment

Only narrow stricture bands may be treated by tracheal resection and anastomosis; but even so, the tension in the repaired incision is such that recurrence of the cicatrix is common. Longer segments of tracheal distortion may be treated by the application of an external prosthesis against which the collapsed cartilage rings are conformed. The prognosis for successful repair of acquired tracheal stenoses is guarded.

## EXTERNAL COMPRESSION AND STENOSIS OF THE TRACHEA

Tracheal compression by extraluminal masses such as lymph node abscesses, lipomas, and mediastinal tumors is an unusual cause of tracheal obstruction. Clinical signs include inspiratory dyspnea and stridor. The diagnosis is achieved by a combination of physical, endoscopic, and radiographic examination. Treatment includes surgical drainage and/or removal, and antibiotic therapy for septic lesions.

## TRACHEAL WOUNDS

Wounds to the trachea may be open or closed. Open wounds can result in fever, respiratory distress, subcutaneous emphysema, and cellulitis. Treatment involves debridement of the wound edges and creation of a pathway for drainage. Healing by secondary intention is usually preferable to attempted primary closure.

Closed wounds are caused by blunt trauma. These result in a rupture or tear of the trachea without any overlying wound. Severe subcutaneous emphysema and edema occur rapidly, and there may be stridor associated with obstruction of the airway by the wound edges. A seroma may be present at the level of the injury. Diagnosis is determined by endoscopic and radiographic examination. Treatment with pressure bandages, combined with antibiotic and anti-inflammatory medication, is often successful. Primary closure of the tracheal wound can be performed in some cases.

The prognosis for tracheal wounds is usually good, provided that appropriate treatment is instituted early. Failure to diagnose and treat the tracheal wound may result in life-threatening pneumomediastinum and pneumothorax as the emphysema tracks down the neck into the chest. Tracheal stenosis may result after large tracheal wounds.

## TRACHEAL NEOPLASIA

Neoplasia of the larynx appears to be very rare. Round cell sarcomas and mastocytomas have been recorded.

## INTRATRACHEAL PROLAPSE OF THE CRICOTRACHEAL MEMBRANE

This is a poorly defined condition where the tracheal mucosa over the cricotracheal membrane is redundant and flaccid, and may be aspirated into the airway during exercise, thereby causing a partial airway obstruction. Treatment by imbrication of the cricotracheal membrane has been proposed.

## TRACHEOBRONCHIAL FOREIGN BODY

The most common form of foreign body that can lodge in the distal trachea and bronchial tree is thorned twigs or brambles. The thorns act as barbs that allow the foreign body to progress distally but prevent it from being coughed up. Clinical signs include a chronic cough and malodorous breath. A mucopurulent nasal discharge may be present.

Diagnosis is confirmed by endoscopic examination. Treatment involves removal of the foreign body, usually using a snare passed through the endoscope (Fig. 13.3). Alternatively, a distal cervical tracheotomy may be made to allow insertion of grasping forceps or a snare. The foreign body may break up as it is being removed (Fig. 13.4), and several separate procedures may be necessary to remove all of the foreign material. Broad spectrum antibiotic therapy should be administered postoperatively.

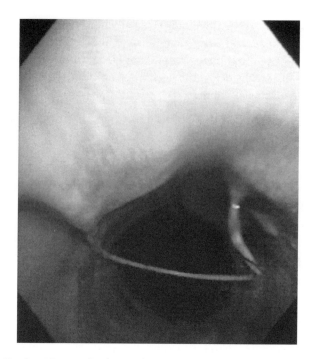

**Fig. 13.3.** Tracheal foreign body in a horse presented for chronic coughing after recovery from pneumonia. The tracheal wash catheter is suspected to have been sheared off into the tracheal lumen during withdrawal of the catheter, as the end of the catheter was embedded in submucusal tissues. The transtracheal wash catheter was removed endoscopically using biopsy forceps.

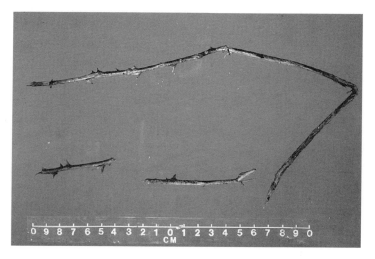

**Fig. 13.4.** Tracheobronchial foreign body (bramble) following removal via a distal cervical tracheotomy. The bramble broke into several fragments as it was retrieved.

## FURTHER READING

Brown, C.M., and Collier, M.A. 1983. Tracheobronchial foreign body in a horse. *J Am Vet Med Assoc* 182:280–281.

Caron, J.P., and Townsend, H.G.G. 1984. Tracheal perforation and widespread subcutaneouis emphysema in a horse. *Can Vet J* 25:339.

Carrig, C.B., Groenendyk, S., and Seawright, A.A. 1973. Dorsoventral flattening of the trachea in a horse and its attempted surgical correction: A case report. *J Am Vet Rad Soc* 14:32–36.

Delanty, D.D., and Georhi, J.R. 1954. A tracheal deformity in a pony. *J Am Vet Med Assoc* 125:42–44.

Freeman, D.E. 1991. Trachea. In *Equine Respiratory Disorders*. J. Beech, ed. Philadelphia: Lea & Febiger, pp 389–402.

Fubini, S.L., Todhunter, R.J., Vivrette, S.L., and Hackett, R.P. 1985. Tracheal rupture in two horses. *J Am Vet Med Assoc* 187:69–70.

Goulden, B.E. 1977. Some unusual cases of abnormal respiratory noises in the horse. *NZ Vet J* 25:389–390.

Honnas, C.M. 1999. Diseases of the trachea. In *Equine Medicine and Surgery*, 5th ed. P.T. Colahan, I.G. Mayhew, A.M. Merritt, and J.N. Moore, eds. St. Louis: Mosby, pp 522–526.

Lane, J.G. 1998. Disorders of the ear, nose and throat. In *Equine Medicine, Surgery and Reproduction*. T. Mair, S. Love, J. Schumacher, and E. Watson, eds. London: W.B. Saunders, pp 81–117.

Mair, T.S., and Lane, J.G. 1990. Tracheal obstructions in two horses and a donkey. *Vet Rec* 126:303–304.

Martin, J.E. 1981. Dorsoventral flattening of the trachea in a pony. *Equine Pract* 3:17–22.

Rakestraw, P.C. 2003. Permanent tracheostomy in standing horses. In *Current Therapy in Equine Medicine*, 5th ed. N.E. Robinson, ed. Philadelphia: W.B. Saunders, pp 396–398.

Robertson, J.T., and Spurlock, G.H. (1986) Tracheal reconstruction in a foal. *J Am Vet Med Assoc* 189:313–314.

Shappell, K.K. 1999. Trachea. In *Equine Surgery*, 2nd ed. J.A. Auer and J.A. Stick, eds. Philadelphia: W.B. Saunders, pp 376–381.

Shappell, K.K., Stick, J.A., Derksen, F.J., and Scott, E.A. 1988. Permanent tracheostomy in equidae: 47 cases (1981–1986) *J Am Vet Med Assoc* 192:939–942.

Tate, L.P., Koch, D.B., Sembrat, R.F., and Boles, C.L. 1981. Tracheal reconstruction by resection and end-to-end anastomosis in the horse. *J Am Vet Med Assoc* 178:253–258.

Tessier, G.J. 1996. Preitracheal abscess as the cause of tracheal compression and severe respiratory distress in a horse. *Equine Vet Educ* 8:127–130.

Urquhart, K.A., and Gerring, E.L. 1981. Tracheobronchial foreign body in a pony. *Equine Vet J* 13:262–264.

Yovich, J.V., and Stashak, T.S. 1984. Surgical repair of a collapsed trachea caused by a lipoma in a horse *Vet Surg* 13:217–218.

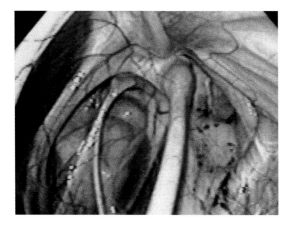

**Fig. 8.1.** Endoscopic view of melanosis of the left guttural pouch. Note the black discolored masses over the external carotid artery and the caudodorsal aspect of the lateral guttural pouch. The stylohyoid bone separates the lateral from medial compartments, and the internal carotid artery can be seen coursing through the caudal aspect of the medial guttural pouch.

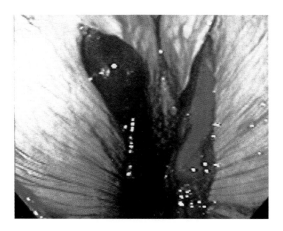

**Fig. 8.2B.** Endoscopic view of the guttural pouch openings in a horse with bilateral hemorrhage originating from the guttural pouch openings.

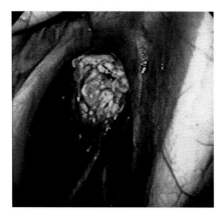
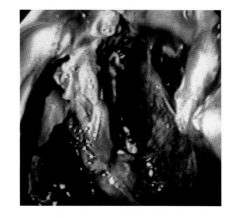

**Fig. 8.8.** Guttural pouch mycosis of the caudodorsal aspect of the medial compartment of the right guttural pouch over the internal carotid artery (left). Note the stylohyoid bone to the right of the mycotic plaque. The endoscopic image (right) demonstrates blood clots interspersed with the mycotic plaque from a horse with an extensive mycotic plaque involving the entire pouch.

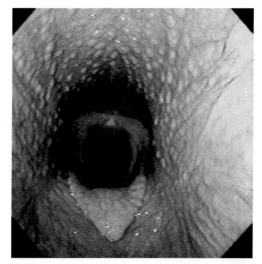

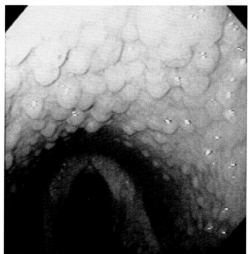

**Fig. 9.2.** Endoscopic view of the pharynx of two young horses with Grade II (top) and Grade III (bottom) lymphoid pharyngeal hyperplasia.

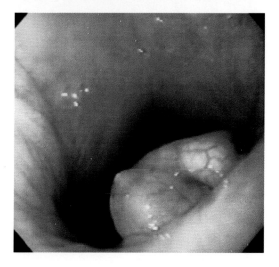

**Fig. 9.4.** Subepiglottic cyst in a 5-day-old foal presenting for dysphagia. The cyst was intermittently visible in the nasopharynx (as seen in this picture), and was primarily hidden under the soft palate in the oropharynx.

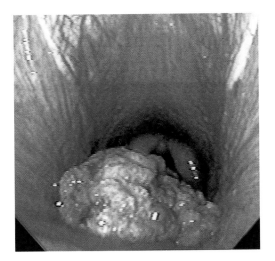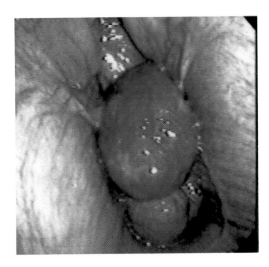

**Fig. 9.5.** Endoscopic views of a squamous cell carcinoma originating from the oral cavity partially obstructing the nasopharynx (left) and a giant cell tumor originating from the dorsal pharyngeal recess completely obstructing the nasopharynx (right). The giant cell tumor is viewed via retrograde examination through the tracheotomy incision. The slits on either side of the mass are the guttural pouch openings.

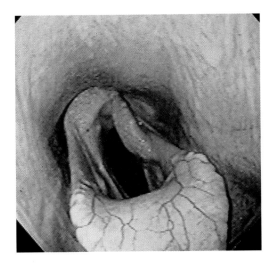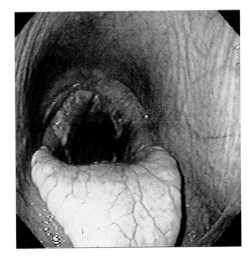

**Fig. 10.1.** Grade 4 left laryngeal hemiplegia prior to surgical correction (left) and after prosthetic laryngoplasty (right). Note the position of the left arytenoid at rest after surgical intervention.

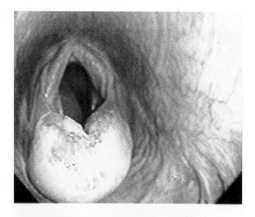

**Fig. 10.3.** Epiglottic entrapment by the aryepiglottic fold. The outline of the epiglottis is visible, but has lost its normal scalloped cartilage border, and superficial blood vessels are obscured by the entrapping mucosa.

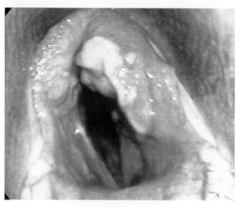

**Fig. 10.4.** Chondritis of the left arytenoid cartilage. Note the granulomatous, exudative, thickened appearance of the affected arytenoid cartilage.

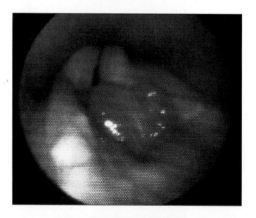

**Fig. 10.6.** Laryngeal lymphosarcoma. A neoplastic mass is obscuring the view of the aditus laryngis.

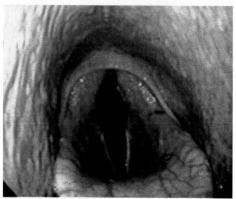

**Fig. 10.7.** Rostral displacement of the palatopharyngeal arch associated with fourth branchial arch defect. The caudal pillars of the soft palate form a hood that partly obscures the corniculate processes dorsally.

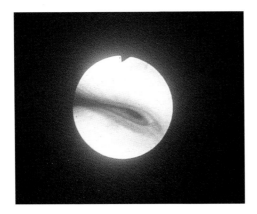

**Fig. 13.1.** Endoscopic view of dorsoventral tracheal collapse in a Shetland pony.

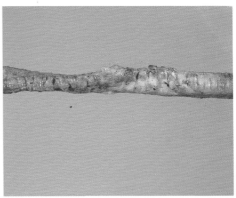

**Fig. 13.2.** Congenital tracheal deformity and stenosis.

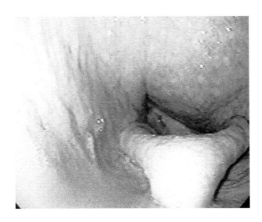

**Fig. 14.1.** Endoscopic view of the nasopharynx in a horse with a retropharyngeal abscess (*S. equi*). The arytenoids and tracheal opening are dorsally compressed and obstructed by the retropharyngeal mass. This image illustrates the source of upper airway obstruction in horses with strangles.

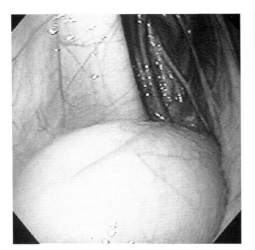

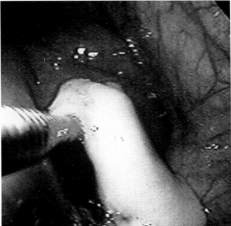

**Fig. 14.3.** Endoscopic examination of retropharyngeal abscesses projecting through the floor of the medial guttural pouch. Left: A large abscess with a thick wall that cannot be lanced via endoscopic manipulation. Right: Lancing of a mature abscess into the guttural pouch.

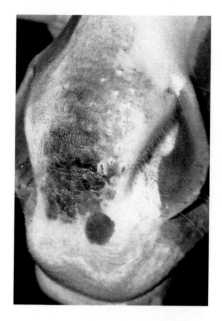

**Fig. 14.4.** The purple discoloration of the muzzle of this 8-year-old Quarter Horse gelding is characteristic of purpura hemorrhagic. When the muzzle is affected, it makes an ideal area for diagnostic skin biopsy.

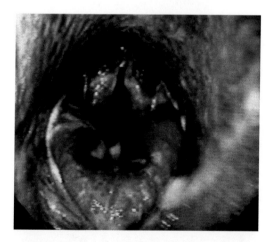

**Fig. 14.6.** Endoscopic view of the larynx and pharynx of a 7-year-old Quarter Horse mare with post-vaccinal purpura hemorrhagica. Note the pharyngeal edema and petechial/ecchymotic hemorrhages on the mucosal surface of the nasopharynx.

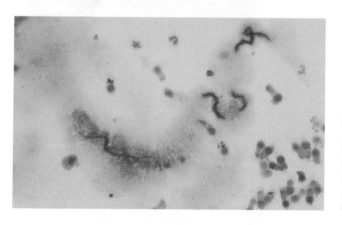

**Fig. 19.2.** Bronchoalveolar lavage cytology from a horse with heaves. Neutrophilic inflammation (76% total cell count) and excessive mucus are consistent with recurrent airway obstruction. Several Curshmann's spirals are odserved. Wright-Giemsa stain, original magnification 140x.

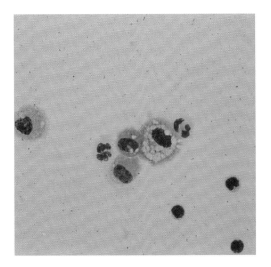

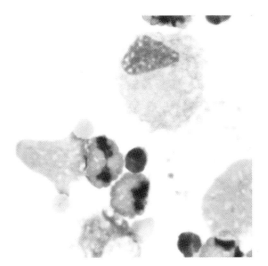

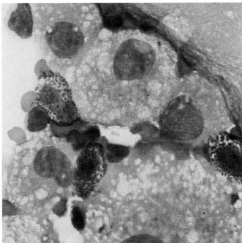

**Fig. 19.6.** Bronchoalveolar lavage cytology from horses with inflammatory airway disease, illustrating the three inflammatory cytologic profiles. Top left: Mixed inflammatory profile with 15% of total cell count neutrophils. Top right: Eosinophilic inflammation with 60% of total cell count eosinophils. Left: Metachromatic inflammation with 5% of total cell count mast cells. Note the cell inflammation. Wright-Giemsa stain, original magnification 168×.

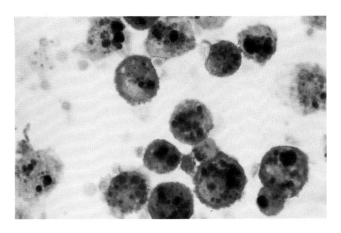

**Fig. 19.8.** Bronchoalveolar lavage cytology from a horse with exercise-induced pulmonary hemorrhage demonstrating hemosiderin-laden macrophages. Perl's Prussian Blue stain, original magnification 140x.

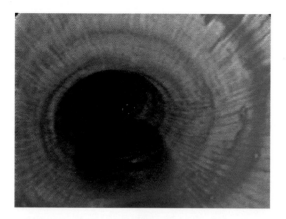

**Fig. 19.9.** Endoscopic examination of the trachea of a horse with exercise-induced pulmonary hemorrhage.

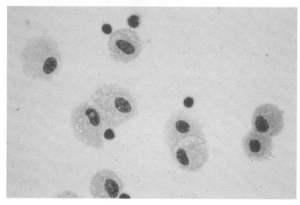

**Fig. 20.2.** Bronchoalveolar lavage cytology from a horse with normal respiratory function. The predominant cell types are macrophages and lymphocytes with neutrophils consisting of less than 5% of the total cell count. Macrophages appear uniform and nonactivated. Wright-Giemsa stain, original magnification 140×.

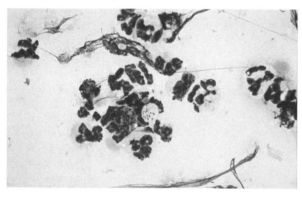

**Fig. 21.6.** Cytologic evaluation of a transtracheal aspirate from a foal with *Rhodococcus equi* pneumonia. Note the Gram-positive, pleomorphic rods within a macrophage. Gram stain, original magnification 40x.

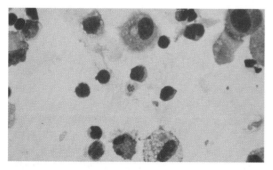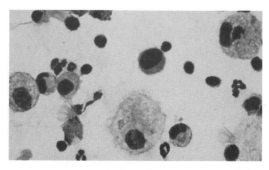

**Fig. 21.7.** Cytologic evaluation of bronchoalveolar lavage sample from a foal with *Pneumoncystis carinii* pneumonia. Note the extracellular (left) and intracellular (right) *Pneumoncystis* cysts. Wright-Giemsa stain.

# Contagious Respiratory Diseases

*Streptococcus equi var equi* is a beta-hemolytic, Gram-positive coccus that is responsible for the highly contagious disease referred to as strangles, distemper, and shipping fever. It is an obligate parasite (requires the horse for survival) and a primary pathogen (capable of primary invasion). Carrier animals are important for interepizootic maintenance and initiation of outbreaks on premises previously free of disease. Persistent nasal shedding for more than 6 months is rare, but the guttural pouch is the likely source in those cases.

Viral respiratory infections are common in horses, and the most notable viral pathogens are equine herpesvirus type 4 (EHV-4, rhinopneumonitis), equine influenza, and equine viral arteritis. The clinical signs of viral respiratory infections are similar, and include serous nasal discharge, fever, submandibular lymphadenopathy, anorexia and cough. In addition to respiratory disease, equine herpesvirus type 1 (EHV-1) can cause abortion and neurologic disease. Equine viral arteritis produces respiratory disease, vasculitis, and abortion. Equine herpesvirus type 2, rhinovirus, and reovirus are ubiquitous viral respiratory pathogens and are minimally pathogenic. Adenovirus pneumonia is most often documented in Arabian foals with severe combined immunodeficiency syndrome. Hendra virus is a newly recognized, zoonotic disease of horses in Australia. The disease is rapidly fatal in horses. Close contact is necessary for transmission to humans, and the virus may cause respiratory disease and encephalitis. African Horse Sickness is a rapidly fatal cardiopulmonary disease that has been eradicated from the United States and Europe.

# Strangles

14

Strangles is a common, highly contagious bacterial infection of the upper respiratory tract caused by *Streptococcus equi*:

- Rupture of the abscessed lymph nodes to the skin (especially submandibular absecsses) or internally to the pharynx or guttural pouches (retropharyngeal abscesses) is generally followed by rapid clinical recovery.
- Long-term asymptomatic carriers of *S. equi* are important sources of infection for susceptible horses.

## ETIOLOGY AND PATHOGENESIS

Strangles is caused by the Gram-positive, Lancefield group C, ß-haemolytic bacterium, *Streptococcus equi* subspecies *equi* (usually known as *Streptococcus equi*). This organism is not a normal inhabitant of the equine respiratory tract, and it acts as a primary pathogen causing a highly contagious respiratory disease. The organism has a worldwide distribution. There are at least two strains of the organism, which vary in pathogenicity. The typical strain is highly virulent, encapsulated, and produces honey-colored mucoid colonies on blood agar. The atypical, less virulent form develops a mat appearance within 24 hours of culture. The atypical form is frequently associated with a milder form of clinical disease ("atypical strangles"). However, other factors, including the immune status of the horse, are likely to be important in determining severity of disease, and some cases of the milder "atypical" strangles are associated with infection with the typical strain. The morbidity rate in outbreaks may reach 100%, but this is highly variable depending on the immune status of the population at risk. Infection occurs via the oral cavity or upper respiratory tract. The source of infection is usually infected discharges or contaminated equipment. The organism adheres to the epithelial cells of the buccal and nasal mucosa and rapidly spreads to the draining lymph nodes of the head and neck, including the submandibular, parotid, and retropharyngeal lymph nodes. The hyaluronic capsule and the M protein (a cell wall protein) both appear to be important features in determining the pathogenicity of the organism. In susceptible horses, the organism can survive in neutrophils following phagocytosis.

## EPIDEMIOLOGY

Chronic guttural pouch empyema and chondroid formation can follow strangles infection, and are a major cause of long-term carriage of S. equi.

The source of infection includes discharges from clinical cases, recovering cases and asymptomatic carriers of S. equi. Transmission can occur by direct horse-to-horse contact or indirectly. Indirect transmission includes contact with fomites (e.g., feed, water buckets, tack, etc.) and premises that have been contaminated with the organism. Human attendants can act as fomites, and the organism can be spread by flies. Although it is said that premises can harbor the infection for up to a year, the exact duration of survival of S. equi in the environment is uncertain. However, it is likely that the organism can survive for prolonged periods if protected from sunlight and disinfectants.

A significant number of horses continue to harbor S. equi after a full clinical recovery from strangles. These horses can excrete the organism in normal nasal secretions and can therefore act as an important source of infection for susceptible animals. Thus infection can be maintained within a herd after the apparent recovery of the last clinical case. In most horses, nasal shedding ceases within 4–6 weeks. Therefore, recovered horses should be considered potential sources of infection for at least 6 weeks after resolution of the purulent discharge.

Although S. equi is no longer detectable in the majority of horses 4–6 weeks after recovery, a small number of horses will maintain the infection for longer. These long-term asymptomatic carriers of S. equi are outwardly healthy, but they continue to excrete the organism and are an important source of infection in the general horse population. This is probably the most important means by which the organism is maintained between outbreaks of strangles. Many of these long-term asymptomatic carriers of S. equi have persistent guttural pouch infections with empyema or chondroids. Guttural pouch empyema can persist for months or years with no overt signs of disease in the affected horse. Identification and treatment of these horses is an important aspect of the control of outbreaks and prevention of strangles in the general horse population.

### Clinical signs
Clinical signs of strangles include the following:

- Pyrexia, bilateral purulent nasal discharge, and lymphadenopathy affecting the lymph nodes of the head are common.
- Abscessation and rupture of affected lymph nodes also is common.
- Pharyngeal compression can cause dyspnea and dysphagia.

Strangles can occur in horses of any age, but is most common in animals between 1 and 5 years old. The incubation period of the disease is 3–14 days, dependent on the immune status of the horse and the infective dose of the bacteria.

The clinical signs are quite variable, depending on the strain of the organism, and the age, immune status, and history of previous infection of the horse. The initial clinical signs include pyrexia (up to 40°C), depression, anorexia, and serous nasal discharge. The nasal discharge rapidly becomes mucopurulent, and then purulent; the submandibular and parotid lymph nodes become enlarged, firm, and painful. Over the next few days, abscesses develop within some or all of the infected lymph nodes. Neck pain may be apparent, and the affected horse may stand with the head and neck outstretched. Distension of the retropharyngeal lymph nodes may cause compression of the nasopharynx, resulting in dyspnea (hence the name "strangles") and/or dysphagia (Fig. 14.1). In a small number of cases, upper airway obstruction may become severe and life-threatening (Fig. 14.2).

Around 1–2 weeks after the initial signs, the abscessed lymph nodes start to fluctuate and then develop sinuses and rupture. The submandibular and paro-

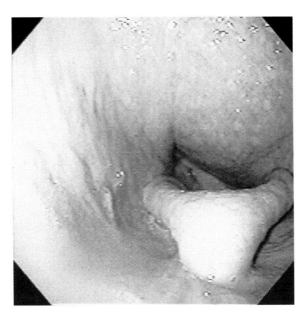

**Fig. 14.1.** Endoscopic view of the nasopharynx in a horse with a retropharyngeal abscess (*S. equi*). The arytenoids and tracheal opening are dorsally compressed and obstructed by the retropharyngeal mass. This image illustrates the source of upper airway obstruction in horses with strangles. *(See also color section.)*

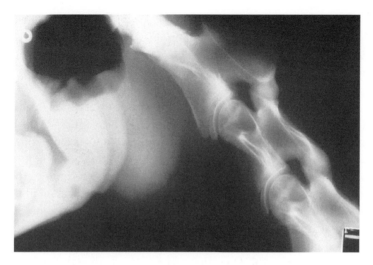

**Fig. 14.2.** Lateral radiographic projection of the guttural pouch and pharynx in a horse with a retropharyngeal abscess (*S. equi*). The abscess projects through the ventral aspect of the guttural pouch and dorsally compresses the larynx and pharynx, obstructing the upper airway.

tid lymph node abscesses usually rupture through the skin in the intermandibular space or parotid region. The retropharyngeal lymph node abscesses typically rupture into the pharynx or guttural pouch (Fig. 14.3). Once rupture of the lymph node abscesses has occurred, the affected horse usually shows rapid clinical improvement and unremarkable recovery. Drainage of the abscesses and the nasal discharge slowly reduce over a period of 3–7 days, followed by healing of the skin. The duration of the clinical syndrome can vary from less than a week in very mild cases, to more than 2 months. Mortality rates of 8–10% have been reported; however, the mortality rate in most outbreaks of well-managed animals is usually much lower.

Other clinical signs that may be observed during the acute stage of the disease include conjunctivitis and purulent ocular discharge, periorbital abscesses and eyelid swelling, agalactia in lactating mares, myocarditis, and aspiration pneumonia. Guttural pouch empyema may develop as a result of rupture of a retropharyngeal lymph node abscess through the wall of the guttural pouch. This may result in the persistence of a nasal discharge after other signs of the disease have regressed. However, some horses may develop chronic empyema of the guttural pouch with few or no overt clinical signs. Inspissation of exudate in the guttural pouch in horses with chronic empyema results in the formation of chondroid material.

The atypical form of strangles is characterized by a milder clinical disease. Lymphadenopathy and abscesses may not develop, and the clinical picture may resemble a mild upper respiratory viral infection.

## Complications and sequela
Complications of strangles occur in approximately 20% of cases:

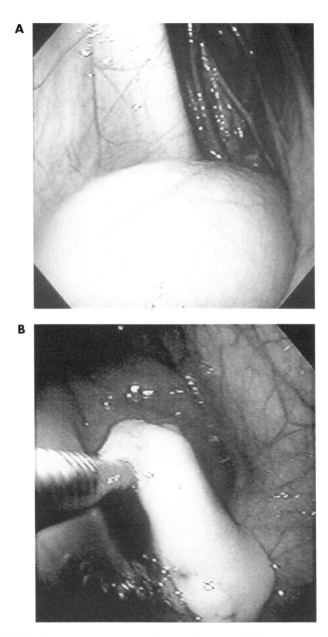

**Fig. 14.3.** Endoscopic examination of retropharyngeal abscesses projecting through the floor of the medial guttural pouch. A. A large abscess with a thick wall that cannot be lanced via endoscopic manipulation B. Lancing of a mature abscess into the guttural pouch. *(See also color section.)*

- Metastatic spread of *S. equi* ("bastard strangles") may result in abscesses elsewhere in the body, most commonly the lungs, mesentery, liver, spleen, kidney, brain, and other lymph nodes.
- Purpura hemorrhagica is a rare, immune-mediated vasculitis observed subsequent to exposure to *S. equi* antigen via natural exposure or vaccination.

The most common complication is bastard strangles, metastatic spread of the infection to lymph nodes and organs other than the nodes of the head. A wide range of organs and lymph nodes may become infected, and the clinical signs will vary depending on the site of infection. The most common sites of metastatic lymph node infection are the cervical, tracheobronchial, prescapular, mediastinal, and mesenteric lymph nodes. Abscess formation can also occur in the lungs, mesentery, liver, spleen, kidney, brain, spinal cord, vertebrae, joints, tendon sheaths, and endocardium. Cutaneous abscesses may develop in the periorbital, perianal, facial, and inguinal areas. Horses with internal abscesses may present with a history of intermittent colic, recurrent pyrexia, inappetence, depression, and weight loss.

Predisposing factors for the development of bastard strangles are uncertain. It has been suggested that inadequate penicillin treatment during the acute stage of strangles may predispose to metastatic spread by virtue of moderation of the immune response. However, there is no conclusive evidence to support this theory, and cases of bastard strangles arise whether or not antibiotic therapy is used.

Purpura hemorrhagica is an immune-mediated vasculitis that can be a serious and life-threatening complication. Purpura hemorrhagica can arise after other respiratory diseases, and is not restricted to cases of strangles. However, it appears to be most common after *S. equi* infection. It is usually seen in older horses and may follow a second natural infection with *S. equi* or following vaccination. The onset of purpura hemorrhagica is usually 2–4 weeks after the respiratory infection. The disease causes an aseptic necrotizing leucocytoclastic vasculitis, and has been associated with precipitation of heavy chain IgA immune complexes in blood vessels. Horses with purpura hemorrhagica have high serum IgA titers to both the M-like protein and other supernatant proteins of *S. equi*.

Clinical signs of purpura hemorrhagica include urticaria, followed by well-demarcated subcutaneous edema of the limbs, ventrum, and head (Fig. 14.4). Edema can progress to exudation, ulceration, crusting, and sloughing of the skin (Fig. 14.5). The mucous membranes show petechiation and ecchymotic hemorrhages (Fig. 14.6). Vasculitis may also affect the muscles, heart, gastrointestinal tract, kidneys, and lungs. Death occurs in severe cases due to circulatory collapse, gastrointestinal disorders, or renal failure.

Other reported complications of strangles include retropharyngeal abscesses, laryngeal hemiplegia, tracheal compression due to mediastinal abscessation, septicemia, and necrotic bronchopneumonia.

## Diagnosis

A presumptive diagnosis of strangles is often determined on the basis of typical clinical signs. Definitive diagnosis requires isolation of *S. equi* via bacterial cultures of respiratory secretions or abscess fluid. Direct smears of exudate may reveal chains of Gram-positive cocci. Appropriate samples for culture include purulent exudates aspirated from lymph nodes and swabs from discharging abscesses. Swabs from the nasal cavity or nasopharynx are used to

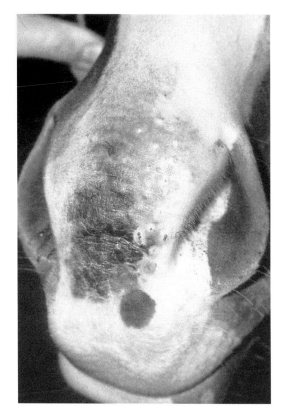

**Fig. 14.4.** The discoloration of the muzzle of this 8-year-old Quarter Horse gelding is characteristic of purpura hemorrhagic. When the muzzle is affected, it makes an ideal area for diagnostic skin biopsy. *(See also color section.)*

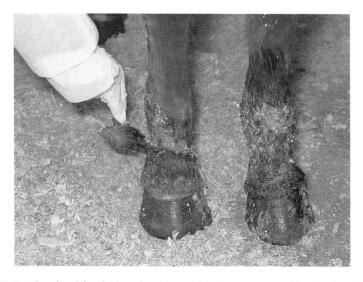

**Fig. 14.5.** The distal forelimbs of a 2-year-old Quarter Horse filly that has sloughed the skin due to severe purpura hemorrhagica. The depth of the defect was sufficient to expose the fetlock joint capsule on the lateral aspect of the left forelimb.

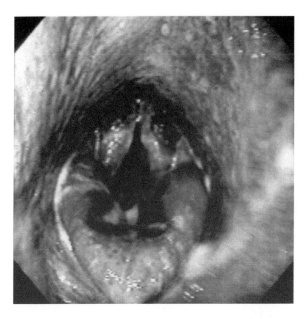

**Fig. 14.6.** Endoscopic view of the larynx and pharynx of a 7-year-old Quarter Horse mare with post-vaccinal purpura hemorrhagica. Note the pharyngeal edema and petechial/ecchymotic hemorrhages on the mucosal surface of the nasopharynx. *(See also color section.)*

identify atypical cases and chronic carriers. The positive culture rate for such samples is probably no better than 50%, and care must be taken in the interpretation of negative results. The background bacterial flora of the nasal cavity and nasopharynx is complex, and *S. equi* may easily become masked by other bacteria in cultures. Likewise, secondary infection of abscesses rapidly occurs, and these other bacteria may overgrow *S. equi*. For these reasons, it is appropriate to assume that "if it looks like strangles, then it probably is strangles." A polymerase chain reaction (PCR) test has recently been developed and can be used in conjunction with standard culture techniques to improve the sensitivity of detection of *S. equi*.

Confirmation of the diagnosis by bacterial culture is difficult in cases where there is no readily available source of exudate. Percutaneous needle aspiration of retropharyngeal abscesses may be possible using ultrasound guidance. Inspissated chondroid material may be present in cases of chronic guttural pouch empyema without nasal discharge. In such cases, lavage of the affected pouch may be performed through an endoscope, and an aspirate submitted for culture.

The diagnosis of internal abscesses may be aided by rectal palpation, thoracic radiography, thoracocentesis, abdominocentesis, and diagnostic ultrasonography, depending on the site of abscessation. A firm diagnosis can be difficult to achieve, and internal abscesses can be difficult to distinguish from neoplasia and other causes of recurrent colic and weight loss. Both abdominal abscesses and neoplasia can result in similar changes to the peritoneal fluid (leucocytosis and increased total protein concentration) and hematological examination may show anemia, leucocytosis, neutrophilia, and hyperfibrinogenemia. Exploratory laparotomy or laparoscopy may be required to confirm the presence of an abdominal abscess.

Purpura hemorrhagica is generally diagnosed on the basis of the typical clinical signs. Vasculitis may be confirmed by biopsy of affected areas of skin or mucosa, and immunohistological techniques can be used to demonstrate immune complex deposition.

### Treatment

In most cases, symptomatic treatment and nursing care are all that is required. The affected animals should be kept in a clean, dry environment and offered soft and palatable feed. Abscesses are encouraged to mature and rupture by use of poultices and hot packs. Surgical lancing of submandibular abscesses can be performed, but only when the abscess is mature (Fig. 14.7).

Once the abscesses have ruptured, lavage with 3–5% povidone-iodine solution will facilitate resolution of discharge. Nonsteroidal anti-inflammatory drugs, especially phenylbutazone (4.4 mg/kg/day) or flunixin meglumine (1.1 mg/kg/day), are helpful to reduce pain, pyrexia, and inflammation, and to improve the overall demeanor. These drugs should be used cautiously in dysphagic horses that may develop dehydration.

In horses that are dysphagic or unwilling to eat, enteral feeding via nasogastric intubation should be provided, and particular attention should be paid to maintaining adequate hydration. Temporary tracheotomy may be necessary in horses with severe dyspnea due to upper airway obstruction.

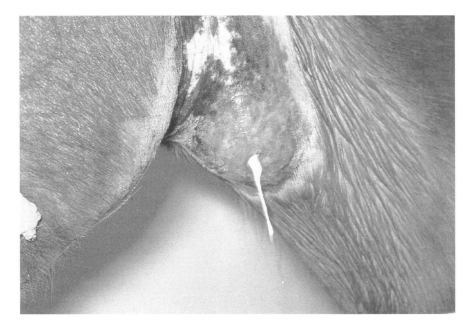

**Fig. 14.7.** Purulent exudate draining from a subcutaneous abscess (*S. equi*) that has been lanced to facilitate rapid resolution of disease.

The use of antibiotics in the treatment of uncomplicated strangles cases is controversial. The organism is susceptible to a wide range of commonly used antibacterial drugs. Although it has been suggested that antibiotic treatment may increase the risk of bastard strangles, there is no supportive evidence. However, in the majority of cases, antibiotics appear to offer little benefit in the treatment, and should probably be avoided once lymph node swelling and abscess formation has begun. Antibiotic usage at this stage of the disease will probably slow maturation of abscesses and prolong the course of the disease.

Some clinicians advocate the use of antibiotics, usually penicillin, in the early stages of infection, prior to the development of lymphadenopathy. It is proposed that antibiotics can arrest the development of the disease when used at this stage. This may instil a false sense of security that the animal is not infected, not contagious, and will not develop typical disease. Unfortunately, many horses treated in this manner will subsequently develop strangles when antibiotic therapy is discontinued, either because the infection has not been completely eliminated, or due to reinfection from the environment. Treatment in the very early stages will prevent development of a protective immune response and the horse remains susceptible to reinfection.

Prophylactic antibiotic treatment for horses exposed to strangles, but not yet demonstrating clinical signs of infection, has also been proposed. While this treatment is likely to prevent infection from becoming established in the treated horses, those horses will remain susceptible to infection when antibiotic therapy is discontinued.

Treatment with antimicrobials is indicated in horses with severe disease and horses with complications. Procaine penicillin (22000 IU/kg im q12 hours) is the antibiotic of choice, although ceftiofur (5 mg/kg im q12 hours) and potentiated sulphonamides (15 mg/kg po q12 hours) may be effective.

Treatment of bastard strangles involves drainage of abscesses, when possible, and prolonged antibiotic therapy. Additional treatments are used as indicated by the individual case. Treatment of purpura hemorrhagica should be early and aggressive. Corticosteroids are administered for their anti-inflammatory and immunosuppressive effects. Systemic dexamethasone (0.04–0.16 mg/kg iv or im q24 hours) is most effective. Treatment is continued at the clinical response dose for 2–3 days, and then reduced over 7–14 days. Corticosteroid treatment may be switched from dexamethasone to oral prednisolone (1 mg/kg q24 hours) after a clinical response is achieved. Concurrent treatment with antibiotics (penicillin) is recommended, although there is a theoretical worry that this might promote bacterial cell death and increase the quantities of circulating M-protein available for immune complex formation. Hydrotherapy, leg wraps, and gentle exercise are also helpful for decreasing limb edema.

Appropriate treatment of guttural pouch empyema depends on the consistency and nature of the material within the pouch. The general principles of treatment of guttural pouch empyema are described in Section II, "Noncontagious Diseases of the Upper Respiratory Tract."

## Control of an outbreak

Control measures that are implemented will vary from outbreak to outbreak, and need to be fashioned to the individual circumstances and requirements of the horse owners. In general, there are four separate areas where control measures need to be considered. The objectives of these control measures are

1. Prevent spread of infection to new premises.
2. Prevent infection of new arrivals to the infected premises.
3. Control of the outbreak within the infected premises.
4. Ensure that all horses are free of infection at the end of the outbreak.

Movements of horses onto and off the premises should cease in order to prevent spread of infection to other premises and to prevent infection in new arrivals.

The extent of any control measures that are implemented within the affected premises needs careful consideration. Some clinicians advocate minimum control measures, and suggest that it is preferable to allow the infection to spread among all susceptible horses to build natural immunity. Alternatively, strict isolation and testing procedures can be instituted in an attempt to minimize the spread of *S. equi* within the herd. Isolation areas should be established to house infectious horses and to segregate them from uninfected horses. The "dirty" areas should be physically separated from "clean" areas. If possible, horses in the "dirty" areas are cared for by dedicated staff who do not access "clean" areas. Strict hygiene measures should be introduced, including provision of dedicated equipment and clothing for each area and thorough disinfection and cleaning of stables. All horses demonstrating clinical signs of strangles are isolated within the "dirty" areas. All recovered cases and contacts are subject to at least 3 nasopharyngeal swabs or guttural pouch lavage sampling at weekly intervals for bacterial culture and PCR for *S. equi* to identify asymptomatic carriers. All horses testing positive for *S. equi* are maintained in the "dirty" areas. All recovered cases and other horses that tested positive for *S. equi* should have at least three negative swabs and PCR results before they are returned to the "clean" areas. Such intensive control measures require the dedication and patience of the horses' owners, and it needs to be established at the outset that owners are prepared for the time and cost involved with these procedures.

## Prevention

In order to prevent the introduction of strangles into a herd by virtue of asymptomatic carriers of *S. equi*, all new arrivals should be placed in quarantine and screened for *S. equi* by bacterial cultures of 3 repeated nasopharyngeal swabs or guttural pouch lavages. Any horse that tests positive should remain in quarantine and be investigated for guttural pouch disease. Treatment should be carried out until they test negative for the organism (on three separate occasions).

Several vaccines against strangles are available, but none of them guarantee prevention of infection. The protective immunity afforded by current vaccines is generally poor and short-lived. Both local and systemic reactions appear to be common following vaccination. A live intranasal vaccine is currently available in North America. This type of vaccine should provide better immunity at the mucosal surface (the site of infection) than systemically administered vaccines. The attenuated strain is not temperature-sensitive (inactivated by core body temperature), like the intranasal influenza vaccine. Complications reported with this vaccine include *Strep equi* abscesses at subsequent intramuscular injection sites (live culture on hands), submandibular lymphadenopathy, serous nasal discharge, and purpura hemorrhagica. The veterinarian is encouraged to administer all intramuscular vaccines prior to administration of the intranasal vaccine on a single premise.

## FURTHER READING

Galan, J.E., and Timoney, J.F. 1985. Immune complexes in purpura hemorrhagica of the horse contain IgA and M antigen of *Streptococcus equi*. *J Immunol* 135:3134–3137.

Newton, J.R., Verheyen, HK., Talbot, N.C., Timoney, J.F., Wood, J.L., Lakhani, K.H., and Chanter, N. 2000. Control of strangles outbreaks by isolation of guttural pouch carriers identified using PCR and culture of *Streptococcus equi*. *Equine Vet J* 32:515–526.

Newton, J.R., Wood, J.L.N., and Chanter, N. 1996. Strangles: Long-term carriage of *Streptococcus equi* in horses. *Equine Vet Educ* 9:98–102.

Newton, R., and Chanter, N. 2003. Strangles. In *Current Therapy in Equine Medicine*, 5th ed. N.E. Robinson, ed. Philadelphia: W.B. Saunders, pp 64–68.

Sweeney, C. 1996. Strangles: *Streptococcus equi* infection in horses. *Equine Vet Educ* 8:317–322.

Sweeney, C.R., Whitlock, R.H., Meirs, D.A., Whitehead, S.C., and Barningham, S.O. 1987. Complications associated with *Streptococcus equi* infection on a horse farm. *J Am Vet Med Assoc* 191:1146–1148.

Timoney, J.F. 1993. Strangles. *Vet Clinics N Am Equine Pract* 9:365–374.

Verheyen, K., Newton, J.R., Talbot, N.C., de Brauwere, M.V., and Chanter, N. 2000. Elimination of guttural pouch infection and inflammation in asymptomatic carriers of *Streptococcus equi*. *Equine Vet J* 32:527–532.

# Equine Herpesvirus (Rhinopneumonitis)

Equine herpesvirus 1 (EHV-1) and 4 (EHV-4) comprise two antigenically distinct groups of viruses, and both are ubiquitous in horse populations worldwide. The natural reservoir of both EHV-1 and EHV-4 is the horse. Latent infections and carrier states occur with both viral types. Transmission occurs by direct or indirect contact with infectious nasal secretions. The equine herpesviruses are slightly more stable than equine influenza in the environment, and limited fomite transmission is possible. EHV-4 produces respiratory disease, and EHV-1 is primarily responsible for herpesvirus abortion and herpes myeloencephalitis.

## EQUINE HERPESVIRUS 4 (EHV-4)

Equine herpesvirus 4 produces an acute, febrile respiratory disease in young horses characterized by rhinopharyngitis and tracheobronchitis:

- Viral replication of EHV-4 is limited to the respiratory tract.
- Typical clinical signs include fever, serous nasal discharge, pharyngitis, cough, inappetence, and/or submandibular lymphadenopathy.

Outbreaks of respiratory disease occur annually among weanling foals in areas with concentrated horse populations. The severity of disease in individual horses is determined by viral strain, immune status, and age. Viral replication with EHV-4 infection is restricted to respiratory tract epithelium and associated lymph nodes; therefore, infection of pregnant mares with EHV-4 rarely results in abortion.

The incubation period is 2–10 days, and susceptible horses develop fever

(102–106°F) neutropenia, lymphopenia, serous nasal discharge, malaise, pharyngitis, cough, inappetence, and/or submandibular lymphadenopathy. Secondary bacterial infections are common and manifest with mucopurulent nasal exudates, tracheitis, bronchitis, and pneumonia. The infection is mild or inapparent in horses immunologically sensitized to the virus.

Gross lesions of viral rhinopneumonitis are hyperemia and ulceration of the respiratory epithelium, and multiple, plum-colored foci (< 2 mm) in the lungs. Histologically, there is evidence of inflammation, necrosis, and intranuclear inclusions in the respiratory epithelium and germinal centers' respiratory-associated lymphoid tissue. Pulmonary lesions are characterized by neutrophilic inflammation of the terminal bronchioles, peribronchiolar and perivascular mononuclear cell infiltration, and serofibrinous exudate in the alveoli.

## EQUINE HERPESVIRUS 1 (EHV-1)

EHV-1 strains are endotheliotrophic, with a particular predilection for vascular endothelium of the nasal mucosa, lungs, adrenal glands, thyroid, placenta, and central nervous system:

- Cell-associated viremia allows EHV-1 to access other body systems.
- Endotheliotrophism accounts for the clinical syndromes of abortion and equine herpesvirus encephalomyelitis.

EHV-1 gains access to peripheral tissues via cell-associated viremia. Horses infected with EHV-1 strains often develop a diphasic fever, with cell-associated viremia coinciding with the second temperature peak. Clinical manifestations of systemic EHV-1 infection are abortion and ascending myelitis.

Abortion occurs 2–12 weeks after infection, usually between the seventh and eleventh month of gestation. Aborted fetuses are fresh or minimally autolyzed, and the placenta is expelled shortly after abortion. Mares that abort after infection with EHV-1 seldom display premonitory signs. There is no evidence of damage to the mare's reproductive tract, and subsequent conception is unimpaired. Abortions may be sporadic, isolated events or may be observed as an abortion storm within a herd.

Mares exposed to EHV-1 late in gestation may not abort, but give birth to live foals with fulminating viral pneumonitis, icterus (hepatitis), and marked neutropenia (bone marrow destruction). Neonatally, EHV-infected foals are susceptible to secondary bacterial infections and usually die within hours or days.

Outbreaks with specific strains of EHV-1 infection result in neurologic disease. Clinical signs vary from mild incoordination and posterior paresis to severe posterior paralysis with recumbency, loss of bladder and tail function, and loss of sensation to the skin in the perineal and inguinal areas. In exceptional cases, the paralysis may be progressive and culminate in quadriplegia and death. Prognosis depends on severity of signs and the period of recumbency. Neurologic disease associated with EHV-1 is thought to occur more commonly in mares after abortion storms, but has been reported in barren mares, stallions, geldings, and foals after an outbreak of EHV-1 respiratory infection.

Typical gross fetal lesions associated with EHV-1 abortion include interlobular pulmonary edema, pleural effusion, necrosis of lymphoreticular tissue (liver, bone marrow, thymus), and petechiation of the myocardium, adrenal gland, and spleen. Intranuclear inclusions are found in lung, liver, and adrenal gland via routine histopathology or immunohistochemistry.

Horses with EHV-1–associated neurologic disease may have no gross lesions, or only minimal evidence of hemorrhage in the meninges, brain, and spinal cord parenchyma. Histological lesions are discrete lymphocytic vasculitis with endothelial cell damage and perivascular cuffing, thrombus formation, and hemorrhage, and in advanced cases, areas of malacia. Lesions are most common in the spinal cord, but may occur in the brain and brain stem.

## Diagnosis

Equine viral rhinopneumonitis cannot be differentiated from equine influenza or other common equine respiratory infections solely on the basis of clinical signs. Serologic testing (neutralizing antibody) of acute and convalescent sera will demonstrate a fourfold rise in antibody titer in horses with recent infection. However, diagnosis of equine herpesvirus infections by serology is difficult because many healthy horses have circulating antibody against EHV-1 and EHV-4 (latent infection, subclinical infection, vaccination). Abortion and neurologic disease may occur after the viremic phase; therefore, the fourfold rise in antibody titer may have occurred prior to clinical signs of disease.

Definitive diagnosis is determined by virus isolation from samples obtained via nasopharyngeal swab and citrated blood sample (buffy coat) early in the course of infection. Nasopharyngeal swabs should be placed in virus transport medium and transported (4°C) to the laboratory within 24 hours. Blood in the sample will destroy the virus. In cases of suspect EHV-1 abortion, diagnosis is based on characteristic gross and microscopic lesions in the aborted fetus, virus isolation, and demonstration of viral antigen in fetal tissues (PCR or immunohistochemistry). Lung, liver, adrenal, and lymphoreticular tissues are productive sources of virus. Serologic testing of aborted mares has little diagnostic value.

Diagnosis of herpesvirus myeloencephalopathy depends on demonstration of characteristic vascular lesions in sections of CNS tissue of horses that do not survive. Alternatively, the diagnosis is presumptive, based on clinical signs (urinary incontinence, poor tail tone) and cerebrospinal fluid analysis (xanthochromia, albuminocytologic dissociation).

## Treatment

There is no specific treatment for EHV infection. Rest and nursing care are indicated to minimize secondary bacterial complications. Affected horses should be offered high-quality, palatable feeds and placed in a warm and dry environment. Antipyretics are recommended for horses with a fever >104°F; however, nonjudicial use of NSAIDs may mask the clinical signs of secondary bacterial infection. Antibiotic therapy is instituted if clinical signs of secondary bacterial infection become evident, including purulent nasal discharge or pulmonary disease. Most foals infected prenatally with EHV-1 succumb shortly after birth despite intensive care. The antiviral drug, acyclovir, has been used with limited success in the treatment of neonatal herpes infection. If horses with EHV-1–associated neurologic disease remain ambulatory, or become recumbent for less than 2–3 days, the prognosis is usually favorable. Intensive nursing care is necessary to avoid traumatic injury, ruptured bladder, or bowel atony. Recovery may be complete, but a small percentage of cases have permanent, neurologic sequelae. Affected horses that remain recumbent for longer than 2–3 days generally have a very poor prognosis.

## Prevention

Control of herpesvirus disease is difficult because latent infections and inapparent carriers are common in adult horses, herpesvirus can evade the immune system and infect horses that are appropriately vaccinated, convalescing horses shed infective virus for 2–3 weeks after recovery of clinical signs, and the virus is more stable in the environment than influenza and can be spread by fomites. Little cross-protection occurs between EHV-1 and EHV-4 after primary infection of immunologically naive foals; however, significant cross-protection develops in adult horses after repeated infections with a particular viral type. Most horses are latently infected with EHV-1 and EHV-4, with the potential for recrudescence of disease or shedding of infectious virus with stress or immunosuppression. Immunity to reinfection of the respiratory tract persists for only 3 months, but multiple infections induce sufficient immunity to prevent clinical signs of respiratory disease. Diminished resistance in pregnant mares facilitates cell-associated viremia, which may result in transplacental infection of the fetus.

For prevention and control of EHV-4– and EHV-1–related diseases, management practices to reduce viral spread are recommended. Newly introduced horses are isolated for 3–4 weeks prior to commingling with resident horses, particularly pregnant mares. Management-related stress-inducing circumstances should be avoided to prevent recrudescence of latency. Pregnant mares should be maintained in a group away from weanlings, yearlings, and frequently transported horses. In an outbreak of respiratory disease or abortion, affected horses should be isolated and appropriate measures taken for disinfection of contaminated premises. No horse should leave the premises for 3 weeks after recovery of the last clinical case.

Parenterally administered modified live vaccines are licensed in some countries but banned in others. An inactivated vaccine is the only product currently recommended by the manufacturer for prevention of EHV-1 abortion. Vaccine should be administered during months 3, 5, 7, and 9 of pregnancy. Humoral immunity induced by vaccination against EHV-1 and EHV-4 generally persists for 2–4 months. Antigenic variation within each virus type means that available vaccines do not cover all strains to which horses can be exposed. In particular, the neurotrophic strain of EHV-1 appears particularly unresponsive to vaccination. Vaccination should begin when foals are 8–9 months old and, depending on the vaccine used, a second dose given 4–8 weeks later. Booster vaccinations may be indicated as often as every 3–6 months through maturity. Vaccination programs against EHV-1 are not limited to pregnant mares, but should include all horses on the premises.

## EQUINE HERPESVIRUS 2 (EHV-2)

Equine herpesvirus 2 (EHV-2, cytomegalovirus) is ubiquitously found in normal horses of all ages and is localized in respiratory mucosa, conjunctiva, and white blood cells. The pathogenic significance remains obscure. It has been suggested that EHV-2 is the cause of herpetic keratoconjunctivitis and contributes to pharyngeal lymphoid hyperplasia in young horses.

# Equine Influenza

**16**

Equine influenza is highly contagious and spreads rapidly by direct contact. Infection predisposes horses to secondary bacterial infection by disruption of the mucociliary blanket. Rest (a minimum of 3 weeks) and supportive care constitute the most important treatment principles for equine influenza. Equine influenza is the most economically important contagious respiratory disease of horses. It is classified as an orthomyxovirus (RNA virus) and has two characteristic envelope antigens ("spikes"), neuraminidase and hemagglutinin, which are important for virulence, protective immunity, and virus classification. Virus attaches to epithelial cells via hemagglutinin spikes and enters cells via endocytosis. Virus damages epithelial cells in the respiratory tree resulting in desquamation and focal erosion of the respiratory epithelium, interruption of the protective mucociliary blanket, and impairment of clearance mechanisms. Unlike equine herpesvirus, replication is limited to the respiratory tract, and viremia does not occur.

Equine influenza is highly contagious and rapidly spread among susceptible horses by direct contact. Two immunologically distinct influenza viruses have been found in horse populations worldwide except in Australia and New Zealand. Orthomyxovirus A/Equi-1 has not been isolated since 1980. Orthomyxovirus A/Equi-2 was first recognized in 1963 as a cause of widespread epidemics, and has subsequently become endemic in many countries. Unlike EHV, a carrier state is not recognized for equine influenza.

Clinical disease may vary from a mild, inapparent infection to severe disease in susceptible animals (high morbidity, low mortality). Influenza is rarely fatal except in donkeys, zebras, and debilitated horses. Epidemics arise when one or more acutely infected horses are introduced into a susceptible group assembled for show, sale, training, or racing. Antigenic drift (gradual alteration in HA and NA antigens due to random mutation) is observed with specific strains of

177

A/Equi-2 virus in some parts of the world, and may be due to frequent natural exposure or regular vaccination. Transmission occurs by inhalation of infectious respiratory secretions (direct horse-to-horse transmission), and infectious virus is stable in aerosols over distances of 35 yards or more. Convalescent horses continue viral shedding for up to 10 days. Subclinical viral shedding is possible, but latent infections do not occur. Strenuous exercise increases susceptibility to influenza, due to alteration of the immune system.

The incubation period of influenza is approximately 1–3 days. Clinical signs begin abruptly and include high fever (up to 106°F), serous nasal discharge, submandibular lymphadenopathy, and coughing. Depression, anorexia, and weakness are frequently observed. Clinical signs usually last <3 days in uncomplicated cases. Coughing induced by influenza is dry, harsh, and nonproductive, and is a significant feature of this disease. Influenza replicates within respiratory epithelial cells, resulting in destruction of tracheal and bronchial epithelium (and mucociliary apparatus). A cough develops early in the course of infection and may be inducible by tracheal palpation for several weeks. Nasal discharge, although scant and serous initially, may become mucopurulent due to secondary bacterial infection. Mildly affected horses recover uneventfully in 2–3 weeks; severely affected horses may convalesce for up to 6 months. Recovery is hastened by complete restriction of strenuous physical activity. Respiratory tract epithelium takes longer to regenerate (approximately 21 days) than clinical signs take to abate. During this time, horses are susceptible to development of secondary bacterial complications, such as pneumonia, pleuropneumonia, and chronic bronchitis. Uncommon complications of influenza infection include vasculitis, myositis, and myocarditis.

## DIAGNOSIS AND TREATMENT

The presence of a rapidly spreading respiratory infection in a group of horses characterized by rapid onset, high fever, depression, and cough is presumptive evidence of equine influenza. Definitive diagnosis of influenza can be determined by virus isolation, influenza A antigen detection, or paired serology (hemagglutination inhibition). Nasopharyngeal swabs are obtained for virus isolation and antigen detection. These samples should be obtained as soon as possible after the onset of illness. Virus isolation in chick embryos is highly specific, but less sensitive for detection of influenza due to bacterial contamination of the sample. Antigen detection is performed using a human influenza A kit, which provides immediate horse-side results that are not affected by bacterial contamination.

Nonsteroidal anti-inflammatory drugs provide antipyretic and anti-inflammatory activity for horses with a fever of >104°F. Antibiotics are indicated when fever persists beyond 3–4 days or when purulent nasal discharge or pneumonia are present. Complications are minimized by restricting exercise, controlling dust, providing appropriate ventilation, and practicing good stable hygiene. Horses require rest and supportive care during the convalescent period. Horses should be rested for 1 week for every day of fever, with a minimum of 3 weeks rest (to allow regeneration of the mucociliary apparatus). Coughing and airway inflammation may persist for weeks to months if return to work is premature.

## PREVENTION OF INFLUENZA

Prevention of influenza requires hygienic management practices and vaccination. Exposure to influenza can be reduced by isolation of newly introduced horses for 2 weeks. Vaccination does not completely eliminate clinical episodes of influenza. There is significant heterogeneity in the response of horses to vaccine and viral challenge. In general, horses with high serum antibody concentrations against influenza results in lower viral shedding post-challenge. Numerous vaccines are commercially available for prevention of equine influenza. An intranasal modified live influenza vaccine, designed to induce mucosal (local) antibody protection, has demonstrated protection against natural challenge. Based on the duration of immunity, booster vaccination is recommended every 6 months. This modified live vaccine is temperature-sensitive and is not capable of replicating beyond the nasal passages. The majority of commercially available influenza vaccines are inactivated, adjuvanted vaccines for intramuscular administration. Because the duration of protection provided by current vaccines is limited, booster injections should be administered every 3–6 months. Vaccine manufacturers monitor antigenic drift to ensure that influenza strain content reflects, as closely as possible, the antigenicity of current strains of field virus.

Foals should not be vaccinated prior to 8 months of age. Undetectable maternal antibody concentrations appear to be protective in weanling foals, and clinical disease is difficult to induce in this age group with natural challenge. In addition, early/aggressive vaccination of foals reduces the immunologic response to vaccine or natural challenge in adulthood.

# Equine Viral Arteritis (EVA)

Equine viral arteritis is caused by an RNA togavirus, and produces clinical signs of respiratory disease, vasculitis, and abortion:

- EVA produces limb swelling, conjunctivitis, and abortion, in addition to the clinical signs typical of viral respiratory infection.
- The most important consequences of this disease are abortion in the mare and establishment of a carrier state in stallions.
- A modified-live vaccine is effective for prevention of disease in at-risk individuals; however, specific considerations regarding transport and breeding must be considered prior to vaccination.

Vasculitis results from direct viral damage to the tunica media of small arteries and venules. The two most important consequences of this disease are abortion in the mare and establishment of a carrier state in semen of actively breeding stallions.

Equine arteritis virus (EAV) is spread by aerosolization of respiratory secretions, fomite contamination with respiratory secretions, and venereal transmission. The incubation period is 7–19 days. Infectious virus is present in respiratory secretions for 2 weeks following recovery from clinical disease. Intact males exposed to the virus after sexual maturity develop a persistent infection in the ampulla of the vas deferens. Carrier stallions are seropositive, and their semen (fresh and frozen) remains infectious for years. Semen quality is unaffected by EAV infection. Mares bred to affected stallions develop respiratory disease (85–100%) and early embryonic death, but do not develop a persistent EVA infection or permanent reproductive consequences. Most cases of EVA are mild or subclinical, and mortality is rare. Clinical signs are most severe in very young and aged horses. Standardbreds have a higher incidence of seropositivity and carrier infections than other breeds.

The typical clinical signs of EVA are fever, anorexia, and depression. The clinical signs associated with the respiratory tract are serous nasal discharge, cough, conjunctivitis, lacrimation, and palpebral and periorbital edema. Edema of the prepuce, scrotum, and limbs is a common manifestation of vasculitis. Limb edema is asymmetric and painful. Clinical signs persist for 2–9 days. Abortion may occur at any point in gestation and occurs during late clinical disease or early convalescent period. The fetus dies due to viral infection and is autolyzed by the time of expulsion.

## DIAGNOSIS AND TREATMENT

Profound lymphopenia during acute disease should increase the clinician's suspicion of equine viral arteritis. Equine viral arteritis is definitively diagnosed by viral detection and serology. Virus isolation and PCR are performed on respiratory secretions and semen samples. A fourfold rise in virus neutralizing antibody between the acute and convalescent (10–14 days apart) samples is consistent with recent infection. Treatment consists of supportive care (support bandages) and NSAIDS for fever and inflammation. Antimicrobial therapy is usually unnecessary, unless the horse develops signs of a secondary bacterial infection.

## PREVENTION OF EVA

The most important viral factor, which makes control of EVA difficult, is the persistent carrier state in the stallion. The risk of venereal transmission can be reduced by administration of a modified-live vaccine prior to the breeding season. Stallions should be vaccinated 60 days prior to breeding and isolated for 21 days after vaccination. Vaccination results in positive serologic testing, which complicates international travel and identification of negative stallions. Therefore, written certification of seronegativity is required prior to vaccination of breeding stallions. Seropositive stallions without written certification must be tested to confirm virus-negative semen prior to export. Ideally, colts should be serotested and vaccinated at <278 days old and isolated for 21 days after vaccine administration. Because the vaccine is modified-live, it should not be administered to pregnant mares or foals <6 weeks old. Mares intended to be bred to a known shedding stallion are vaccinated (and isolated) 21 days prior to breeding and are isolated for 21 days after breeding (first year only). At-risk performance horses should be vaccinated, and vaccinated horses should be isolated from nonvaccinates for 21 days. Infected horses should be isolated for 3 weeks after recovery from disease, and in general, contact between broodmares and young horses should be avoided.

# Other Contagious Respiratory Diseases

## HENDRA VIRUS (EQUINE MORBILLIVIRUS)

Hendra virus (HeV) was first recognized in Hendra, Australia, (a suburb of Brisbane) in 1995 as a new zoonotic disease of horses:

- Hendra virus causes fatal pneumonia and encephalitis in humans and horses.
- The clinical signs of Hendra virus are similar to African Horse Sickness.
- Fruit bats are the reservoir of infection, and disease transmission requires very close contact with infected horses or bat droppings.
- Hendra virus is classified as a Hazard Group 4 pathogen, requiring the highest level of biosecurity procedures.

Hendra is the prototype species of a new genus (*Megamyxovirus*) within the subfamily *Paramyxovirinae*. The viral agent is endemic in specific species of fruit bats (also called flying foxes), and close contact with these bats is suspected to have precipitated transfer of the HeV to horses.

There have been three incidents of equine epizootics. In one outbreak, 14 of 21 horses died. During this outbreak, two caretakers developed influenza-like signs, one of whom did not survive. A morbillivirus cultured from his kidney was identical to the virus isolated from lungs of 5 affected horses. All human cases have been reported in association with equine cases. Morbillivirus is not considered highly contagious. Very close contact is required to transmit the virus among horses and from horses to humans. There was no serological evidence of infection in 157 humans who had had casual contact with infected humans and horses. Grey-headed fruit bats seroconvert and develop subclinical disease when inoculated with HeV; however, widespread subclinical disease or seroconversion is not recognized in horses. Horses are

183

infected by oronasal routes and excrete HeV in urine, saliva, and respiratory secretions. The virions are labile, and infectivity is readily destroyed by heat, lipid solvents, detergents, formaldehyde, and oxidizing agents.

Horses infected with Hendra virus develop severe—and often fatal—respiratory disease, characterized by dyspnea, vascular endothelial damage, and pulmonary edema. Depression, anorexia, fever, respiratory difficulty, ataxia, tachycardia, and frothy, nasal discharge are common clinical signs. Encephalitic signs and subcutaneous edema may be observed in some cases. The incubation period is 8–11 days, and the clinical course of disease is peracute. Death typically occurs from 1–3 days after the onset of clinical signs. The most important differential diagnosis, based on clinical signs of disease, is African Horse Sickness. Diagnosis is based on serologic testing using neutralizing and immunofluorescing antibody, virus isolation in Vero cell culture, and immunofluorescent testing to demonstrate viral antigens in tissues. Due to the zoonotic potential, suspect samples should be collected and transported with caution. The virus is classified as a Hazard Group 4 pathogen, requiring the highest level of biosecurity procedures.

## ADENOVIRUS

Subclinical infections are most common. Racehorses are often seropositive and virus may be isolated from respiratory secretions. Clinical disease is limited to Arabian foals with severe combined immunodeficiency syndrome (SCID).

## AFRICAN HORSE SICKNESS

African Horse Sickness (AHS) is a foreign animal disease and has never been reported in the United States:

- *Culicoides imicola* is the vector for transmission of African Horse Sickness.
- Morbidity and mortality are high in naive populations.
- Clinical syndromes range from fulminate pulmonary edema, subcutaneous edema, and myocardial failure, to "Horse Sickness" depending on the immune status of the horse.

There are four clinical syndromes including peracute, acute, subacute, and mild, and mortality is high in naive populations. The disease manifestation is dependent on the immune status of the horse. African Horse Sickness is caused by a virus in the family *Reoviridae*, genus *Orbivirus* (double-stranded RNA virus), and is related to the causative agent of bluetongue.

African Horse Sickness is endemic in portions of Africa. All equidae are susceptible; however, horses are most prone, followed by mules, donkeys, and zebras. The virus is vector-transmitted, primarily by *Culicoides imicola*. This biting midge prefers habitats with clay-like, moisture-rententive soils, and insect numbers increase 200-fold during years with above average rainfall. This vector is moving further north each year in Europe, purportedly due to global warming. It is unlikely to reach the U.K. in the foreseeable future, but may stretch sufficiently far to bring African Horse Sickness into the range of other competent vectors, which may spread the virus over Europe. Epidemics frequently occur in Middle Eastern countries, and recent outbreaks have occurred in Spain, Portugal, and Morocco. A 1989 outbreak in Portugal was successfully eradicated primarily by vaccination of all Portuguese equines (170,000) at a cost of $1,955,514.

The four basic forms of AHS represent a continuum in disease manifestion, with severity based on the host's susceptibility to the pathogen. The peracute or pulmonary form is most severe, with 95% mortality with a brief incubation period (3–5 days). Clinical signs of peracute AHS include fever, congestions, respiratory difficulty, and blood-tinged, foamy nasal discharge (pulmonary edema). Gross necropsy findings include hydrothorax and pulmonary edema. Acute or mixed AHS is the most common form of the disease, and is characterized by a combination of cardiac and pulmonary signs. The incubation period is slightly more prolonged (5–7 days) than the peracute form and the mortality rate is 50–95%. The clinical signs consist of a mixture of pulmonary disease (cough, pulmonary edema, respiratory distress) and cardiac disease (edema of head and neck). Post-mortem examination characteristically reveals subcutaneous and fascial edema of the head and neck. Horses with the subacute form of AHS display signs of myocardial dysfunction, fever, edema of the head and neck, and depression. Edema of the supraorbital fossa is considered pathognomic for AHS by some authors. The incubation period is 7–14 days and mortality is 50%. Horse Sickness Fever is the mildest form of AHS, and is observed in horses with some degree of immunocompetency against AHS and resistant species (donkeys and zebras). Clinical signs of Horse Sickness Fever include depression, conjunctival edema, and low-grade fever. Mortality is low.

Governmental veterinary officials should be contacted if a veterinarian suspects AHS. A definitive diagnosis is determined by serology and virus isolation. An inactivated viral vaccine (serotype 4) provides full protection against experimental AHS challenge and is used in endemic areas to prevent losses. During an epidemic, the first approach to management of disease outbreak is to eradicate disease through quarantine, vector control, and euthanasia of exposed horses. If eradication efforts fail, perimeter vaccination is used to limit the spread.

## FURTHER READING

Balasuriya, U.B., Leutenegger, C.M., Topol, J.B., McCollum, W.H., Timoney, P.J., and MacLachlan, N.J. 2002. Detection of equine arteritis by real-time Taqman reverse transcription-PCR assay. *J Virol Methods* 101(1–2):21–28.

Barclay, A.J., and Paton, D.J. 2000. Hendra (equine morbillivirus). *Vet J* 160(3): 169–176.

Del Pirero, F. 2000. Equine viral arteritis. *Vet Pathol* 37(4):287–296.

Folsom, R.W., Littlefield-Chabaud M.A., French D.D., Pourciau S.S., Mistric L., and Horohov D.W. 2001. Exercise alters the immune response to equine influenza virus and increases the susceptibility to infection. *Equine Vet J* 33(7):664–669.

Glass, K., Wood, J.L., Mumford, J.A., Jesset, D., and Grenfell, B.T. 2002. Modelling equine influenza 1: A stochastic model of within-yard epidemics. *Epidemiol Infect* 128(3):491–502.

House, J.A. 1998. Future international management of African Horse Sickness vaccines. *Arch Virol Suppl* 14:297–304.

Meiswinkel, R. 1998. The 1996 outbreak of African Horse Sickness in South Africa— The entomological perspective. *Arch Virol Suppl* 14:69–83.

Mumford, E.L., Traub-Dargatz, J.L., Carman, J., Callan, R.J., Collins, J.K., Goltz, K.L., Romm, S.R., Tarr, S.F., and Salman, M.D. 2003. Occurrence of infectious upper respiratory tract disease and response to vaccination in horses on six sentinel premises in northern Colorado. *Equine Vet J* 35(1):72–77.

Portas, M., Boinas, F.S., Oliveira, E., Sousa, J., and Rawlings P. 1999. African Horse Sickness in Portugal: A successful eradication programme. *Epidemiol Infect* 123(2): 337–346.

Townsend, H.G., Penner, S.J., Watts, T.C., Cook, A., Bogdan, J., Haines, D.M., Griffin, S., Chambers, T., Holland, R.E., Whitaker-Dowling, P., Youngner, J.S., and Sebring, R.W. 2001. Efficacy of cold-adapted, intranasal, equine influenza vaccine: Challenge trials. *Equine Vet J* 33(7):637–643.

Wittmann, E.J., and Baylis, M. 2000. Climate change: Effects on culicoides—transmitted viruses and implications for the UK. *Vet J* 160(2):107–117.

# Noninfectious Pulmonary Diseases and Diagnostic Techniques

**IV**

Respiratory disease is the second most common cause of lost training days and premature retirement in performance horses. In a series of 300 referral cases of respiratory disease, a noninfectious etiology was implicated in approximately 80% of the cases. Recurrent airway obstruction was the most common noninfectious pulmonary disease, followed by exercise-induced pulmonary hemorrhage, lungworms, eosinophilic pneumonitis, and pulmonary neoplasia. Nearly 60% of horses presenting for poor exercise tolerance (without overt signs of respiratory disease) have primary pulmonary disease diagnosed as the source of poor performance. Cough is the most reliable indicator of lower respiratory tract disease in horses, whereas, nasal discharge is a less consistent clinical sign. Pulmonary and tracheal auscultation are insensitive techniques for identifying and/or characterizing noninfectious respiratory disease, although, performing a rebreathing procedure does improve the ability to detect abnormal lung sounds. The most common diagnostic tests performed in horses with suspected pulmonary disease include endoscopic examination, cytologic evaluation of transtracheal wash and bronchoalveolar lavage samples, arterial blood gas analysis, and thoracic radiographic examination.

# Noninfectious Pulmonary Diseases

## RECURRENT AIRWAY OBSTRUCTION (HEAVES)

Recurrent airway obstruction (RAO or heaves) is a common, performance-limiting, allergic respiratory disease of horses characterized by chronic cough, nasal discharge, and respiratory difficulty:

- Clinical signs of disease are induced in sensitive horses by exposure to organic dusts.
- There is a broad range of clinical manifestation in affected horses, from exercise intolerance to dyspnea at rest.
- Average age of onset is 9 years, with approximately 12% of mature horses affected with some degree of allergen-induced airway inflammation.
- No breed or gender predilection has been shown.

Alternative terms for heaves include *chronic obstructive pulmonary disease (COPD)*, *emphysema*, and *broken wind*; however, the terms *emphysema* and *COPD* have fallen out of favor because the pathogenesis of heaves differs from these human conditions. Episodes of airway obstruction are usually observed when horses are stabled, bedded on straw, and fed hay; elimination of these inciting factors results in remission or attenuation of clinical signs. The pathophysiology of heaves is small airway inflammation (neutrophilic), mucus production, and bronchoconstriction in response to allergen exposure. The most common environmental entity to precipitate an episode of airway obstruction in heaves-affected horses is the organic dust present in hay and straw.

As mentioned earlier, the average age of onset of RAO is 9 years of age. Approximately 12% of mature horses have some degree of allergen-induced lower airway disease, and over 50% of horses that present for evaluation of respiratory disease are diagnosed with heaves. There is no breed or gender predilection; however, there does appear to be a heritable component to the etiology of this condition. As with human asthmatics, there is a broad spectrum of sensitivity to antigens and severity of clinical signs.

Horses with classic heaves present with flared nostrils, tachypnea, wheezes, and a heave line. The typical breathing pattern is characterized by a prolonged, labored expiratory phase of respiration. The abdominal muscles are recruited to assist with expiration, and hypertrophy of these muscles produces the classic heave line (Fig. 19.1). Characteristic auscultatory findings include a prolonged expiratory phase of respiration, wheezes, tracheal rattle, and overexpanded lung fields. Wheezes are generated by airflow through narrowed airways, and are most pronounced during end expiration. Crackles may be present and are associated with excessive mucus production. Mild to moderately affected horses may present with minimal clinical signs at rest; however, coughing and exercise intolerance are noted during exercise. Horses with heaves are not typically febrile unless secondary bacterial pneumonia has developed.

## Diagnosis

The diagnosis of classic heaves is determined in most horses on the basis of history and characteristic physical examination findings:

- Thoracic radiography is indicated in horses that fail to respond to standard therapy.
- Bronchoalveolar lavage can identify pulmonary inflammation in horses with mild to moderate disease.

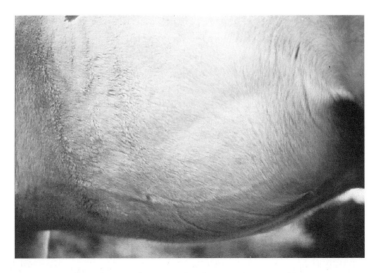

**Fig. 19.1.** Heave line from a horse with chronic (>1 month) recurrent airway obstruction.

Hematology and serum chemistry results are unremarkable. Thoracic radiographic examination should be performed in horses that fail to respond to standard treatment for heaves after 14 days of therapy. Thoracic radiography should be performed immediately in horses that have more difficulty on inspiration than expiration (restrictive breathing pattern), which may be indicative of interstitial disease or pulmonary fibrosis. Fever is also an indication for thoracic radiography to identify the presence of primary or secondary infectious (bacterial, fungal) pulmonary disease. Thoracic radiographic findings in horses with heaves are peribronchial infiltration and overexpanded pulmonary fields (flattening of the diaphragm). Thoracic radiographs are of little benefit in confirming the diagnosis of heaves, but may be helpful in identifying the most important differential diagnoses, including interstitial pneumonia, pulmonary fibrosis, or bacterial pneumonia.

Bronchoalveolar lavage is rarely required for diagnosis of fulminant heaves, and is not necessarily innocuous in horses that are dyspneic at rest. Bronchoalveolar lavage is indicated in horses with mild to moderate disease and poor performance and coughing during exercise. The protocol for performing BAL appears in Chapter 20. Neutrophilic inflammation (20–70% of total cell count) confirms the presence of lower airway inflammation and differentiates horses with heaves from horses with eosinophilic pneumonitis, fungal pneumonia, or lungworm infestation. Curschmann's spirals (Fig. 19.2) may be observed on cytologic evaluation and represent inspissated mucus/cellular casts from obstructed small airways. Transtracheal wash provides little assistance in differentiating heaves from infectious respiratory disease. Both conditions

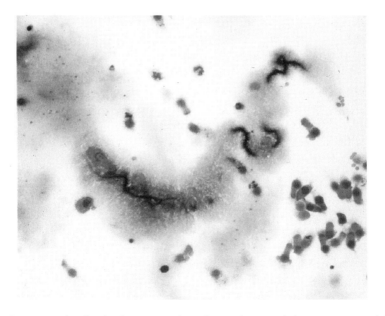

**Fig. 19.2.** Bronchoalveolar lavage cytology from a horse with heaves. Neutrophilic inflammation (76% total cell count) and excessive mucus are consistent with recurrent airway obstruction. Several Curshmann's spirals are observed. Wright-Giemsa stain, 140x. *(See also color section.)*

have neutrophilic inflammation, and bacterial culture of tracheal aspirates from heaves-affected horses often recovers opportunistic pathogens, including *Streptococcus zooepidemicus* and *Actinobacillus equuli*.

## Treatment

The single most important treatment for heaves is environmental management to reduce allergen exposure:

- Reduction of environmental allergen exposure is the key to long-term management of horses with heaves.
- Medical therapy will improve the clinical signs of disease during an episode of airway obstruction.
- Corticosteroid therapy reduces pulmonary inflammation.
- Bronchodilator therapy provides relief of bronchoconstriction (symptomatic therapy).

Medication will alleviate clinical signs of disease; however, respiratory disease will return after medication is discontinued if the horse remains in the allergen-challenged environment. The most common offending allergens are organic dusts, present in hay and straw, consisting of mold spores and endotoxin. Hay does not have to appear overtly musty to precipitate an episode in a sensitive horse. If possible, horses should be maintained at pasture with fresh grass as the source of roughage and supplemented with pelleted feed. Round bale hay is particularly allergenic and a common cause of treatment failure for horses on pasture. Horses that remain stalled should be maintained in a clean, controlled environment. A complete commercial feed eliminates the need for roughage in the diet. Hay cubes and hay silage are acceptable, low-allergen alternative sources of roughage and may be preferred (more palatable) by horses over the complete feeds. Soaking hay with water prior to feeding may control clinical signs in mildly affected horses, but is unacceptable for highly sensitive horses. Although horses with heaves are not allergic to "dust," their airways are hyperreactive to nonspecific stimuli, and they should not be pastured near a dry, dusty road or paddock. Horses maintained in a stall should not be housed in the same building as an indoor arena, hay should not be stored overhead, and straw bedding should be avoided.

Medical treatment of horses with clinical signs of heaves consists of combination therapy using bronchodilators and corticosteroids (Table 19.1). Corticosteroids reduce pulmonary inflammation, and bronchodilators provide symptomatic relief of airway obstruction. Corticosteroid therapy does not relieve clinical signs of airway obstruction for several days, therefore, bronchodilator therapy will provide immediate relief of airway obstruction until clinical signs of disease are controlled by corticosteroids. It is inappropriate to treat heaves with bronchodilators as solo therapy; bronchodilators do not ad-

**Table 19.1.** Corticosteroids and bronchodilators for treatment of horses with heaves during disease exacerbation

| | Mechanism | Dose | Onset | Duration | Comments |
|---|---|---|---|---|---|
| **Corticosteroid Therapy** | | | | | |
| **Systemic** | | | | | |
| dexamethasone | anti-inflammatory | 0.1 mg/kg, IV, SID | 24–72 hr | 2–4 d | Marked adrenal suppression, recovers 2–4 d |
| triamcinolone | anti-inflammatory | 0.09 mg/kg, IM | <1 wk | 4 wk | Single dose, prolonged adrenal suppression |
| **Aerosolized** | | | | | |
| beclomethasone | anti-inflammatory | 500 mg, BID | 24 hr | 2 d | Equine Aerosol Delivery Device |
| beclomethasone | anti-inflammatory | 3750 mg, BID | 72 hr | <1 wk | MDI and Equine AeroMask |
| fluticasone | anti-inflammatory | 2000 mg, BID | ND | ND | MDI and Equine AeroMask |
| mometasone | anti-inflammatory | 1.6 mg BID | ND | ND | MDI and Equine AeroMask |
| **Bronchodilator Therapy** | | | | | |
| **Systemic** | | | | | |
| clenbuterol | $\beta_2$ agonist | 0.8–3.2 mg/kg BID | 30–60 min | 10 hr | |
| aminophylline | phosphodiesterase inhibitor | 6 mg/kg, PO, BID | ND | ND | May delay fatigue of mm of respiration |
| atropine | anticholinergic | 5–7 mg/450 kg, IV | 10 min | 6–8 hr | Single dose, significant adverse effects |
| **Short-Acting Aerosolized** | | | | | |
| albuterol | $\beta_2$ agonist—short | 360 mg | 5 min | 1–3 hr | Equine Aerosol Delivery Device |
| pirbuterol | $\beta_2$ agonist—short | 600 mg | 5 min | 1–4 hr | Equine Aerosol Delivery Device |
| fenoterol | $\beta_2$ agonist—short | 2–3 mg/kg | ND | 4–6 hr | MDI and Equine AeroMask |
| **Long-Acting Aerosolized** | | | | | |
| salmeterol | $\beta_2$ agonist—long | 210 mg | ND | 8–10 hr | MDI and Equine AeroMask |
| ipratropium | antimuscarinic | 90–180 mg | ND | 4–6 hr | MDI and Equine AeroMask |
| ipratropium | antimuscarinic | 2–3 mg/kg | <1 hr | 4–6 hr | Ultrasonic nebulizer |
| ipratropium | antimuscarinic | 4 mg/kg | 15 min | >1 hr | Dry powder inhaler |

dress the underlying inflammatory process, and tolerance develops rapidly to $\beta_2$-adrenergic agents (5 days) when administered alone to horses with heaves. Corticosteroid therapy prevents and/or reverts tolerance to $\beta_2$ adrenergic drugs by preventing down-regulation of $\beta_2$ receptors and inducing formation of new $\beta_2$ receptors on pulmonary cells. Nonsteroidal anti-inflammatory drugs, antihistamines, and leukotriene-receptor antagonists have failed to demonstrate therapeutic benefit in horses with heaves.

## RESPIRATORY DISTRESS AT REST

Horses with respiratory difficulty at rest should be treated with systemic corticosteroid drugs and aerosolized bronchodilators:

- Systemic corticosteroid administration is recommended in severely affected horses.
- Short-acting, aerosolized bronchodilators are used for immediate relief of airway obstruction (rescue therapy).
- Long-acting bronchodilators are used to provide prolonged relief of airway obstruction.

Pulmonary distribution of aerosolized preparations is poor in the presence of severe airway obstruction, therefore, administration of surface-active, corticosteroid drugs via inhalation is inappropriate for horses or humans that are markedly dyspneic at rest. However, aerosolized bronchodilators typically remain effective, regardless of the severity of disease. Aerosolized bronchodilator therapy can be used to provide relief of airway obstruction until systemic corticosteroids control the clinical signs of disease. In patients with poor asthma control, optimal control of clinical signs is obtained by addition of a bronchodilator rather than increasing the dose of corticosteroid. Increasing the dose of corticosteroid does not provide equivalent improvement in therapeutic efficacy in human asthmatics or heaves-affected horses, and is typically not effective in stabilizing clinical signs in patients with severe disease. Dose-dependent therapeutic effects of steroids are not typically observed beyond the recommended dosage range; however the risk of adverse side effects is dose-dependent.

### Systemic corticosteroid therapy
Systemic corticosteroid preparations are inexpensive and easy to administer; however, therapeutic drug concentrations are capable of inducing adverse effects in horses, and conservative dosing regimens are recommended. Therapeutic benefit of systemic corticosteroids may not be detected for 24–72 hours in heaves-affected horses.

Triamcinolone is one of the most potent systemic corticosteroid preparations. Triamcinolone acetonide (0.09 mg/kg, IM, single dose) relieves airway obstruction for up to 4 weeks; however, adrenal suppression is evident for 4 weeks following administration. Repeated administration of triamcinolone has produced iatrogenic Cushing syndrome, adrenal insufficiency, and laminitis. Because of the risk of adverse side effects, administration of triamcinolone for treatment of heaves is limited to salvage efforts.

Dexamethasone (0.1 mg/kg, IV, SID) improves clinical signs of heaves by day 3 of administration, and the maximal response is obtained by day 7. After cessation of treatment, some therapeutic benefit can be detected 7 days later. Improvement in lung function is paralleled by decreased inflammation, as reflected by a reduction in the number of neutrophils in bronchoalveolar lavage fluid. Administration of dexamethasone produces marked suppression of endogenous cortisol production, which persists approximately 3 days after discontinuation of drug. Adrenal responsiveness to ACTH is not affected by a 7-day treatment regimen of dexamethasone. A long-acting intramuscular form of dexamethasone (dexamethasone 21-isonicotinate; Voren, Boehringer Ingelheim; 0.04 mg/kg, q3d) reduces airway obstruction by day 3, and maximal effect is achieved by day 7. The efficacy of orally administered dexamethasone preparations has not been evaluated. Because of the possibility of adrenal suppression, the dose and frequency of administration of potent steroids should be reduced gradually to doses sufficient to maintain disease remission.

Oral prednisone (1.0–2.2 mg/kg, PO, SID) is frequently used as an anti-inflammatory agent in horses because of its ease of administration, minimal cost, and reduced risk of laminitis (perceived). Despite widespread use, there is no supporting information on the pharmacokinetics or clinical benefits of prednisone. Clinical improvement in heaves-affected horses treated with oral prednisone has not been documented using objective parameters. Pretreatment of heaves-susceptible horses with prednisone fails to prevent the onset of airway obstruction when horses are stabled in an allergen-challenged environment. Coupling prednisone with environmental management provides no additional benefit in pulmonary function over environmental management alone. Prednisone administration reduces pulmonary neutrophilia at 3 and 7 days post-administration, but this finding does not translate to improved pulmonary function. The reason for lack of efficacy of prednisone is presently unknown. Oral bioavailability of prednisone appears to be poor, evidenced by minimal to undetectable serum prednisolone (active metabolite) concentrations after administration of oral prednisone. The short duration of the anti-inflammatory effect of prednisolone may make it ineffective when administered only once daily to horses with heaves.

## Bronchodilator therapy

Aerosolized, short-acting ß$_2$ adrenergic agonists (albuterol, pirbuterol, fenoterol) are rapid and powerful bronchodilators, and serve as "rescue therapy" for horses with respiratory distress at rest. A description of aerosol delivery devices for horses appears in the techniques portion of this chapter. Albuterol sulfate (360 µg) improves pulmonary function by 70% within 5 minutes of administration. To overcome poor drug distribution in horses with severe airway obstruction, albuterol (salbutamol) may be administered every 15 minutes for 2 hours to provide sequential bronchodilation. Unfortunately, the beneficial effects of the short-acting $\beta_2$ agonists last approximately 1 hour in severely obstructed horses, which necessitates addition of a long-acting bronchodilator to provide prolonged relief of airway obstruction. Concurrent administration of corticosteroids prevents $\beta_2$ tolerance and may induce formation of new $\beta_2$ receptors.

The long-acting bronchodilators are inappropriate to provide rescue therapy in horses with severe airway obstruction due to the delayed onset of action and slightly diminished magnitude of response in comparison to albuterol. However, twice to three times daily administration of long-acting bronchodilators are indicated to provide prolonged relief of airway obstruction, after rescue therapy has been achieved with a short-acting bronchodilator. The most popular long-acting bronchodilators are salmeterol xinafoate and ipratropium bromide.

Salmeterol xinafoate is a long-acting $\beta_2$ agonist that is a chemical analog of albuterol, with the addition of an elongated (aliphatic) side chain. The side chain is thought to bind to an exosite proximal to the region of the $\beta_2$ adrenoceptor, which allows salmeterol to repeatedly contact the $\beta_2$ receptor while anchored adjacent to the receptor site. Salmeterol has higher lipophilicity (prolonged pulmonary residence time), $\beta_2$ affinity, $\beta_2$ selectivity (safety), and potency (tenfold) than albuterol. Salmeterol xinafoate (210 µg) improves pulmonary function by 55% within 60 minutes of aerosol administration, and the duration of action is approximately 8 hours in severely affected horses.

Ipratropium bromide is a surface-active, antimuscarinic agent with little to no systemic absorption (quaternary ammonium structure) from the respiratory or gastrointestinal system. Ipratropium (90–180 µg) improves pulmonary function by 50% within 1 hour, and the duration of effect is approximately 4–6 hours in severely affected horses. Few adverse effects are attributed to ipratropium due to minimal systemic absorption, and unlike atroprine, ipratropium does not inhibit mucociliary clearance.

Atropine (5–7 mg/450 kg horse, IV) is a rapid and powerful antimuscarinic bronchodilator in horses with heaves. The adverse effects of systemic administration (ileus, CNS toxicity, tachycardia, increased viscosity of mucus secretion, impaired mucociliary clearance) limit use of atropine in horses with heaves to a single "rescue therapy" dose for horses with severe airway obstruction.

Horses with severe disease may develop secondary bacterial infection, which contributes to respiratory compromise. Horses with heaves with marked exudate production, fever, and/or abnormal hematologic findings should be treated with antimicrobial therapy in addition to corticosteroids and bronchodilators. The antimicrobials of choice in most instances are potentiated sulfonamides based on common pathogens, ease of administration, and pulmonary penetration.

Horses with severe airway obstruction should begin breathing more comfortably within 24–72 hours after initiation of therapy. When clinical signs of airway obstruction begin to abate, systemic corticosteroid therapy may be replaced with aerosolized corticosteroids to avoid the adverse effects of systemic corticosteroid administration (laminitis, immunosuppression, PU/PD). Aerosolized bronchodilators should be administered several minutes prior to aerosolized corticosteroid administration to improve pulmonary distribution of the surface-active corticosteroids.

## MILD TO MODERATE AIRWAY OBSTRUCTION

Treatment of mild to moderate airway obstruction includes corticosteroids and bronchodilators:

- Corticosteroids may be administered via inhalation or systemic administration.
- Long-acting bronchodilators may be administered via inhalation or systemic administration to provide prolonged relief of airway obstruction and prevent exercise-induced bronchoconstriction.

### Aerosolized corticosteroids

Aerosolized corticosteroids are effective in horses with mild to moderate airway obstruction with clinical signs ranging from exercise intolerance to horses with moderate increased effort of respiration at rest. Aerosolized drugs reduce the total therapeutic dose and allow direct delivery of the drug to the lower respiratory tract, but are generally more expensive. There are three aerosolized corticosteroid preparations available in MDI formulation for administration to horses via the Equine AeroMask or Equine Haler: beclomethasone dipropionate, fluticasone propionate, and flunisolide. The relative potency of these surface-active corticosteroids is fluticasone > beclomethasone > flunisolide = triamcinolone. Using dexamethasone as the standard (1), the relative glucocorticoid receptor affinity of common corticosteroids is flunisolide = 1.9, triamcinolone = 2.0, beclomethasone = 13.5, and fluticasone propionate = 18.0.

Of the commercially available aerosolized corticosteroid preparations, fluticasone is the most potent and the most expensive. Fluticasone is highly lipophilic, and consequently has the longest pulmonary residence time. Due to its low oral bioavailability (<2%) and extensive first-pass metabolism (99%), fluticasone has the least potential for adverse systemic effects and the most favorable therapeutic index of all of the aerosolized corticosteroids.

In heaves-affected horses, fluticasone (2000 μg, BID, Equine AeroMask, Canadian Monaghan, Ontario, Canada) reduces pulmonary neutrophilia, improves parameters of pulmonary function, and reduces responsiveness to histamine challenge during an episode of airway obstruction. In normal horses, fluticasone propionate reduces serum cortisol concentrations by 40% after

1 day of therapy and 65% after 7 days. Serum cortisol concentrations return to pretreatment values within 1–2 days after discontinuation of drug.

Beclomethasone is first-line of therapy for moderate to severe allergic airway disease in human patients. Beclomethasone (500–1500 µg, BID, Equine Aerosol Delivery Device, Boehringer Ingelheim Vetmedica) reduces pulmonary inflammation, improves parameters of pulmonary function, and improves ventilation imaging of horses with recurrent airway obstruction. There is no immediate (15-minute) therapeutic effect; however, clinical signs and pulmonary function begin to improve within 24 hours of administration. Administration of beclomethasone (3750 µg, BID) using the Equine AeroMask, improves parameters of pulmonary function and arterial oxygen tension for a 2-week treatment period. Clinical signs of airway obstruction, pulmonary neutrophilia, and pulmonary function return to pre-treatment levels 3–7 days after discontinuation of beclomethasone. Short-term administration of inhaled beclomethasone without minimizing environmental allergen exposure is not expected to provide prolonged anti-inflammatory benefit for horses with recurrent airway obstruction.

Endogenous cortisol production is suppressed by approximately 35–50% of baseline values within 24 hours of administration of high-dose beclomethasone (>1000 µg, BID) to horses. After a 7-day treatment period, serum cortisol concentrations drop to 10–20% of baseline values. However, serum cortisol concentrations recover approximately 2 days after discontinuation of drug, and adrenal responsiveness to exogenous ACTH administration is not affected by a 7-day treatment period. The threshold for adrenal suppression in normal and heaves-affected horses is approximately 500 µg of beclomethasone administered twice daily. Therapeutic efficacy of this minimally adrenosuppressive dose of beclomethasone is equivalent to the efficacy of doses in excess of 1000 µg twice daily.

Flunisolide is the least potent of the synthetic, topically active corticosteroids. The primary advantage of flunisolide is cost. It is the least lipophilic resulting in the shortest pulmonary residence time. Flunisolide has relatively high oral bioavailability (21%) and is extensively absorbed from the respiratory tract as unchanged drug. Flunisolide is similar to triamcinolone in terms of potency, lipophilicity, and clinical efficacy. Much higher dosages are required to achieve therapeutic effects similar to fluticasone or beclomethasone, and adverse effects (adrenal suppression) occur more frequently in human patients with flunisolide. Despite its limitations, the therapeutic index of flunisolide is superior to systemically administered corticosteroids. In fact, initiation of flunisolide therapy as replacement of oral prednisone allows recovery of the hypothalamic-pituitary-adrenal axis and superior asthma control in patients with steroid-dependent asthma. The safety and efficacy of aerosolized flunisolide has not been evaluated in heaves-affected horses.

## Adrenal suppression

Considering the safety of long-term administration (years) of inhaled beclomethasone in human patients at higher relative doses, marked suppression of endogenous cortisol production within 1 day in horses indicates horses are more sensitive to the adrenosuppressive effects of aerosolized corticosteroids than human patients. Documentation of systemic absorption (adrenal suppression) of inhaled beclomethasone and fluticasone raises concern that other systemic glucocorticoid effects may occur with aerosolized corticosteroid administration. Administration of adrenosuppressive doses (>1600 µg/day) of beclomethasone to asthmatic patients does not produce other complications of systemic gluco-corticoid administration. Adrenal suppression is the most sensitive indicator of systemic absorption of inhaled corticosteroids and does not necessarily correlate with other systemic effects. Clinical signs of iatrogenic Cushing syndrome, such as laminitis, secondary bacterial infection, polydipsia, and polyuria have not been observed in horses receiving beclomethasone or fluticasone. Recognition of systemic absorption and activity should alert the clinician to use inhaled corti-costeroids judiciously by administering the lowest effective dose.

## Long-acting bronchodilator therapy

Horses with mild to moderate airway obstruction will benefit from administra-tion of a long-acting, aerosolized bronchodilator. Preliminary data indicates that the duration of bronchodilation is more prolonged in horses with mild to mod-erate disease, as compared to the duration of activity in horses with severe airway obstruction. Ipratropium and salmeterol can be administered twice daily prior to aerosolized corticosteroid administration and 30 minutes prior to work to avert an episode of bronchoconstriction induced by exercise or nonspecific irritants.

Oral clenbuterol (0.8–1.6 µg/kg, PO, BID; Ventipulmin, Boehringer Ingel-heim Vetmedica) is the systemic alternative to the aerosolized, long-acting bron-chodilators for management of horses with mild to moderate disease. Terbu-taline was previously considered to be an acceptable systemic bronchodilator in horses; however, the bioavailability has recently been demonstrated to be neg-ligible in horses, and clinical efficacy has not been demonstrated. Aminophyl-line and theophylline (phosphodiesterase inhibitors) are alternative systemic bronchodilators for horses with airway obstruction; however, the therapeutic index is relatively narrow, and the magnitude of bronchodilation is less than that of the ß$_2$ agonists. The phosphodiesterase inhibitors delay fatigue of the muscles of respiration and may be valuable in horses with severe airway ob-struction with impending respiratory failure due to fatigue.

## Maintenance therapy

Maintenance therapy for mild to moderate airway obstruction includes long-term, low-dose aerosolized corticosteroids and offers the following results:

• May prevent episodes of airway obstruction
• May provide progressive improvement in pulmonary function

Horses in apparent "remission" from heaves may improve exercise toler-ance and performance by being maintained on low-dose, long-term, aerosolized corticosteroids. Asthmatic patients with "acceptable pulmonary function" (in the patient's opinion) have progressive improvement in forced expiratory volume and exercise tolerance for 6 months after initiation of daily, low-dose corticosteroid therapy. In addition, maintenance aerosolized corticosteroid therapy in asthmatic patients prevents episodes of airway obstruction and reduces (often eliminates) the need for intermittent, symptomatic bronchodilator therapy. The adverse effects of systemic corticosteroids preclude their use for long-term, daily administration for maintenance therapy. The safety and efficacy of daily, long-term aerosolized corticosteroids have not been objectively investigated in horses with recurrent airway obstruction or inflammatory airway disease; however, clinical use of these drugs in this manner is widespread.

During low-dose maintenance therapy, dose timing has a pivotal effect on the safety profile and consequently the risk/benefit ratio of inhaled corticosteroids. In humans, maximum adrenal suppression occurs with administration of aerosolized corticosteroids in the early morning hours (3:00 a.m.), whereas endogenous cortisol production is least disrupted by administration in the afternoon. The longer the terminal elimination half-life of the drug, the earlier in the afternoon it should be administered. For example, the adrenosuppressive effects of flunisolide ($t_{1/2}$ = 1.5 hr) are minimized when a single daily dose is administered at 7:00 p.m., whereas the optimum time for administration of fluticasone ($t_{1/2}$ = 6 hr) is 4:00 p.m. In addition to safety concerns, afternoon drug administration provides superior control of the clinical signs of nocturnal asthma. The safety and efficacy of once-daily administration (afternoon/evening) of aerosolized corticosteroids in horses has not been evaluated.

## Response to therapy

There is no long-term cure for heaves, and the primary goal of therapy is to prevent episodes of airway obstruction by avoiding allergen exposure. Horses with heaves should be breathing more comfortably within 2–5 days of initiation of medical management and environmental change. Failure to demonstrate improvement in clinical signs within 7 days warrants reassessment of the therapeutic plan and environmental management. Failure to respond to therapy within 14 days indicates that the diagnosis of heaves should be reevaluated, and the clinician should consider interstitial pneumonia or lungworm infestation as potential differential diagnoses.

## Stable hygiene

There are three approaches to decreasing exposure to organic dusts for horses with heaves that must be maintained in confinement housing:

1. Reduce allergen load by controlling source material (hay, silage, shavings).
2. Decrease organic dust dispersion by changing the presentation of source materials (wetting hay, hay cubes).
3. Increase the rate of organic dust removal via improved ventilation systems.

Ventilation systems that provide 5 air-changes/hour were previously considered effective for reducing allergen load based on in-stall particle collectors. However, investigations with personal particle collectors have revealed that the aeroallergen load in the "breathing zone" of horses is not adequately reflected by standard stall detectors, and ventilation systems are not capable of reducing allergen loads to acceptable levels when horses are eating hay. Organic dust concentrations are 35-fold higher in the "breathing zone" in horses bedded on straw and offered hay than for horses bedded on shavings and fed a pelleted feed. The combination of grass silage and wood shavings provides acceptable control of clinical signs in horses with heaves. Wetting the hay does not provide acceptable control of clinical signs for most horses with heaves. Therefore, controlling the source material is the most effective method to reduce aeroallergen exposure for sensitive horses that must be maintained in a confined housing environment.

Aerosolized endotoxin potentiates clinical signs of airway obstruction induced by allergen exposure in sensitive horses. Total airborne endotoxin concentrations in most conventional stables exceeds that which can induce pulmonary inflammation and bronchial hyperresponsiveness in normal humans, and exceeds levels which induce bronchoconstriction in humans with preexisting pulmonary inflammation. A hay- and straw-free environment (grass silage/wood shavings) has 10 times less respirable endotoxin concentrations compared to a conventional hay and straw environment.

Although a low-dust, controlled environment provides acceptable respiratory comfort and remission of overt clinical signs, pasture is the ideal environment for horses with heaves. Horses maintained in a pasture environment have the lowest exposure to respirable aeroallergens and endotoxins. Horses that are apparently in remission from heaves (based on standard pulmonary function testing and clinical signs) will maintain some degree of pulmonary inflammation in the low-dust, controlled environment evidenced by persistent pulmonary neutrophilia, increased alveolar clearance rates, and hyperreactivity to bronchoprovocation challenge.

## SUMMER PASTURE-ASSOCIATED OBSTRUCTIVE PULMONARY DISEASE

Summer pasture-associated obstructive pulmonary disease (SPAOPD) is a syndrome very similar to recurrent airway obstruction (heaves). The primary difference in these two conditions is the environment that triggers an episode of airway obstruction:

- Seasonal (hot, humid) episodes of airway obstruction are triggered by a pasture environment.
- Clinical signs, diagnostic findings, and medical therapy are similar to heaves.
- Management of disease requires relocation to a clean, confined environment.

Unlike heaves, the clinical signs of airway obstruction become apparent when SPAOPD-affected horses are on pasture in hot and humid climates, rather than induced by confinement housing and exposure to hay and straw. Summer pasture-associated obstructive pulmonary disease occurs most frequently in the Gulf Coast States of the United States and in England, and manifests during late spring, summer, and early autumn. The etiology is thought to be pulmonary hypersensitivity to molds on grasses or seasonal pollen. Similar to heaves, there is no breed or gender predilection, and the average age of onset is 10–13 years. Approximately 10% of heaves-affected horses also suffer from SPAOPD, and approximately half of SPAOPD-affected horses also demonstrate sensitivity to moldy hay and straw.

Typical clinical signs are indistinguishable from heaves-affected horses and commonly include serous nasal discharge, cough, tachypnea, tachycardia, labored expiratory effort, flared nostrils, and abnormal thoracic auscultation (wheezes and crackles). Most affected horses demonstrate marked severity in clinical disease, and mild to moderate airway obstruction is rarely reported. Serum chemistry and hematology are typically unremarkable in affected horses. Thoracic radiographic findings include a moderate interstitial pattern, variable peribronchial infiltration, and pulmonary overinflation. During disease exacerbation, cytologic evaluation of BAL fluid reveals findings similar to heaves (nondegenerate neutrophils), and histologic evaluation of pulmonary parenchyma demonstrates accumulation of mucus and neutrophils within the small airways, metaplasia of bronchiolar goblet cells, and mild peribronchial infiltrate. Gross necropsy reveals overinflation of lungs due to air trapping, as described in horses with heaves.

The most important treatment consideration for horses with SPAOPD is environmental management to reduce allergen exposure. Unlike heaves, horses affected with SPAOPD are best managed in a confined environment to reduce exposure to allergens at pasture. Approximately half of SPAOPD-affected horses are also sensitive to hay and straw; therefore, precautions should be taken to reduce allergen content in the barn environment. Medical therapy for treatment of an acute exacerbation of SPAOPD is similar to that of heaves, consisting of corticosteroids and bronchodilating agents.

## INTERSTITIAL PNEUMONIAS

The interstitial pneumonias are a poorly defined, heterogenous category of sporadic respiratory diseases in adult horses:

- Interstitial pneumonia may result from various etiologies, including hypersensitivity, drug reaction, plant toxicity, and silicosis.
- Diagnosis is based on thoracic radiography and percutaneous lung biopsy.
- Horses are generally unresponsive to treatment and the prognosis is poor.

The interstitial pneumonias of foals appear to be a separate clinical entity, and are discussed in Chapter 21. The etiology is undetermined in the majority of cases; however, hypersensitivity pneumonitis, plant toxicity, silicosis, and drug reaction have been confirmed to cause interstitial disease in horses. *Perilla frutescens* has been reported to cause interstitial pneumonia experimentally in ponies, and croton weed, *Eupatorium adenophorum*, causes chronic interstitial pneumonia in horses in Australia and Hawaii.

Regardless of etiology, the clinical signs of interstitial pneumonia include weight loss, exercise intolerance, fever (inconsistent), and progressive respiratory distress. Cyanosis will be apparent with end-stage disease. Depending on the stage of disease, most horses with interstitial pneumonia will have leukocytosis characterized by mature neutrophilia and increased fibrinogen concentration. Pulmonary auscultation reveals crackles and wheezes, although absent breath sounds may be noted in severely affected horses. The pattern of respiration in horses with interstitial pneumonia differs from that of heaves. Interstitial pneumonia is a restrictive pulmonary disease; therefore, affected horses have a prolonged inspiratory phase of respiration, abbreviated expiratory phase and breathe at low lung volumes. Horses with heaves have a prolonged expiratory phase of respiration and an abbreviated inspiratory phase, and breathe at high lung volumes. Pulmonary compliance is reduced due to pulmonary fibrosis and interstitial inflammation (stiff lungs). Pulmonary hypertension and cor pulmonale are common with end-stage disease.

Cytologic evaluation of BAL fluid from horses with interstitial pneumonia are nonspecific and include high cellularity and chronic, nonseptic mixed inflammation (neutrophilia, lymphocytosis, monocytosis). Nonetheless, cytologic evaluation of BAL fluid may be indicated to rule out potential differential diagnoses, including infectious and neoplastic disorders. Bacterial culture of transtracheal wash and/or bronchoalveolar lavage generally reveals no significant growth.

Thoracic radiography is a more valuable tool than cytologic evaluation of respiratory secretions for diagnosis and monitoring disease in most instances of interstitial pneumonia. Characteristic radiographic findings include diffuse interstitial infiltration with discrete and diffuse nodularity (Fig. 19.3). The degree of radiographic changes may not correlate with the severity of respiratory compromise, and prognosis should ultimately be determined via histopathologic evaluation of lung biopsy.

Lung biopsy is the most reliable diagnostic aid to definitively diagnose interstitial pneumonia and determine the extent of pulmonary fibrosis. The technique for percutaneous lung biopsy is described in Chapter 20. In the acute phase of disease, there is alveolar septal necrosis, fibrin exudation, and hyaline membrane formation within alveolar spaces. With chronicity, the alveolar walls and supporting stroma become affected, and type II pneumocytes proliferate, producing loss of the functional alveolar-capillary unit. Interstitial inflammation is often granulomatous in the subacute stages of disease and eventually progresses (irreversibly) to pulmonary fibrosis.

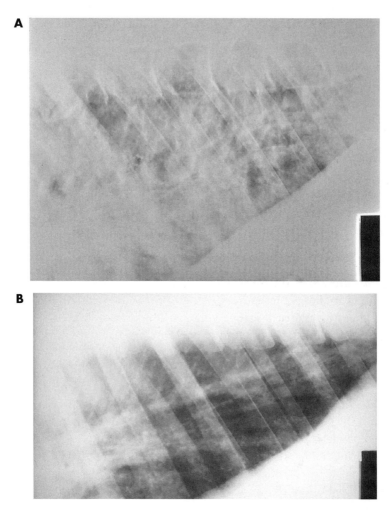

**Fig. 19.3.** Lateral thoracic radiographs of the caudodorsal lung fields from two horses with interstitial pneumonia. A. Marked interstitial pattern from a horse with pulmonary fibrosis. B. Interstitial and miliary pattern from a horse with pulmonary fibrosis and interstitial granuloma formation.

Horses with interstitial pneumonia are generally unresponsive to antimicrobial and nonsteroidal anti-inflammatory therapy. Treatment with corticosteroids, dimethyl sulfoxide, and furosemide is also ineffective unless instituted early in the disease process. Treatment with corticosteroids and nonsteroidal anti-inflammatory therapy should be attempted in horses with acute or subacute interstitial pneumonia based on lung biopsy. The prognosis for return to athletic function is very poor, regardless of the etiology or stage of disease. The prognosis for survival is poor in horses with cyanosis, cor pulmonale, and/or pulmonary fibrosis.

Development of interstitial pneumonia after intravenous administration of purified mycobacterial cell wall extract (nonspecific immunostimulant) has been reported in four horses. The clinical signs include cough, fever, tachypnea, lethargy, and leukocytosis. The pulmonary lesion is progressive, multifocal granulomatous pneumonitis, bronchiolitis, and pulmonary fibrosis. Thoracic radiographic examination reveals diffuse interstitial infiltrate, and cytologic examination of bronchoalveolar lavage fluid reveals lymphocytic inflammation. A marked local reaction can be elicited by intradermal injection of mycobacterial cell wall extract in affected horses.

Silicosis is a form of interstitial pneumonia in horses caused by inhalation of particulate inorganic silicon dioxide. The majority of horses with pulmonary silicosis originate from the Monterey-Carmel Peninsula of midcoastal California. Definitive diagnosis is determined by identification of intracytoplasmic silicate crystals in alveolar macrophages on cytologic evaluation of respiratory secretions. Transtracheal aspiration has been used more frequently than BAL to diagnose silicosis in horses; however, serial transtracheal aspirates may be required to identify the characteristic intracellular crystals. Cytologic evaluation of BAL fluid has been used for identification of silicate crystals and is a more sensitive procedure for diagnosis of pulmonary silicosis. Thoracic radiographic examination reveals a marked interstitial pattern with miliary, reticulonodular, or linear patterns. Lung biopsy or necropsy evaluation is characterized by multifocal, granulomatous pneumonia with areas of pulmonary fibrosis. The prognosis for survival is poor.

## LUNGWORMS

The lungworm, *Dictyocaulus arnfeldi*, produces clinical signs of lower airway obstruction in horses that may be indistinguishable from heaves:

- Coughing and lower airway obstruction are common clinical findings.
- Patent infections are rare in adult horses.
- Larvae may be identified in respiratory secretions.
- Diagnosis may be based on a combination of historical exposure to the natural host and eosinophilic pulmonary inflammation.
- Ivermectin is an effective anthelmintic for treatment of lungworms.

Lungworm infestation should be suspected in cases of a "herd outbreak" of heaves in horses with historical exposure to donkeys and/or donkey crosses. Mules, asses, and donkeys are the natural hosts of *D. arnfeldi* and rarely develop clinical evidence of infestation. Coughing is a prominent feature of the disease and clinical evidence of lower airway obstruction (expiratory difficulty) is common. Clinical signs of disease are typically observed in late summer and early fall in geographic areas with cold winter months.

Horses with lungworm infestation may have peripheral eosinophilia, and eosinophils are the predominant inflammatory cell type in BAL fluid or transtracheal aspirates. Eosinophilic BAL fluid is not pathognomonic for lungworm infections; however, identification of eosinophilia should prompt the clinician

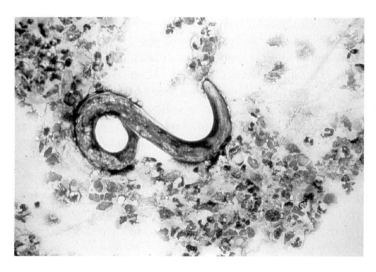

**Fig. 19.4.** Lungworm larvae identified during cytologic evaluation of a bronchoalveolar lavage sample from a horse infested with *Dictyocaulus arnfeldi*. Wright-Giemsa stain, 140x.

to determine exposure to donkeys and mules and perform Baermann fecal examination on the patient and potential reservoir hosts. Larvae may be observed in respiratory secretions (Fig. 19.4) from horses with lungworms and provide definitive evidence of infestation. Adult horses rarely develop a patent infection (2%); therefore, negative findings on Baermann fecal examination does not preclude a diagnosis of lungworms. Foals may develop a patent lungworm infection, in the absence of clinical signs. Eosinophilic pneumonitis is an important differential diagnosis (see the next section "Inflammatory Airway Disease (IAD)") for horses with peripheral eosinophilia and eosinophilic inflammation in respiratory secretions. Ivermectin (200 µg/kg PO) is effective against both mature and immature stages of the parasite and is the drug of choice for treatment of donkeys and horses with lungworm infection.

## INFLAMMATORY AIRWAY DISEASE (IAD)

Inflammatory airway disease (IAD) occurs in 22–50% of Thoroughbred and Standardbred racehorses, and is a common cause of impaired performance and interruption of training:

- Inflammatory airway disease is a common cause of exercise intolerance in racehorses and pleasure-performance horses.
- Physical examination findings of IAD-affected horses at rest are mild to undetectable.
- Inflammatory airway disease likely represents a clinical syndrome resulting from multiple etiologies.

The terms *lower respiratory tract inflammation (LRTI)* and *small airway inflammatory disease (SAID)* have also been used to describe the condition. The most common clinical signs in horses with IAD are chronic cough and mucoid to mucopurulent nasal discharge. Fever and auscultable pulmonary abnormalities are rarely observed. Horses with IAD demonstrate poor exercise tolerance at race speed and perform several seconds slower than previous performances. Endoscopic examination reveals mucopurulent exudate in the pharynx, trachea, and bronchi. Identification of excess mucus in large airways is associated with poor race performance and low arterial oxygen tension during maximal exercise. Thoracic radiographic examination in horses with IAD may reveal mild to moderate bronchial, bronchointerstitial, or interstitial pulmonary patterns; however, the severity of diffuse pulmonary disease in racehorses is poorly correlated to radiographic findings.

Proposed etiologies of IAD in racehorses include allergic airway disease, recurrent pulmonary stress, deep inhalation of particulate matter, noxious gases ($H_2S$, $NH_3$), atmospheric pollutants (ozone), and/or persistent respiratory viral infections. Chronic IAD often develops following overt viral respiratory tract infection and may result from inability of the immune system to fully eliminate virus or bacteria from small airways. *Streptococcus pneumoniae* has been isolated from horses with IAD; however, the role of *S. pneumoniae* in the pathophysiology is unclear, because this population of horses is largely unresponsive (or transiently responsive) to antibiotic therapy.

## Diagnosis

Diagnosis of IAD is based on poor race performance, clinical signs of mild respiratory disease, and identification of mucopurulent exudates in the trachea and bronchi (Fig. 19.5):

- Endoscopic identification of exudate in the lower airway indicates that IAD is likely present.
- Bronchoalveolar lavage confirms the diagnosis and identifies the inflammatory cell type, which directs the therapeutic plan.

Bronchoalveolar lavage should be performed to characterize the type of inflammation present in the lung. The protocol for performing BAL appears in Chapter 20 . Cytologic evaluation of BAL fluid in horses with IAD will reveal one of the following inflammatory profiles:

- Mixed inflammation with high total nucleated cells, mild neutrophilia (15% of total cells), lymphocytosis, and monocytosis (Fig. 19.6A)
- Eosinophilic inflammation (5–40% of total cells) (Fig. 19.6B)
- Increased metachromatic cells (mast cells >2% of total cells) (Fig. 19.6C)

High total nucleated cell count in BAL fluid is associated with arterial hypoxemia during maximal exercise, and the degree of exercise intensity is positively correlated to the degree of increase in nucleated cell count.

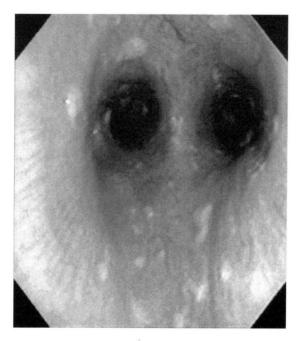

**Fig. 19.5.** Endoscopic examination of the distal trachea and carina from a horse with inflammatory airway disease and excessive mucus in the lower respiratory tract.

A

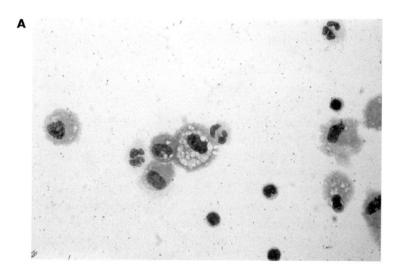

**Fig. 19.6.** Bronchoalveolar lavage cytology from horses with inflammatory airway disease, illustrating the three inflammatory cytologic profiles. A. Mixed inflammatory profile with 15% of total cell count neutrophils.

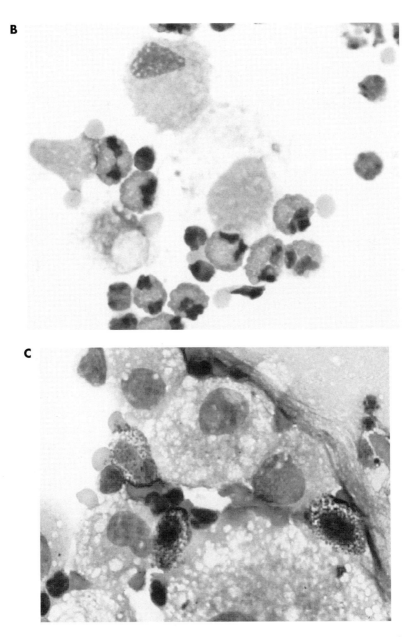

**Fig. 19.6.** *(continued)* B. Eosinophilic inflammation with 60% of total cell count eosinophils. C. Metachromatic inflammation with 5% of total cell count mast cells. Note the activated, vacuolated macrophages with mast cell inflammation. Wright-Giemsa stain, 168x. *(See also color section.)*

**Treatment**

The type of inflammation in BAL fluid from horses with IAD will dictate the therapeutic plan:

- The most appropriate treatment for horses with IAD is dependent on cytologic evaluation of BAL fluid.
- A mixed inflammatory cytologic profile is treated with immunostimulant or immunomodulatory drugs.
- An eosinophilic or mast cell cytologic profile is treated with a combination of anti-inflammatory or immunosuppressive drugs.

In horses with a mixed inflammatory cytologic profile, administration of low-dose natural human interferon-alpha reduces exudate in the respiratory tract, lowers total cell counts in BAL fluid, and converts the differential cell count to a noninflammatory cytologic profile. Interferon-alpha (IFN-alpha) is a proximal mediator of immunomodulation and antiviral activity. The specific mechanism of therapeutic benefit of IFN-alpha in horses with IAD is unknown. The pathway for dissemination of the biologic effects—with oral administration—may be activation of natural defense systems originating in oropharyngeal-associated lymphoid tissue that involves cellular communication and amplification of the biologic response. Lymphocytes exposed to IFN-alpha can transfer enhanced biologic effects to naive lymphocytes in the absence of IFN-alpha. It is hypothesized that lymphocytes recruited to antiviral activity by IFN-alpha in the oral cavity can enter the circulation and rapidly confer antiviral capability to cells at distant sites. The process would not require continued presence of IFN-alpha and may represent a major amplification mechanism. This mechanism allows the biologic effects of IFN-alpha to reach tissues accessible to mobile lymphocytes, in which penetration of IFN-alpha might be poor, such as the surface of the respiratory tract, gastrointestinal tract, and the eye.

Clinical signs observed in horses with eosinophilic BAL fluid are indistinguishable from those in other IAD-affected horses. Eosinophilic BAL fluid is associated with poor exercise performance, high total nucleated BAL fluid cell counts, and airway hyper-responsiveness, and may be accompanied by systemic eosinophilia. The pathophysiology of pulmonary inflammation likely represents an immune-mediated pulmonary response consistent with Type I hypersensitivity reaction. Affected horses typically have a moderate to strong interstitial pattern on thoracic radiography (Fig. 19.7), and eosinophilic pulmonary granulomas are often identified at post-mortem examination of horses with pulmonary eosinophilia. If eosinophilic BAL fluid is identified, the clinician should investigate parasitic pulmonary disease, including ascarid migration and lungworm infection, in addition to hypersensitivity pneumonitis. Horses with eosinophilic BAL fluid do not respond favorably to IFN-alpha therapy. Aerosolized corticosteroid administration is recommended for horses with eosinophilic BAL fluid; however, this treatment has not yet been investi-

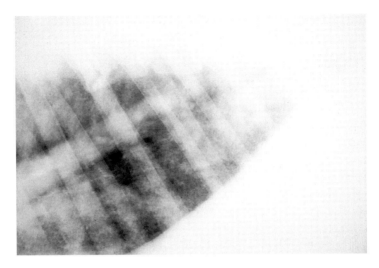

**Fig. 19.7.** Lateral thoracic radiograph of the caudodorsal lung fields of a horse with eosinophilic pneumonitis. Note the diffuse interstitial pattern with coalescing miliary densities consistent with granuloma formation.

gated under conditions of a controlled, randomized clinical trial in racehorses. In this author's experience, eosinophilic pneumonitis responds slowly and incompletely to immunosuppressive therapy.

Diagnosis of metachromatic inflammation requires identification of >2% of the total cell count as mast cells. Clinical signs include poor race performance, chronic cough, and airway hyperreactivity. Identification of mast cells in BAL fluid cytologic preparations is facilitated by use of cationic dyes, such as toluidine blue stain. Mast cells are thought to play an important role in the pathophysiology of early-stage allergic lung disease in humans through release of inflammatory mediators following antigen exposure. Metachromatic inflammation likely represents a local pulmonary hypersensitivity response and may represent an early form of recurrent airway obstruction. In IAD-affected horses with elevated metachromatic cells in BAL fluid, aerosol administration of sodium cromoglycate (200 μg/day) or nedocromil sodium improves the clinical signs of respiratory disease and stabilizes mast cell histamine release.

## EXERCISE-INDUCED PULMONARY HEMORRHAGE (EIPH)

Exercise-induced pulmonary hemorrhage (EIPH) occurs in the majority of racehorses and is observed sporadically in many other sports that require strenuous exercise for short periods of time:

- EIPH is suspected to occur in the vast majority of horses that perform at maximal speed.

- Hemorrhage originates from the pulmonary vascular system.
- Investigators and clinicians do not agree on the effect of EIPH on exercise performance.

Epistaxis occurs only in a small proportion (approximately 5%) of horses with EIPH. Blood in the tracheobronchial tree is identified in 44–75% of racehorses via endoscopic examination, and hemorrhage is detected by cytologic examination of bronchoalveolar lavage in 93% of racehorses. The condition has been identified in three-day event horses, polo ponies, barrel racing horses, and pulling horses, but has not been observed in horses performing low-intensity endurance events. Investigators agree that the incidence of EIPH in racehorses is high, however, the pathophysiology, therapeutic approach, and impact on race performance is controversial. Horseman and track veterinarians generally believe EIPH adversely affects performance, and one epidemiologic investigation demonstrated positive correlation between poor finishing position and endoscopic identification of blood in the airway. However, most investigations fail to identify a direct relationship between pulmonary hemorrhage and poor race performance. Conflicting data regarding the impact of EIPH on race performance may reflect the difficulty in defining performance and individual performance potential.

Proposed pathophysiologic mechanisms for pulmonary hemorrhage include high pulmonary vascular pressures during maximal exercise, neovascularization secondary to pulmonary inflammation, coagulation dysfunction, and intrathoracic shear forces generated during running. Some research suggests that EIPH is a physiologic process, rather than a pathologic process, resulting from failure of the pulmonary system to accommodate a massive increase in cardiac output to meet the demands of high intensity exercise.

Rapid acceleration to high-intensity exercise results in equally rapid increases in pulmonary arterial and capillary pressures. Pulmonary capillary pressures are suspected to exceed the capacity of the pulmonary system to maintain vascular integrity, resulting in "stress failure" of capillaries and hemorrhage from the pulmonary vascular system. Several studies have confirmed that the source of hemorrhage originates from the pulmonary vascular system and have demonstrated stress failure of pulmonary capillaries, including disruption of capillary endothelium and alveolar epithelium, accumulation of red blood cells in the alveolar wall interstitium and alveolar spaces, and interstitial edema. High pulmonary capillary pressures are suspected to result from failure to accommodate massive increases in cardiac output, high left-atrial pressures, and poor compliance of the left ventricle. An extension of the stress failure theory is disruption of capillaries due to shear stress within pulmonary tissue resulting from compression of the chest by the forelimbs during maximal exercise.

Some investigators believe EIPH occurs secondary to IAD. It is proposed that a focus of pulmonary inflammation, secondary to infectious disease, results in proliferation of vessels originating from bronchial circulation. The region of neovascularization is suspected to be fragile and prone to rupture during maximal exercise. However, this cause-and-effect relationship between pulmonary hemorrhage and inflammation may be misinterpreted. Instillation of autologous blood into the pulmonary parenchyma initiates an inflammatory response characterized by airway hyperreactivity, parenchymal fibrosis, and parenchymal inflammation. Repeated episodes of EIPH may create self-perpetuating lower respiratory tract inflammation and hemorrhage. It has been recently proposed that pulmonary capillaries rupture as the result of high pulmonary vascular pressures, and blood in the pulmonary parenchyma initiates airway inflammation, bronchiolitis, and proliferation of bronchial circulation. Lower respiratory tract inflammation and bronchial novascularization may be the result—rather than the cause—of EIPH.

## Diagnosis

In most instances of EIPH, pulmonary hemorrhage originates in the caudodorsal lung fields, and although EIPH is not a diffuse pulmonary disease, BAL remains a useful diagnostic technique:

- Endoscopic examination is performed 30–90 minutes after exercise; however, failure to identify blood in the airway does not preclude a diagnosis of EIPH.
- Thoracic radiography demonstrates alveolar or mixed alveolar-interstitial opacities in the caudodorsal lung fields.
- Identification of hemosiderin-laden macrophages via BAL aids in the diagnosis, but may overestimate the number of affected horses.
- Quantitative evaluation of red blood cells in BAL fluid after exercise is arguably the most reliable technique to document disease severity.

The protocol for performing BAL appears in Chapter 20. Blind passage usually wedges the lavage catheter in the right caudodorsal lung fields. Identification of hemosiderin-laden macrophages via cytologic evaluation of BAL fluid (Fig. 19.8) is more sensitive for documentation of pulmonary hemorrhage than endoscopic visualization of blood in the airway after exercise (Fig. 19.9). Serial endoscopic examinations improve the ability to detect pulmonary hemorrhage, but there is no correlation between the amount of visible hemorrhage in the trachea, the percentage of hemosiderophages on cytologic examination, or the concentration of red blood cells in BAL fluid. The optimal time for identification of EIPH via endoscopic examination is 30–90 minutes after exercise, whereas the time period between breezing and diagnostic BAL is not critical. Some degree of hemosiderin-laden macrophages can be identified in BAL fluid from nearly all racehorses; therefore, merely observing the presence or absence of hemosiderin in alveolar macrophages will overestimate the number of EIPH-positive horses. Determination of the number of red blood cells in BAL fluid has improved the ability to objectively determine the severity of pulmonary hemorrhage.

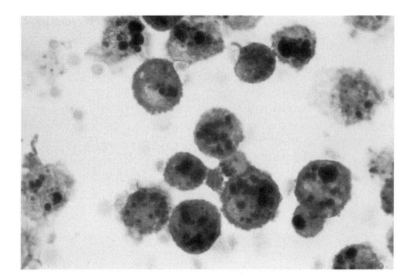

**Fig. 19.8.** Bronchoalveolar lavage cytology from a horse with exercise-induced pulmonary hemorrhage demonstrating hemosiderin-laden macrophages. Perl's Prussian Blue stain, 140x. *(See also color section.)*

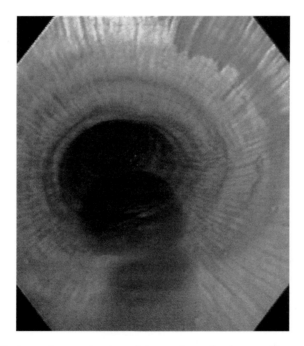

**Fig. 19.9.** Endoscopic examination of the trachea of a horse with exercise-induced pulmonary hemorrhage. *(See also color section.)*

Radiographic examination of the thorax appears to have little impact on the diagnosis or management of EIPH (Fig. 19.10) In horses with well-documented EIPH, thoracic radiography occasionally demonstrates alveolar or mixed alveolar-interstitial opacities in the caudodorsal lung fields.

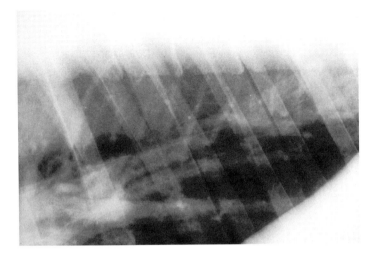

**Fig. 19.10.** Lateral thoracic radiograph of the caudodorsal lung fields of a horse with exercise-induced pulmonary hemorrhages. Note the area of pulmonary consolidation consistent with the site of hemorrhage.

## Treatment

Furosemide has been advocated for treatment of EIPH for more than 20 years, and its use preceded identification of the lung as the site of hemorrhage:

- Furosemide appears to decrease the severity of hemorrhage.
- Furosemide may be performance-enhancing, via mechanisms unrelated to EIPH.
- Nasal dilator bands reduce red blood cell counts in BAL fluid by 33%.
- Alternative treatments have failed to demonstrate therapeutic benefit.

Furosemide does not appear to prevent pulmomary hemorrhage, but there is increasing evidence that it reduces the severity of hemorrhage in a given episode. Several investigators have demonstrated a reduction in red blood cell counts in BAL after furosemide administration. Improved race performance (approximately 1 second) has been demonstrated with furosemide administration; however, it has not been definitively determined that improved performance is due to reduction in pulmonary hemorrhage. Horses with and without EIPH demonstrate equal improvements in race performance after furosemide administration, therefore, furosemide may be performance-enhancing, via mechanisms unrelated to EIPH status.

The mechanism of enhanced performance with furosemide is unknown. Furosemide decreases pulmonary arterial, pulmonary artery wedge, and pulmonary capillary pressures. It is likely that the hemodynamic effects of furosemide are dependent on reduction of plasma and blood volumes. Lower pulmonary vascular pressures should lower the transmural force exerted across pulmonary capillary walls. Reduced pulmonary capillary pressure is suspected to be beneficial in reducing volume of hemorrhage in horses with EIPH. Reduction of pulmonary vascular pressures is suspected to be prostenoid-mediated ($PGE_2$); however, definitive evidence has not been demonstrated. Because the therapeutic effect of furosemide is hypothesized to be prostenoid-mediated, concurrent administration of non-steroidal anti-inflammatory drugs may negate the beneficial effect. There are conflicting results regarding inhibition of beneficial effects with concurrent administration of nonsteroidal anti-inflammatory drugs, and further investigation is indicated.

Alternative treatments have been investigated including procoagulant agents (vitamin K, oxalic acid, conjugated estrogens, aminocaproic acid), antihypertensive drugs (enalapril, nitric oxide donors/analogues), rheologic agents (pentoxyphylline), bronchodilators (clenbuterol, albuterol, ipratropium), and anti-inflammatory drugs (corticosteroids, cromolyn sodium). None of these treatments have demonstrated therapeutic benefit in horses with EIPH. In addition, prolonged periods of rest from strenuous exercise have not reduced the severity of bleeding in affected horses. Dietary supplements (hepseridin-citrus bioflavinoids) to improve capillary strength have not been successful in reducing the severity of EIPH or enhancing performance.

Corticosteroids may be the most likely alternative therapy to benefit horses with EIPH. Lower respiratory tract inflammation, bronchiolitis, and bronchial neovascularization may result from repeated episodes of EIPH. Repeated episodes may create self-perpetuating lower respiratory tract inflammation and hemorrhage. Administration of corticosteroids via aerosolization allows local delivery of anti-inflammatory therapy to the pulmonary system while minimizing systemic side effects. Although corticosteroids will not prevent pulmonary capillary rupture during exercise, they may prevent or reduce the airway inflammation, airway hyperreactivity, and neovascularization that accompanies EIPH.

Application of nasal dilator bands (Flair Strip, CNS, Inc.) has been demonstrated to reduce red blood cell counts in BAL fluid from affected horses by 33%. The strip is purported to stabilize unsupported tissue overlying the area between the nostril and the nasomaxillary notch. This tissue is suspected to collapse during inspiration at high flow rates, creating higher negative inspiratory pressures, and increasing the airway component of transmural pressure. Furosemide has considerable greater efficacy for reduction in BAL fluid red cell counts than the nasal dilator strip.

It is unlikely that an ideal therapeutic agent for EIPH (eliminate pulmonary hemorrhage without impairing race performance) will be developed until the pathogenesis of disease is understood. At this point, it appears that EIPH results from "stress failure" of the pulmonary vascular system, and the presence of blood in the pulmonary parenchyma stimulates a self-perpetuating inflammatory response. Given the universal occurrence of EIPH in horses that exert a maximal level of effort, it is unlikely that a single agent will completely eliminate the problem in horses that perform high-intensity exercise.

## THORACIC NEOPLASIA

Neoplasia of the thoracic cavity is rare (<1% of cases of respiratory disease), and is most commonly reported in older horses:

- The clinical signs of thoracic neoplasia are dependent on tumor location and cell type.
- Mediastinal tumors present with clinical signs reflecting large volume pleural effusion, such as rapid, shallow respiration and pectoral edema.
- Intrapulmonary tumors present with exercise intolerance, weight loss, cough, and potentially epistaxis.
- Lameness, due to bone infiltration and lysis, is frequently observed in horses with metastatic pulmonary neoplasia.

Thoracic neoplasias are divided into mediastinal and intrapulmonary tumors. Intrapulmonary tumors are usually metastatic in origin, whereas primary pulmonary neoplasias are exceedingly uncommon. Mediastinal neoplasia may be metastatic or primary.

Lymphoma is the most common mediastinal tumor and accounts for approximately 50% of thoracic neoplasia. Multisystemic involvement is common in horses with mediastinal lymphoma; however, the most obvious clinical signs are associated with the mediastinal mass. There are many single case studies reporting a wide variety of thoracic neoplasms; however, squamous cell carcinoma, melanoma, fibrosarcoma, and hemangiosarcoma appear to be the most common metastatic mediastinal/pleural cavity tumors. Mediastinal neoplasms often produce a large volume of malignant pleural effusion. Therefore, presenting clinical signs are likely to reflect large volume effusion, such as rapid and shallow respiration, tachycardia, weight loss, pectoral edema, and distended jugular veins. Thoracic auscultation reveals muffled heart and lung sounds in the ventral lung fields, and ultrasonographic examination reveals a large volume of hypoechoic fluid with minimal cellularity and few fibrin tags. Pleural fluid recovered from horses with mediastinal neoplasia will appear straw-colored and transluscent to slightly serosanguinous, with the exception of hemangiosarcoma, in which the pleural fluid is often hemorrhagic. Neoplastic effusions typically have low to moderate cellularity (5,000–40,000 cells/μl) characterized by reactive mesothelial cells, lymphocytes and macrophages, and a high total protein (3.5–6.5 mg/dl). Some mediastinal tumors may be exfoliative, and neoplastic cells are readily apparent on cytologic evaluation (melanoma, squamous cell carcinoma, hemangiosarcoma). The absence of neoplastic cells in malignant effusions, however, is not uncommon.

Granular cell myoblastoma is the most common primary intrapulmonary tumor, although adenocarcinoma and bronchogenic carcinoma have been reported in horses. Granular cell myoblastoma is of mesenchymal origin derived from myoblasts. Presenting clinical signs include paroxysmal cough and exer-

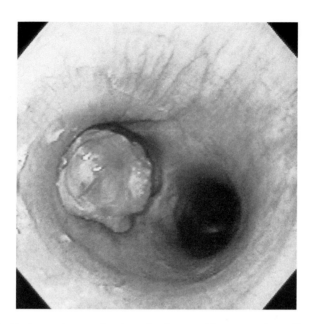

**Fig. 19.11.** Endoscopic examination of a horse with a granular cell myoblastoma. The tumor obstructs the entire right mainstem bronchus.

cise intolerance. Pulmonary auscultation is unremarkable. The tumor usually consists of multiple, well-defined nodules associated with a major bronchus, and a portion of the mass may be seen on endoscopic examination of the carina (Fig. 19.11). The majority of the mass is intrapulmonary and often involves the cranial lung lobes. Thoracic radiographs may reveal cranioventral opacity. Other intrapulmonary neoplasms are likely metastatic and originate from adenocarcinoma (renal, ovarian, thyroid), melanoma, or undifferentiated sarcoma. Examination of other body systems may reveal evidence of multisystemic infiltration or may identify the primary neoplastic mass. Definitive diagnosis of intrapulmonary neoplasia is determined by cytologic evaluation of bronchoalveolar lavage fluid or histopathologic evaluation of endoscopic or percutaneous lung biopsy. Granular cell tumors have been treated by lung lobe resection; however there is no successful treatment for metastatic intrapulmonary neoplasia.

Pulmonary neoplasia can be a primary predisposing condition for development of hypertrophic osteopathy (Marie's disease, hypertrophic pulmonary osteoarthropathy) in horses. The syndrome is characterized by symmetric proliferation of subperiosteal bone along the diaphyses and metaphyses of long bones of the appendicular skeleton. Affected horses have symmetric, firm limb swelling of all four limbs and shifting leg lameness. The pathophysiology of bony proliferation is unclear; however, hormonal, hemodynamic, and neurogenic theories have been proposed. Intrathoracic disease is present in the majority of cases of hypertrophic osteopathy and should be investigated in horses displaying these unusual clinical signs.

## SMOKE INHALATION

Smoke inhalation produces edema, congestion, and necrosis of both the upper and lower respiratory tract:

- Smoke inhalation injury is the major cause of death among fire victims, and is a stronger determinant of mortality than severity of cutaneous burns.
- Smoke inhalation damages both the upper and lower respiratory tracts via thermal and chemical (toxic) mechanisms.
- There are three stages in the progression of disease: acute pulmonary insufficiency, pulmonary edema, and bronchopneumonia.

Upper respiratory tract injury primarily results from thermal injury due to inhalation of air and particles heated to 150°C. Thermal damage to the lower respiratory tract is less common, but can occur due to inhalation of super-heated particles (<5 μm). The majority of lower respiratory tract damage results from inhalation of toxic chemicals. The severity of lower airway injury is dependent on duration of exposure, solubility of the chemicals, and size of the chemicals in smoke. Highly water-soluble gases—such as aldehydes, ammonia, chlorine, hydrogen chloride, and sulfur dioxide—produce rapid pulmonary injury, whereas insoluble gases—nitrogen and phosgene oxide—cause delayed pulmonary injury. Carbon monoxide toxicity, common with smoke inhalation, does not cause direct airway damage, but exacerbates tissue hypoxia by impairing oxygen delivery and utilization.

Clinical signs of respiratory injury are often immediate; however, some horses may not exhibit signs for 2–3 days and should remain under close observation for at least 72 hours. There are three stages to the progression of smoke inhalation injury: acute pulmonary insufficiency, pulmonary edema, and bronchopneumonia. Acute pulmonary insufficiency occurs during the first 36 hours, and is attributed to thermal injury to the upper respiratory tract (6–18 hours after exposure), carbon monoxide toxicity (immediate), and chemical injury to the tracheobronchial tree and parenchymal tissue. Thermal injury to the upper respiratory tract peaks at 18–24 hours after exposure, and may result in upper airway edema to the point of obstruction (inspiratory stridor) necessitating emergency tracheotomy. Carbon monoxide toxicity is difficult to detect clinically because blood remains a bright red color (carboxyhemoglobin); therefore, the clinician must anticipate carbon monoxide toxicity in smoke inhalation patients. Irritation from soluble gases causes bronchoconstriction, mucosal edema of central airways, and degradation of pulmonary surfactant.

The second stage of inhalation injury begins at approximately 24 hours, and is characterized by pulmonary edema, which develops as a result of the inflammatory response initiated by chemical injury. Clinical signs include tachypnea, dyspnea, paroxysmal coughing, and nasal discharge. Increased pulmonary microvascular permeability results via release of cytotoxic, vasoactive, and chemotaxic factors from injured tissue and release of oxygen-free radicals.

In instances of severe mucosal injury, a psuedomembranous cast, consisting of cellular debris, fibrin, and proteinaceous exudate, may form in large- to medium-sized airways at 24–72 hours. Necrotizing bronchiolitis, intraalveolar hemorrhage, thrombus formation, pneumothorax, and massive pulmonary edema are potential sequelae. The presence of subcutaneous emphysema indicates pneumothorax and/or pneumomediastinum due to ruptured pulmonary bullus.

The third stage of smoke inhalation injury is bronchopneumonia, which may develop as early as 5–7 days after exposure; however, the window of opportunity for development of bacterial infection may last up to 2 weeks. The primary predisposing factor is impaired pulmonary defense mechanisms, including loss of mucociliary clearance, impaired alveolar macrophage function, and denuded respiratory epithelium. Clinical signs include continued cough and nasal discharge and development of fever and depression.

## Diagnosis

Endoscopic examination of the upper and lower respiratory tract is the most sensitive indicator of smoke inhalation injury. Thoracic radiography may be useful to monitor progression of pulmonary edema and consolidation, detect development of bronchopneumonia, and identify pneumothorax or pneumomediastinum. Thoracic radiography may also identify pulmonary fibrosis and scarring in patients that have suffered severe inhalation injury several months after recovery. Serial blood gas analysis can be performed to monitor respiratory function, and carboxyhemoglobin concentrations should be determined to detect carbon monoxide toxicity. Transtracheal wash may be performed during the bronchopneumonia (third) stage of smoke inhalation injury to identify opportunistic pathogens. *Pasteurella, Streptococcus,* and *Pseudomonas* spp are common isolates in horses with smoke inhalation injury.

## Treatment

Treatment for horses with smoke inhalation injury includes the following:

- Supplemental oxygen to facilitate gas exchange and combat carbon dioxide toxicity
- Tracheostomy to create a patent airway in horses with severe upper airway damage
- Bronchodilation with systemic or aerosolized bronchodilators
- Furosemide administered in patients demonstrating signs of pulmonary edema
- Although controversial, administration of corticosteroids, prophylactic antibiotics, and intravenous fluid therapy

Supplemental oxygen is indicated in horses with smoke inhalation injury to facilitate removal of carbon monoxide and improve pulmonary gas exchange. Fractional concentrations of 40% oxygen can be achieved with flow rates of

50–100 ml/kg. Administration of greater than 50% oxygen for more than 24 hours may exacerbate pulmonary damage. Tracheostomy may be necessary in horses with severe injury/edema of the upper airway. Indication for tracheostomy is determined by the presence of a marked inspiratory stidor. In addition to providing a patent airway, tracheostomy may facilitate removal of fibinous casts from the lower respiratory tract.

Bronchodilator therapy should be administered as early as possible (stage 1 bronchoconstriction) to horses with smoke inhalation injury. In addition to bronchodilation, ß$_2$ agonists stimulate surfactant production and combat pulmonary edema by stimulating active sodium transport within the alveolar epithelium, which is the primary mechanism driving alveolar fluid clearance. Aerosolized albuterol is the most powerful, rapid-acting bronchodilator and should be paired with a long-acting aerosolized (salmeterol) or oral (clenbuterol) ß$_2$ agonists. The majority of bronchoconstriction associated with smoke inhalation injury is vagally mediated; therefore, addition of a parasympatholytic agent is valuable. Atropine can be administered in an emergency, single-dose basis, and aerosolized ipratropium can be used for subsequent maintenance therapy.

Furosemide (1–2 mg/kg) will reduce pulmonary edema via diuretic and non-diuretic mechanisms and is indicated upon development of clinical signs of pulmonary edema. Fluid, electrolyte, and acid-base balance should be monitored with repeated administration of furosemide.

Corticosteroid therapy has been used successfully in equine patients with smoke inhalation injury to combat pulmonary edema and maintain surfactant production. However, the immunosuppressive effects of corticosteroids may unnecessarily predispose patients to bronchopneumonia, and studies in humans and animals with smoke inhalation have failed to identify therapeutic benefit of corticosteroid administration. Corticosteroids appear to be particularly detrimental in patients with surface burns, and therefore, use should be limited to patients with smoke inhalation injury alone. Dimethyl sulfoxide has demonstrated therapeutic benefit in some smoke inhalation patients and is thought to reduce inflammation and edema via free-radical scavenging. Nonsteroidal anti-inflammatory drugs may be an alternative to corticosteroids to reduce pulmonary inflammation.

Intravenous fluid therapy in patients with smoke inhalation is controversial. Clinicians must strike a careful balance between maintaining adequate plasma volume for the shocky patient and exacerbating pulmonary edema during phase 1 injury. Intravenous fluid therapy is now considered an essential component of treatment in human patients with severe pulmonary injury and cardiovascular shock, and intravenous fluid therapy has been successfully used in equine patients with severe smoke inhalation injury.

Prophylactic antibiotic therapy is particularly controversial. Indiscriminant prophylactic use of antibiotics in human patients leads to the development of resistant strains of bacteria and has not reduced mortality in burn patients. Nonetheless, most equine clinicians consider administration of prophylactic antibiotics standard care in equine patients with severe pulmonary injury, and particularly in cases requiring tracheostomy.

The long-term prognosis for horses with smoke inhalation injury is uncertain. Some horses appear to recover uneventfully without detectable evidence of pulmonary impairment, whereas other horses suffer from chronic exercise intolerance due to pulmonary fibrosis and bronchoconstriction.

## IMMUNOSTIMULANT THERAPY

The primary indication for immunostimulant administration to horses is treatment of chronic, bacterial or viral respiratory infection:

- Immunostimulants are indicated for treatment of chronic, low-grade respiratory infections rather than acute, fulminant infection.
- Exogenous immunostimulant preparations are derived from bacterial, viral, or plant sources.
- Mechanism of action of exogenous products is macrophage activation and production of cytokines, which induce a strong Th1-biased immune response.
- Immunostimulant activity of killed bacterial products may be triggered by repetitive sequences (CpG motifs) of bacterial DNA.

The indications for immunostimulant therapy in horses are relatively specific, and these compounds are not intended to treat a broad spectrum of respiratory conditions. The proposed mechanism of action of nonspecific immunostimulation is activation of macrophages to induce production of proinflammatory cytokines. Immunostimulant therapy may not be effective in patients with acute, fulminant infections, because the immune response is likely maximally stimulated by the pathogens. Horses with primary immunodeficiency syndromes, such as severe combined immunodeficiency syndrome of Arabian foals, are incapable of responding to immunostimulant therapy. Immunostimulant therapy is indicated in horses with chronic bacterial or viral respiratory infections due to immunosuppression or immunotolerance to the organism. Prophylactic administration of immunostimulant preparations prior to stressful events—such as weaning or long-distance transportation—may decrease morbidity and mortality associated with acute infection. The benchmark of nonspecific immunomodulation is protection against a 50% lethal bacterial challenge in laboratory animals.

The majority of veterinary immunostimulants are relatively crude, exogenous immunostimulants derived from bacterial, viral, or plant sources. Immunostimulant particles are phagocytized by macrophages, which induces cellular activation and cytokine production, particularly IFN-alpha, IL-1, tumor necrosis factor, and interleukins. Bacterial DNA appears to be responsible for the immunostimulatory effects of bacterial extracts. Unmethylated CpG oligodeoxynucleotides (ODN) are specific, repetitive, DNA sequences, which appear in noncoding sequences of bacterial DNA. These CpG motifs are detected by innate immune defense pattern recognition receptors and trigger a "danger signal," which stimulates immune reponses. Unmethylated CpG motifs induce strong Th1-biased innate and acquired immune responses in murine, bovine, and human immune cells. Purified CpG ODN demonstrate promise as vaccine adjuvant, and eventually may be an important component of antineoplastic and atopic therapies.

Endogenous immunostimulants, such as interferons, interleukins, and growth factors are derived from the mammal genome and are intended to augment the innate immune response. Newer-generation recombinant cytokines have selective effects on specific components of the immune system. Extensive immunopharmacological evaluation of immunomodulatory preparations has revealed that these products demonstrate substantial divergence from conventional pharmacology, particularly in terms of the pharmacodynamics relating to dosage schedules, therapeutic drug concentrations, and biologic activity.

## BACTERIAL AND VIRAL PRODUCTS

Bacterial and viral products include *Propionibacterium acnes* and *mycobacterium*.

### *Propionibacterium acnes*
Inactivated *Propionibacterium acnes* (EqStim, Neogen Inc.) is a popular nonspecific immunostimulant labeled for treatment of chronic respiratory disease:

- Indicated as adjunct therapy for chronic, exudative respiratory disease
- Prophylactic administration recommended prior to stressful events
- Administered intravenously, every 48–72 hours for 3 treatments

Inactivated *Propionibacterium acnes* (EqStim, Neogen Inc.) is a popular nonspecific immunostimulant labeled for treatment of chronic respiratory disease. The *P. acnes* organism was formerly known as *Corynebacterium parvum*, and its immunomodulatory activity has been recognized for more than 30 years. The DNA sequence of *P. acnes* contains repetitive CpG motifs, which may be responsible for its immunostimulatory activity. In laboratory animals, administration of *P. acnes* stimulates macrophage function, natural killer cytotoxicity, and cytokine production (IL-1, IFN-gamma), and provides prophylactic protection against lethal bacterial and viral challenge. Stimulation of systemic immunity can be documented in laboratory animals for 4–5 days after intravenous or intraperitoneal administration; however, prolonged immunostimulant activity is not anticipated.

In equine medicine, *Propionibacterium acnes* is recommended for treatment of chronic, exudative respiratory disease that is unresponsive to conventional antibiotic treatment. In addition, it is recommended for prophylactic administration prior to stressful events that may impair pulmonary defense mechanisms, including weaning and long-distance transport. *Propionibacterium acnes* is considered an adjunct to antibiotic therapy and is labeled for intravenous administration every 2–3 days for three treatments. Clinical signs of naturally occurring, infectious respiratory disease (cough, fever, nasal discharge) improve within 14 days of treatment in 96% of horses treated with *P. acnes*, compared to 35% of horses treated with conventional therapy. Administration of *P. acnes* prior to long distance transport (390–2300 miles) reduces the incidence of infectious respiratory disease from 60.9% in nontreated controls to 18% in treated horses during the 7-day period after shipment (n = 450 horses).

Immunostimulation has been documented after intravenous administration of *P. acnes* in horses. Administration of *P. acnes* to healthy, yearling horses using the recommended dosage regimen increases the number of CD4+ lymphocytes and enhances lymphokine-activated killing activity and nonopsonized phagocytic activity. Total white blood cell count, neutrophil count, and serum fibrinogen concentrations are not affected. Cellularity of bronchoalveolar lavage is reduced after *P. acnes* administration and is predominately related to a reduction in lymphocytes. The reduction in cellularity of bronchoalveolar lavage fluid may reflect migration of pulmonary lymphocytes into adjacent lymphoid tissues or resolution of subclinical infection.

Fever, anorexia, and lethargy may occur 12–24 hours after administration of the first or second injection, presumably due to increased IL-1 production. Therefore, administration is not recommended immediately prior to an athletic event. Subsequent injections usually elicit milder reactions.

In addition to equine respiratory disease, *P. acnes* has been anecdotally recommended for treatment of endometritis, osteomyelitis, papillomatosis, abdominal abscess, fistulous withers, and sarcoid skin tumors. In this author's experience, administration of *P. acnes* is effective for treament of viral papillomatosis, whereas efficacy for treatment of sarcoid skin tumors (intralesional and intravenous) is less consistent.

In humans, *P. acnes* has been used as a sclerosant agent for treatment of malignant pleural effusion. Intrapleural infusion of *Propionibacterium acnes* induces pleurodesis in 90% of the patients, a rate superior to that induced by tetracycline or talc. The volume of effusion is reduced within days of intrapleural infusion, and survival time is prolonged. Prolonged survival has been attributed to stimulation of local antitumor activity, although the effect has not been definitively demonstrated.

## Mycobacterium

Mycobacterial products have long been recognized as potent stimulators of nonspecific immunity:

- Is used as solo therapy in single-dose, intravenous administration for treatment of equine herpesvirus infection

- Improves clinical recovery from respiratory disease resulting from stress, transportation, bacteria and/or viral infections
- May cause adverse pulmonary effects as a result of overzealous administration

The bacillus Calmette-Guerin (BCG) vaccine was developed from a strain of *Mycobacterium bovis* that had been attenuated through serial passage in culture. Live BCG, whole-inactivated BCG, and mycobacterial cell wall fractions have been used as nonspecific immunostimulant agents, and all three preparations demonstrate adjuvancy when administered with antigen. The mechanism of action is macrophage activation and subsequent release of interleukin-1, tumor necrosis factor, and colony stimulating factors. Whole, inactivated BCG preparations induce tuberculin sensitivity; therefore, deproteinized mycobacterial cell wall products (muramyl dipeptide and lipoarabinomannan) have been developed to prevent induction of tuberculin positivity in treated animals. Purified muramyl dipeptides are the smallest subunit of the mycobacterial cell wall that retains immunostimulant activity. In equine medicine, mycobacterial cell wall products are used to treat infectious respiratory disease (Equimune) and sarcoid skin tumors (Regressin).

Purified mycobacterial cell wall extract is labeled for single-dose, intravenous administration, as solo therapy for treatment of equine herpesvirus infection. Administration of purified mycobacterial cell wall extract improves clinical recovery of horses with respiratory disease resulting from stress, transportation, and bacterial and/or viral infections. Response to treatment in a randomized, double-blind investigation was determined by monitoring clinical signs (fever, cough, anorexia, nasal discharge, abnormal auscultation, poor performance) and laboratory indices of inflammation (complete blood count, differential, acute phase protein concentration). Eighty-three percent of the horses treated with mycobacterial cell wall extract became clinically normal within 7 days after administration of a single, intravenous (1.5 ml) dose, whereas only 36% of horses receiving a placebo injection were without clinical signs. Extra-label use of this product in horses has been anecdotally recommended as adjunct therapy for treatment of equine protozoal myelitis.

In human medicine, live BCG immunotherapy is used for treatment of superficial transitional cell carcinoma. Instillation of live BCG organisms into the bladder prevents recurrence or progression of superficial bladder tumors, and the response is superior to intravesical administration of chemotherapeutic agents. Stimulation of both local and systemic immune function has been documented after intravesical BCG therapy in patients with urinary bladder carcinoma. Mycobacterial cell wall fractions have been used to induce hematopoiesis and recover bone marrow function following cancer chemotherapy through macrophage production of colony stimulating factor.

Suspected adverse pulmonary reactions to intravenous purified mycobacterial cell wall extract have been reported in horses. Adverse reactions occurred after multiple intravenous administrations of the product. Pulmonary lesions include multifocal granulomatous pneumonitis, bronchiolitis, and progressive pulmonary fibrosis, and the clinical signs are cough, fever, tachypnea, lethargy, and leukocytosis. Thoracic radiographic examination reveals diffuse interstitial infiltration. Cytologic examination of bronchoalveolar lavage fluid reveals increased total cell counts and marked lymphocytic inflammation. A marked local reaction (20–40 cm) is elicited by intradermal injection of mycobacterial cell wall extract in affected horses. A similar adverse pulmonary reaction (interstitial pneumonitis with disseminated pulmonary granulomas) occurs in approximately 1% of patients after intravesical BCG therapy. In human patients, pulmonary lesions are suspected to result from either a pulmonary hypersensitivity reaction against the proteineic component of BCG, or BCG mycobacteremia resulting in pulmonary infection. Mycobacterial organisms are rarely recovered from the pulmonary lesions; therefore, hypersensitivity reaction is considered to be the most likely origin of these pulmonary lesions.

### Parapoxvirus ovis

Inactivated, purified parapoxvirus ovis (Baypamune), a viral-based immunostimulant, is

- The etiologic agent of contagious ecthyma in sheep
- Recommended for prophylaxis, metaphylaxis, and treatment of infectious diseases, and prevention of stress-induced diseases in horses
- Administered intramuscularly 2–4 doses at 48-hour intervals

Metaphylaxis is defined as administration of immunostimulant at approximately the same time as exposure to a pathogen. The immunostimulant properties of poxvirus were first noted after routine smallpox vaccination. Some patients receiving the vaccine experienced spontaneous tumor regression and resolution of chronic viral and bacterial infections. Poxvirus-mediated immunostimulation is independent of viral replication, and the immunostimulative components are located within the viral envelope. Parapoxvirus ovis is the etiologic agent of contagious ecthyma or "orf" in sheep. Intraperitoneal administration of inactivated parapoxvirus ovis in mice increases natural killer cytotoxicity 10–16 hrs after treatment. In addition, parapoxvirus administration stimulates macrophage activation and interferon production, and protects mice against experimental lethal viral infection. The commercial product has demonstrated efficacy against viral and bacterial disease in livestock and companion animal species.

In horses, inactivated parapoxvirus ovis has predominately been used for prophylaxis and treatment of viral respiratory disease. The recommended dosage schedule is 2–44 doses at 48-hour intervals, and the immunostimulant activity is reported to occur within hours of administration. The maximum duration of immunostimulatory activity after parapoxvirus ovis administration is 8 days. Intramuscular administration of inactivated parapoxvirus ovis reduces the severity of respiratory disease caused by equine herpesviruses 1 and 4. Prophylactic administration of inactivated, parapoxvirus ovis, 4 and 6 days prior to weaning reduces the incidence of respiratory disease in foals (7.9%) compared to placebo-treated foals (24%). Administration of the product after weaning (3 doses) reduces the clinical signs of viral respiratory disease in foals subjected to long-distance transport and commingling (natural viral exposure). The incidence of disease in newborn foals is reduced by administration of parapoxvirus ovis immediately after birth and at 24 or 48 hours of life. Unlike its efficacy with equine respiratory disease, intralesional administration of inactivated parapxovius ovis is no more effective for treatment of sarcoid skin tumor than intralesional placebo.

## SYNTHETIC IMMUNOSTIMULANTS

Synthetic immunostimulants include levamisole phosphate and interferon-alpha.

### Levamisole phosphate
A synthetic anthelmintic, levamisole phosphate is

- Basic Child PsychiatryLabeled for treatment of nematode infection in cattle
- A stimulant to host defenses impaired by aging, stress, or immaturity of the immune system
- Anecdotally recommended for treatment of chronic infectious respiratory disease and heaves

Levamisole phosphate appears to have little or no effect on humoral or cell-mediated immunity in healthy animals. The effects of levamisole are more apparent in immuno-compromised individuals, because it stimulates depressed cell-mediated immunity and neutrophil mobility, phosphodiesterase activity, adherence, and chemotaxis.

In humans, levamisole enhances lymphoproliferative responses in postoperative patients and reduces viremia in patients with chronic hepatitis B infection. Levamisole improves cell-mediated immune responses and lymphocyte cytotoxicity in children suffering from severe protein-calorie malnutrition and chronic respiratory infection, and is reported to be an effective adjunct treatment for rheumatoid arthritis and chronic bronchitis.

Controlled investigation of the immunostimulatory effects of levamisole in healthy or immuno-compromised horses has not been reported. However, favorable clinical response has been reported in horses with chronic infectious pulmonary disease and heaves. Levamisole has been anecdotally recommended as adjunct treatment of equine protozoal myelitis.

### Interferon-alpha
Interferon-alpha is an endogenous immunostimulant with antiviral, immuno-modulatory, and antiproliferative activity:

- A low dose, orally administered, of interferon-alpha is recommended for treatment of inflammatory airway disease in young horses.
- Interferon-alpha is ineffective for treatment of acute viral respiratory infection or fulminant respiratory disease.

Endogenous interferon production is induced by viral infection, and is an early, nonspecific antiviral defense mechanism. Interferon-alpha induces an antiviral state in target host cells by stimulating production of enzymes that inhibit viral protein synthesis and degrade viral RNA. In mice, administration of IFN-alpha stimulates peripheral T-lymphocytes to produce IFN-gamma and activate the Th1 cell response, promoting natural killer cell cytotoxicity, macrophage activation, and cytokine production.

Oral administration of interferon-alpha reduces pulmonary inflammation in racehorses with chronic IAD. Inflammatory airway disease occurs in 22–50% of racehorses, and is a common cause of poor race performance. Typical clinical findings include mucopurulent exudate in the lower respiratory tract, nasal discharge, and cough. Affected horses have a high total cell count in bronchoalveolar lavage fluid characterized by neutrophilia (15%), lymphocytosis, and monocytosis. Arterial oxygen tension is low during exercise in affected horses. Low-dose (50–150 IU), natural, human IFN-alpha reduces exudate in the respiratory tract, lowers total cell counts in BAL fluid, and converts the differential cell count to a noninflammatory cytologic profile. Interferon-alpha does not improve the clinical signs of disease or BAL cytology in horses with IAD characterized by eosinophilic or mast cell inflammation. Because the etiology of IAD is unknown, the mechanism of therapeutic benefit of IFN-alpha is undetermined. Interferon may reduce pulmonary inflammation via immunomodulation or elimination of persistent viral infection.

The pathway for dissemination of the biologic effects of IFN-alpha following oral administration does not occur via small intestinal absorption and peripheral circulation of IFN; IFN-alpha is degraded by digestive enzymes and cannot be detected in peripheral blood after enteral administration. In fact, detection of circulating interferon may not be a prerequisite for activation of systemic defense mechanisms. It is likely that interferons are not intended to be circulatory proteins; they are therapeutic agents, which act outside the realm of classic pharmacologic mechanisms. Oral administration appears to activate unique natural defense systems originating in oropharyngeal-associated lymphoid tissue that involves cellular communication and amplification of the biologic response. Lymphocytes exposed to IFN can transfer enhanced biologic effects to naive lymphocytes in the absence of IFN. This process requires direct cell-to-cell contact, does not involve a soluble mediator, and does not require continued presence of IFN. Cellular transfer of the antiviral state to naive cells permits low to undetectable concentrations of IFN-alpha to produce potent antiviral activity, and possibly represents a major mechanism for amplification and dissemination of endogenous IFN-alpha activity.

Interferon administration is not beneficial in the treatment of acute, fulminant viral respiratory infection in horses. Oral administration of low-dose (0.22–2.2 IU/kg bwt) recombinant IFN-alpha-2a does not diminish the severity of clinical disease or duration of viral shedding in horses with experimental equine herpesvirus 1 infection. Treatment failure in this model is attributed to the overwhelming nature of the viral infection.

Treatment failure in human patients can occur after prolonged administration due to production of anti-IFN antibody or down regulation of IFN receptors. The conformational structure of recombinant IFN-alpha is more likely to induce neutralizing antibody production than natural IFNs. Production of neutralizing antibodies to recombinant IFN-alpha correlates with treatment failure in human cancer patients, and anti–IFN-alpha antibody has been identified in calves following treatment with the recombinant product.

In equine medicine, use of exogenous and endogenous immunomodulatory preparations is increasing for prevention and treatment of infectious respiratory disease and neoplastic disorders. As the mechanisms of secondary immunosuppression are elucidated, immunomodulatory preparations that target particular immunologic functions will likely be developed, allowing the equine clinician to identify more specific indications for use of individual preparations.

## FURTHER READING

Berry, C.R. 1991. Thoracic radiographic features of silicosis in 19 horses. *J Vet Intern Med* 5:248–256.

Britt, D.P., and Preston, J.M. 1985. Efficacy of ivermectin against *Dictyocaulus arnfeldi* in ponies. *Vet Rec* 116:343–345.

Bruce, E.H. 1995. Interstitial pneumonia in horses. *Comp Cont Ed Pract Vet* 17:1145–1153.

Buergelt, C.D. 1995. Interstitial pneumonia in the horse: A fledgling morphological entity with mysterious causes. *Equine Vet J* 27(1):4–45.

Cormack, S., Alkemade, S., and Rogan, D. 1991. Clinical study evaluating a purified mycobacterial cell wall extract for the treatment of equine respiratory disease. *Equine Pract* 13(8):18–22.

Costa, L.R.R., Seahorn, T.L., and Moore, R.M., et al. 2000. Correlation of clinical score, intrapleural pressure, cytologic findings of bronchoalveolar fluid, and histopathologic lesions of pulmonary tissue in horses with summer pasture-associated obstructive pulmonary disease. *Am J Vet Res* 61(2):167–173.

Dixon, P.M., Railton, D.I., and McGorum, B.C. 1995. Equine pulmonary disease: A case control study of 300 referred cases. Part I. Examination techniques, diagnostic criteria, and diagnoses. *Equine Vet J* 27:416–421.

Dixon, P.M., Railton, D.I., and McGorum, B.C. 1995. Equine pulmonary disease: A case control study of 300 referred cases. Part II. Details of animals and of historical and clinical findings. *Equine Vet J* 27:422–427.

Dixon, P.M., Railton, D.I., and McGorum, B.C. 1995. Equine pulmonary disease: A case control study of 300 referred cases. Part III. Ancillary diagnostic findings. *Equine Vet J* 27:428–435.

Evans, D.R., Rollins, J.B., and Huff, G.K., et al. 1988. Inactivated *Propionibacterium acnes* as adjunct to conventional therapy in the treatment of equine respiratory diseases. *Equine Pract* 10(6):17–21.

Flaminio, M.J.B.F., Rush, B.R., and Shuman, W. 1998. Immunologic function in horses after non-specific immunostimulant administration. *Vet Immunol Immunopathol* 63:303–315.

Garber, J.L., Reef, V.B., and Reimer, J.M. 1994. Sonographic findings in horses with mediastinal lymphosarcoma: 13 caes (1985–1992). *J Am Vet Med Assoc* 205(10): 1432–1436.

Geor, R.J., and Ames, T.R. 1991. Smoke inhalation injury in horses. *Comp Cont Ed Pract Vet* 13(7):1162–1169.

Hare, J.E., and Viel, L. 1998. Pulmonary eosinophilia associated with increased airway responsiveness in young racing horses. *J Vet Intern Med* 12:163–170.

Hinchcliff, K.W. 1999. Effects of furosemide on athletic performance and exercise-induced pulmonary hemorrhage in horses. *J Am Vet Med Assoc* 212:630–635.

Hoffman, A. 1997. Inhaled medications and bronchodilator use in the horse. *Vet Clin North Amer Eq Pract* 13(3):519–530.

Hoffman, A.M., Mazan, R.M., and Ellenberg, B.S. 1998. Association between bronchoalveolar lavage cytologic features and airway reactivity in horses with a history of exercise intolerance. *Am J Vet Res* 59(2):176–181.

Kemper, T., Spier, S., Barratt-Boyes, D.M., et al. 1993. Treatment of smoke inhalation in five horses. *J Am Vet Med Assoc* 202(1):91–94.

Klei, T.R. 1986. Other parasites: Recent advances. *Vet Clin North Amer Eq Pract* 2(2):329–336.

Klimczak, C. 1992. Immunostimulant quickly aids weanling ERDC cases. *Equine Vet Sci* 12(2):68–69.

Langsetmo, I., Fedde, M.R., and Meyer, T.S. 2000. Relationship of pulmonary arterial pressure to pulmonary haemorrhage in exercising horses. *Equine Vet J* 32:379–383.

Lavoie, J.P. 2001. Update on equine therapeutics: Inhalation therapy for equine heaves. *Comp Cont Ed Pract Vet* 475–477.

Mair, T.S. 1996. Obstructive pulmonary disease in 18 horses at summer pasture. *Vet Rec* 138(4):89–91.

Mair, T.S., Dyson, S.J., Fraser, J.A., et al. 1996. Hypertrophic osteopathy (Marie's disease) in Equidae: A review of twenty-four cases. *Equine Vet J* 28(3):256–262.

McGorum, B.C., Ellison, J., and Cullen, R.T. 1998. Total and respirable airborne dust endotoxin concentrations in three equine management systems. *Equine Vet J* 30(5):430–434.

Moore, B.R., Krakowka, S., Cummins, J.J., et al. 1996. Changes in airway inflammatory cell populations in Standardbred racehorses after interferon-alpha administration. *Vet Immunol Immunopathol* 49:347–358.

Nestved, A. 1996. Evaluation of an immunostimulant in preventing shipping related respiratory disease. *J Equine Vet Sci* 16:78–82.

Parker, G.A., Novilla, M.N., Brown, A.C, et al. 1979. Granular cell tumour (myoblastoma) in the lung of a horse. *J Comp Path* 89:421–430.

Poole, D.E., Kindig, C.A., Fenton, G., et al. 2000. Effects of external nasal support on pulmonary gas exchange and EIPH in the horse. *J Equine Vet Sci* 20(9):579–585.

Rush, B.R., Krakowka, S., Cummins, J.M., and Robertson, J.T. 1996. Changes in airway inflammatory cell populations in Standardbred racehorses after interferon-alpha administration. *Vet Immunol Immunopathol* 49:347–358.

Rush, B.R., Krakowka, S., Robertson, J.T., and Cummins, J.M. 1995. Cytologic evaluation of bronchoalveolar lavage fluid obtained from Standardbred racehorses with
inflammatory airway disease. *Am J Vet Res* 56(5):562–568.

Seahorn, T.L., and Beadle, R.E. 1993. Summer pasture-associated obstructive pulmonary disease in horses: 21 cases (1983–1991) *J Am Vet Med Assoc* 202(5):779–782.

Sweeney, C.R., and Gillette, D.M. 1989. Thoracic neoplasia in equids; 35 cases
(1967–1987). *J Am Vet Med Assoc* (3)195:374–197.

Vail, C.D., Nestved, A.J., Martins, J.B., et al. 1990. Adjunct treatment of equine respiratory disease complex (ERDC) with the Propionibacterium acnes, Immunostimulant, EqStim. *J Equine Vet Sci* 10(6):399–403.

Vandenput, S., Duvivier, D.H., Votion, D., et al. 1998. Environmental control to maintain stabled COPD horses in clinical remission: Effect on pulmonary function.
*Equine Vet J* 30(2):93–96.

Viel, L., and Kenney, D. 1993. Suspected adverse pulmonary reactions to Equimune
I.V. in four horses presented to the Ontario Veterinary College. In *12th Veterinary
Respiratory Symposium*. Pennsylvania: Kennett Square.

Woods, P.S.A., Robinson, N.E., Swanson, M.C., et al. 1993. Airborne dust and aeroallergen concentration in a horse stable under two different management systems.
*Equine Vet J* 25:208–213.

Ziebell, K.L., Kretzdorn, D., Auer, S., et al. 1997. The use of Baypamun N in crowd-
ing associated with infectious respiratory disease: Efficacy of Baypamun N (freeze
dried product) in 4 to 10 month old horses. *J Vet Med B* 44:529–534.

# Techniques: Noninfectious Lower Respiratory Tract

Techniques for evaluation of noninfectious lower respiratory tract disease include endoscopic examination, arterial blood gas evaluation, bronchoalveolar lavage, and lung biopsy.

## ENDOSCOPIC EXAMINATION OF THE LOWER RESPIRATORY TRACT

Endoscopic examination is an essential technique for evaluation of upper and lower respiratory tract disease in equine practice. Based on a report of evaluation of 300 respiratory cases, endoscopic examination of the trachea is more sensitive for detection of lower respiratory tract inflammation than thoracic auscultation. Accumulation of mucus in the lower airway is detected in the majority of horses with recurrent airway obstruction (heaves) and inflammatory airway disease (see Chapter 19, Fig. 19.5). In addition, endoscopic examination of the trachea is more sensitive for identification of EIPH than observation of epistaxis (see Chapter 19, Fig. 19.9). However, endoscopic examination is less reliable than bronchoalveolar lavage (BAL) fluid red blood cell count for quantification of the severity of hemorrhage. Determination of the severity of an EIPH episode based on the volume of blood in the trachea is unreliable because it is affected by head position, timing of examination, and coughing. Endoscopic examination can be a valuable technique to identify less common conditions of the lower respiratory tract including pulmonary neoplasia, particularly granular cell myoblastoma.

Most equine practitioners use a 9.5–12 mm diameter, 1 meter endoscope. The carina can be visualized with a 1 meter long endoscope in an average-to-small horse. A 1.8–2.0 meter endoscope must be used to perform bronchoscopy or obtain a bronchoalveolar lavage sample. Evaluation of laryngeal function is usually performed without sedation; however, endoscopic examination of the lower respiratory tract is facilitated by sedation. Horses without respiratory inflammation will cough minimally during endoscopic examination of the lower respiratory tract; however, endoscopic examination may trigger paroxysmal coughing in horses with tracheobronchial inflammation. Sedation with detomidine (0.01 mg/kg bwt) or the combination of xylazine (0.3–0.5 mg/kg bwt) and butorphanol tartrate (0.02 mg/kg bwt) will suppress coughing, reduce examination time, and reduce patient discomfort.

Tracheal exudate samples are easily obtained through the biopsy port of most endoscopes; however, these samples are less informative for cytologic evaluation than BAL samples and less reliable for bacterial culture than transtracheal aspirates. Satisfactory samples for bacterial culture can be obtained using a guarded sheath technique, although isolation of *Pseudomonas* sp. and anaerobic bacteria must be viewed as potential contaminants from the endoscope. Cytologic evaluation of BAL fluid is more reliable than tracheal aspirate samples for interpretation of lower respiratory tract inflammation. However, BAL via bronchoscopy has two disadvantages:

- The endoscope is more rigid than a BAL tube, with greater potential to traumatize the bronchial wall (iatrogenic hemorrhage).
- The endoscope lacks an inflatable cuff, which typically ensures that only distal lung segments are lavaged.

However, bronchoscopy may improve identification of pulmonary disease in horses with focal or regional pulmonary disease. Moreover, bronchoscopy allows the examiner to visualize the airway and select a particular bronchus for sampling in horses with focal lung disease.

Identification of the affected segment of lung and selective passage into that affected area is challenging. Two independent researchers (Sweeney et al., Smith et al.) have documented an endoscopic map of the equine bronchial tree to assist clinicians with the technique of bronchoscopy. In most horses, the clinician can examine approximately 34 cm from the carina within the right and left caudal lobar bronchi. There are approximately 17 explorable branches from the caudal and principal lobar bronchi of the left lung and 18 explorable branches from the caudal and principal lobar bronchi of the right lung. The branching patterns are fairly consistent. A complete description of endobronchial anatomy of the horse is beyond the scope of this book and the authors refer interested readers to the references cited for a detailed description.

## ARTERIAL BLOOD GAS EVALUATION

Arterial blood evaluation is a readily available technique to assess pulmonary function in horses. Arterial blood gas samples may be obtained from the transverse facial artery or the carotid artery (lower 1/3 of the neck) in adults, and from the femoral artery or the greater metatarsal artery in foals. A heparinized sample should be obtained using a 22 (adults) or 25 (foals) gauge needle. Manual pressure should be applied to the sampling site for 2–5 minutes to prevent hematoma formation. Excess gas bubbles are eliminated from the syringe, and the syringe is secured with an airtight seal (i.e., rubber stopper over the needle). If the sample is not analyzed within 10 minutes, it can be stored on ice for up to 90 minutes. The patient's rectal temperature should be recorded at the time of sampling and arterial blood gas values corrected for temperature.

Hypoxemia is defined as $PaO_2$ <85 mmHg while breathing room air, and hypercapnia is defined as $PaCO_2$ >46 mmHg. The results of arterial blood gas evaluation and response to supplemental oxygen allow the clinician to categorize a hypoxemic disorder into one of five basic pathophysiologic mechanisms:

- Ventilation-perfusion mismatch
- Hypoventilation
- Right-to-left shunt
- Diffusion disorder
- Insufficient fraction of inspired oxygen

Most equine respiratory diseases incorporate more than one of these pathophysiologic mechanisms. However, identification of the predominant cause of low arterial oxygen tension may provide etiologic information and may dictate appropriate therapy to resolve or ameliorate hypoxemia. In addition to pulmonary function, blood gas analysis (arterial or venous) can determine the acid-base status of the patient, and may reveal a non-respiratory cause for tachypnea, such as metabolic acidosis.

Mismatching of ventilation and blood flow (V-Q mismatch) is the most common cause of hypoxemia, and is characterized by unequal distribution of alveolar ventilation and blood flow. Pulmonary regions that are overperfused in relation to ventilation (low V-Q ratio) contribute disproportionate amounts of blood with low arterial oxygen content to the systemic circulation. Respiratory diseases characterized by low V-Q ratios include heaves, pulmonary atelectasis, and consolidation. If ventilation exceeds perfusion (high V-Q ratio), the ventilated pulmonary units are inefficient for elimination of $CO_2$ and $O_2$ uptake. Conditions associated with high V-Q ratios include pulmonary thromboembolism and shock (low pulmonary artery pressure). The ventilatory drive to maintain normal $PaCO_2$ is powerful; therefore, patients with V-Q mismatch often have normal arterial $PCO_2$. Oxygen supplementation will increase $PaO_2$ in patients with V-Q mismatch. However, elevation in arterial $O_2$ is delayed as compared to hypoventilation and in some instances may be incomplete.

The hallmark of hypoventilation (by definition) is hypercapnia. The elevation in $PaCO_2$ is inversely proportional to the reduction in alveolar ventilation; halving alveolar ventilation will double $PaCO_2$. The relationship between the fall in $PO_2$ and rise in $PCO_2$ can be predicted because the reduction in arterial oxygen tension is nearly directly proportional to the increase in carbon dioxide. For instance, if $PaCO_2$ increases from 40–80 mmHg, the $PaO_2$ would decrease from 100 to 60 mmHg. Therefore, the hypoxemia resulting from hypoventilation is rarely life-threatening. Hypercapnea constitutes respiratory failure. Acidosis due to hypercapnia is the most significant clinical feature of hypoventilation, and may threaten the life of the patient. Oxygen supplementation is effective in abolishing hypoxemia due to pure hypoventilation. However, the primary goal of treatment of hypoventilation must address more than hypoxemia. The clinician must improve alveolar ventilation via institution of positive pressure ventilation or elimination of the source of hypoventilation. Hypoventilation can result from failure of central drive (barbituates, cerebral edema, head trauma, hypoxic ischemic encephalopathy), metabolic alkalosis, failure of the muscles of respiration (botulism, nutritional muscular dystrophy, phrenic nerve dysfunction), inability to expand chest (flail chest, pneumothorax, diaphragmatic hernia, restrictive pulmonary disease), and upper airway obstruction.

A right-to-left shunt is defined as venous blood ($PO_2$ = 40 mmHg), which enters the arterial system without traversing ventilated regions of the lung. Addition of a small amount of poorly oxygenated blood to arterial blood will dramatically reduce the resulting oxygen tension in the admixture of blood due to the slope of the oxygen/hemoglobin dissociation curve at this point. Hypoxemia cannot be abolished by administration of 100% oxygen to the patient. The shunt fraction is never exposed to the added $O_2$, the shunt fraction continues to depress $PO_2$ on the flat portion of the dissociation curve, and the hemoglobin exposed to the increased $O_2$ is already fully saturated. Offering 100% oxygen to the patient is a very sensitive test to detect a shunt. Shunt does not produce hypercapnia, even though the shunted blood is rich in $CO_2$. The chemoreceptors sense an elevation of arterial $PCO_2$ and respond by increasing ventilation until $PCO_2$ is normal. Shunts usually result from a cardiac defect or may be an extreme form of V-Q mismatch (physiologic shunt).

Diffusion impairment is the least common cause of hypoxia in equine medicine. Gas exchange between the alveolus and capillary occurs by passive diffusion, which is driven by the property of molecules to randomly move from an area of high concentration to one of low concentration. Factors that determine the rate of gas exchange include

- Concentration gradient between the alveolus and capillary blood
- Solubility of the gas
- Surface area available for diffusion
- Width of the air-blood barrier

Supplemental oxygen therapy is effective in the treatment of hypoxemia due to diffusion impairment because it creates a more favorable concentration gradient and increases the driving pressure of oxygen to move from the alveolus into the blood. Transport of $CO_2$ is less affected by diseases of diffusion impairment because of its greater solubility (20 times) as compared to $O_2$; therefore, hypercapnia is not observed. Diffusion impairment can occur with pulmonary fibrosis, interstitial pneumonia, silicosis, or edema due to increased width of the barrier or decreased surface area available for gas exchange. The clinician should recognize that the major component of hypoxemia for these conditions is V-Q mismatch; however, diffusion impairment can contribute to the severity of hypoxemia.

Low inspired oxygen fraction ($FIO_2$) results in reduced alveolar oxygen content. If $FIO_2$ is reduced to 50 mmHg (high altitude, iatrogenic) pulmonary capillary $PO_2$ may be 20 mmHg and alveolar $PO_2$ will be 50 mmHg. The driving pressure for diffusion (alveolar $PO_2$ minus pulmonary $PO_2$) is reduced from 60 mmHg to 30 mmHg. Additionally, the rate of rise of pulmonary $PO_2$ is slower for a given increase in $O_2$ due to the shape of the $O_2$ dissociation curve. Hypercapnia is not observed in patients with low inspired oxygen fraction, and supplemental oxygen obviously corrects hypoxemia.

## BRONCHOALVEOLAR LAVAGE

BAL was first adapted for horses in 1980, and has become increasingly popular for diagnosis of noninfectious equine pulmonary disease. Cytologic evaluation of BAL fluid often dictates subsequent therapeutic plans. The diagnostic indications for performing BAL in horses include

- Investigation of poor exercise performance
- Assessment of diffuse pulmonary disease

Bronchoalveolar lavage is primarily indicated for characterization of noninfectious pulmonary disease, but may be useful for diagnosis of select infectious diseases, such as fungal pneumonia or *Pneumocystis carinii*. In most instances, BAL is not appropriate for diagnosis of bacterial pneumonia. The procedure is inexpensive and easily performed under field conditions. Cytologic evaluation of BAL fluid is more consistent among normal horses than transtracheal wash cytology, and good correlation has been demonstrated between BAL fluid cytologic analysis and pulmonary histopathology.

The most appropriate diagnostic indication for bronchoalveolar lavage in horses is cytologic evaluation of diffuse pulmonary disease. Cytologic evaluation of BAL fluid represents only the pathologic process present in the lavaged lung segments, and may not adequately reflect the severity of pulmonary inflammation, or may be normal in horses with segmental pulmonary disease. Additionally, BAL fluid is not as valuable as transtracheal aspiration for obtaining samples for bacteriologic culture. Pathogenic organisms may be isolated from BAL fluid if the pneumonic segment of lung is lavaged using a sterile technique. However, it may be impossible to identify the pneumonic segment of lung during the lavage procedure, and contamination of BAL samples with proximal airway commensal organisms is difficult to differentiate from pathogenic bacteria without guarded bronchoscopy, ensheathment of the BAL catheter, or quantitative culture. Transtracheal aspiration provides a representative sample of the bacterial population from the entire lower airway.

## Technique

Bronchoalveolar lavage is routinely performed in standing, sedated horses (xylazine hydrochloride 0.4–0.8 mg/kg, IV) restrained with a nose twitch. The technique can be performed using a bronchoalveolar lavage catheter (Bivona Inc., Gary, IN) or a flexible fiberoptic endoscope (1.8–2.0 meters). Equine BAL catheters are 3 meters long, 10 mm in diameter, and have an inflatable cuff (Fig. 20.1). The catheter is passed blindly through the nasal passages, larynx, trachea, and lower airway until it becomes wedged in a third or fourth generation bronchus, and the cuff is inflated with air. Overzealous inflation of the cuff may produce bronchial mucosal pressure necrosis or overdistension of the distal airways with lavage fluid. Because the BAL catheter is passed blindly, the examiner cannot select a particular segment of lung for evaluation; therefore, this technique is limited to investigation of diffuse pulmonary disease. A blindly passed BAL catheter will enter the right caudodorsal lung field the majority of the time.

Bronchoalveolar lavage via bronchoscopy may improve identification of pulmonary disease in horses with focal or regional pulmonary disease, but the examiner must be familiar with the endoscopic anatomy and map of the equine bronchial tree. Bronchoscopy allows the examiner to visualize the airway and select a particular bronchus for sampling in horses with focal lung disease. Admittedly, identification of the affected segment of lung during the

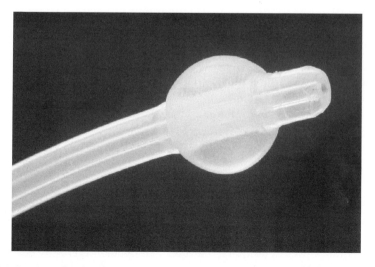

**Fig. 20.1.** Bronchoalveolar lavage catheter with inflatable cuff. Catheters are 3 m long and 10 mm in diameter.

lavage procedure and selective passage into that affected area is challenging. Additionally, it is difficult to obtain a seal in the airway without an inflatable cuff, and the rigid end of the endoscope may traumatize the bronchial wall and produce iatrogenic hemorrhage.

Most clinicians infuse 100–300 ml of a warmed, sterile, isotonic, crystalloid solution, and recover lavage fluid by manual aspiration (60 ml syringes) or vacuum suction (600 mm Hg). Approximately 50–80% of the infused volume is recovered. Gross examination of lavage fluid should be performed to detect flocculent debris and/or discoloration. Cytologic analysis of BAL should include total and differential cell counts, morphologic description of cells, and identification of pharyngeal contamination. Samples that cannot be immediately processed (within 1 hour) should be stored on ice.

Total cell counts are determined using a Unopette microcollection system and a hemocytometer. Coulter counter quantification may significantly underestimate the number of cells. In most instances, total nucleated cell counts are less than 300 cells/μl. Slides are prepared for cytologic examination by cytocentrifugation, although this technique may result in lower lymphocyte counts. Selective loss of lymphocytes may be prevented using centrifugation on microscope glass covers or the millipore filtration system. Differential cell determination is performed by examination of 200 consecutive leukocytes (Wright-Giemsa stain). Toluidine blue stain preparations improve detection of metachromatic granules, and Perl's Prussian Blue stain should be used to quantify hemosiderin content. The predominant cell types in BAL obtained from adult horses are macrophages and lymphocytes, which constitute 30–60% and 30–70% of the total cell count, respectively. Macrophages appear uniform, with minimal cytoplasmic vacuolization (Fig. 20.2). Neutrophils constitute

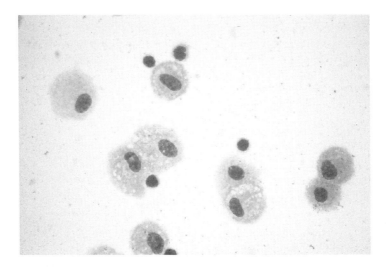

**Fig. 20.2.** Bronchoalveolar lavage cytology from a horse with normal respiratory function. The predominant cell types are macrophages and lymphocytes with neutrophils consisting of less than 5% of the total cell count. Macrophages appear uniform and nonactivated. Wright-Giemsa stain, 140x. *(See also color section.)*

less than 5% of the total cells, and occasional eosinophils and mast cells are observed in normal horses. Identification of squamous epithelial cells or feed material in cytologic preparations indicates pharyngeal contamination.

## Complications

It is not necessary to add antibiotics to the lavage solution, and aftercare is not routinely indicated. Focal pulmonary neutrophilic influx occurs in the lavaged segment of lung for at least 48 hours after the procedure. Frequent serial lavage for research or clinical purposes should be performed in distant segments of lung. There is no evidence of diffuse pulmonary inflammation or long-term focal inflammation following BAL in horses. Some horses can manipulate the BAL catheter into their oral cavity during passage of the catheter. If a horse begins to chew during the procedure, immediate abortion of the technique is recommended to avoid damage to the catheter or, ultimately, loss of the distal aspect of the catheter in the trachea.

## LUNG BIOPSY

Lung biopsy is rarely performed in horses due to limited indications and perceived risk of complications associated with the procedure. Because there are many other diagnostic tests available to evaluate the respiratory system, biopsy is often unnecessary. Lung biopsy is typically performed when less invasive techniques have failed to establish a diagnosis, or confirmation of a poor prognosis is required prior to euthanasia. Radiographic identification of a pulmonary miliary pattern is the most common indication for performing percutaneous lung biopsy, which may provide definitive histologic evidence of interstitial pneumonia, silicosis, or pulmonary neoplasia. In cases of interstitial pneumonia, lung biopsy also provides prognostic information, specifically the presence and severity of pulmonary fibrosis. Contraindications to lung biopsy include pneumonia, pulmonary abscessation, pleuropneumonia, and EIPH.

### Technique

The site for percutaneous lung biopsy is determined via ultrasound guidance. If pulmonary disease is diffuse, the preferred site is the 7th or 8th right intercostal space, approximately 8 cm above a horizontal line through the olecranon. Most clinicians do not routinely perform a clotting profile prior to lung biopsy, unless a hemostatic disorder is specifically suspected in an individual patient. The site should be clipped, surgically prepared, and infiltrated with local anesthetic solution. Horses should be lightly sedated during the procedure. A stab incision is made, and a biopsy needle inserted at the cranial aspect of the rib. Automated biopsy instruments are preferable to manual biopsy instruments. The biopsy needle should be advanced approximately 2 cm into the parenchyma using ultrasound guidance.

A thorascopic technique has been described to obtain a wedge resection from the caudal border of the lung. This technique yields approximately a 2 cm x 8 cm sample of lung, and allows direct visualization of the site to monitor post-resection complications. An automated stapling device with a double row of staples prevents leakage of air or blood from the site. Although iatrogenic injury to the diaphragm was reported in one horse, the technique is well-tolerated by normal and heavy horses.

## Complications

The most common complication reported to occur after percutaneous lung biopsy is epistaxis/hemoptysis. Less commonly reported complications include tachypnea, respiratory distress, hemothorax, pneumothorax, collapse, and sudden death. Sudden death occurs rapidly after biopsy and is thought to result from air embolism, rather than pneumothorax or hemothorax. Inadvertent biopsy of bowel and secondary peritonitis has been reported after attempting percutaneous lung biopsy without ultrasound guidance. The majority of clinicians warn horse owners of potential complications prior to performing percutaneous lung biopsy and reserve the procedure as a final effort to obtain a diagnosis/prognosis.

## ADVANCED RESPIRATORY TECHNIQUES

Pulmonary function testing, bronchoprovocation challenge, and nuclear imaging are primarily research tools for evaluation of horses with recurrent airway obstruction and inflammatory airway disease. Of these advanced techniques, bronchoprovocation challenge is the most readily available at referral institutions for clinical evaluation of horses with poor performance or chronic, low-grade respiratory disease.

Standard pulmonary function testing typically refers to determination of the maximal change in pleural pressure, pulmonary resistance, and dynamic compliance. These tests are relatively insensitive for evaluation of horses with mild to moderate airway disease. If the patient is breathing comfortably at rest, standard pulmonary function testing is likely to reveal normal values for these parameters. For horses with respiratory distress, pulmonary function testing is an accurate method to quantify the severity of airway obstruction. Maximal change in pleural pressure provides a measure of the overall work of breathing. Pulmonary resistance evaluates the severity of bronchoconstriction, and dynamic compliance assesses stiffness of the lung. Determination of standard pulmonary function testing requires an esophageal balloon, a face mask fitted with a pneumotachograph, and a pulmonary function computer.

Bronchoprovocation testing is an indicator of nonspecific airway responsiveness or airway reactivity. This evaluation requires horses to be exposed to sequentially higher doses of aerosolized methacholine or histamine followed by serial pulmonary function testing. The dose of irritant required to reduce dynamic compliance by 35% (standard pulmonary function) or increase respiratory system resistance by 75% (forced oscillatory mechanics) from baseline indicates the severity of airway reactivity. Bronchoprovocation challenge is indicated in horses with mild to moderate airway inflammation and is usually performed in horses with poor exercise performance. Bronchoprovocation challenge is not indicated in horses that have increased respiratory effort at rest or abnormal baseline values during standard pulmonary function testing. Hyperreactivity to aerosolized irritants has been consistently documented in horses with pulmonary eosinophilia or metachromatic inflammation, and in heaves-affected horses in apparent clinical remission, but with persistent pulmonary neutrophilia.

Nuclear imaging of the lower respiratory tract of horses can be used to assess the distribution of pulmonary ventilation, pulmonary perfusion, or pulmonary inflammation. Nuclear imaging requires administration of a radioactive tracer to the patient, a gamma camera, and a computer equipped with nuclear medicine software to provide visual representation of the tracer. Ventilation imaging, in particular, requires a closed system for aerosol delivery to prevent exposure of personnel to radionuclide. Nuclear imaging is typically performed in standing horses with little to no sedation. After completion of the study, horses must be maintained in an isolated area for 24–48 hours to allow decay and excretion of radiopharmaceutical.

Ventilation scanning is used to assess pulmonary ventilation in horses with recurrent airway obstruction, and is more sensitive for detection of mild airway obstruction than standard pulmonary function testing. Ventilation scanning requires inhalation of radioactive pharmaceutical ($^{99m}$technetium-DTPA or $^{99m}$technetium-nanocolloid of human albumin) prepared in small-sized inhalation particles (1–2 µm). Distribution of radionuclide to ventilated pulmonary regions is determined immediately by standing the horse next to a camera that detects gamma-emission. Horses with normal pulmonary function will have uniform, diffuse distribution of radioactivity in all pulmonary fields, whereas horses with obstructed small airways will have patchy distribution of radionuclide with central deposition in larger airways (Fig. 20.3). In addition to assessment of airway obstruction, ventilation scanning has been used to determine qualitative and quantitative pulmonary distribution of aerosolized drugs and various administrative devices.

Perfusion scanning in horses is performed using macroaggregates of human serum albumin labeled with $^{99m}$technetium. The agent is injected into the jugular vein and the relatively large radioactive particles (>10 µm) are trapped in the pulmonary vascular bed (first-pass) in a distribution pattern proportional to regional blood flow. This procedure has no detectable adverse effect on pulmonary mechanics or gas exchange. Perfusion scanning is used primarily to detect pulmonary thromboembolism in human and small animal medicine. Combined ventilation/perfusion studies have been performed in horses and allow calculation of V/Q ratios to define and quantify the origin of mismatching of blood flow and pulmonary ventilation.

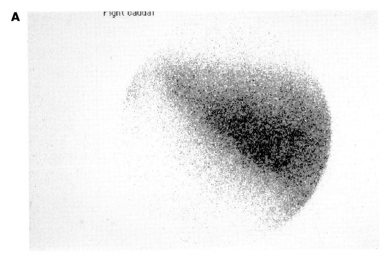

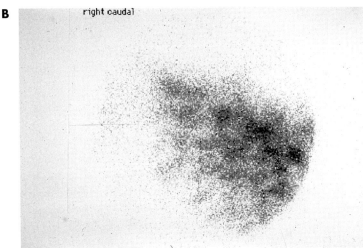

**Fig. 20.3.** Lateral ventilation images of the caudodorsal lung fields from a horse with normal respiratory function (A) depicting uniform distribution of radiopharmaceutical and a horse with heaves (B) illustrating patchy distribution of radiopharmaceutical with excessive deposition in central airways.

Pulmonary epithelial permeability, and hence inflammation, can be determined by the clearance rate of inhaled radiopharmaceuticals from the lungs. $^{99m}$Technetium-DTPA deposited in alveolar regions by nebulization slowly diffuses through the tight intercellular junction of the alveolar-capillary barrier. The rate of disappearance of $^{99m}$technetium-DTPA from the lung increases proportionately with pulmonary inflammation due to alveolar epithelial damage. Determination of alveolar clearance rate is a particularly sensitive technique for detection of subclinical airway inflammation in horses and humans.

## AEROSOL DELIVERY DEVICES

Administration via inhalation improves drug safety and efficacy by reducing the total therapeutic dose, minimizing drug exposure to other body systems, and allowing direct delivery of the drug to the lower respiratory tract. In most instances, the response to aerosolized drug administration is more rapid than systemic drug administration. The equine patient is an ideal candidate for inhalation therapy based on large tidal volume, high inspiratory flow rates, and obligate nasal breathing. However, the initial devices designed for delivery of aerosolized drugs to the lower respiratory tract of horses were cumbersome, expensive, and marginally efficacious. Today, efficient systems for delivery of aerosolized drugs to horses are being rapidly developed and inhalation therapy has become increasingly popular for treatment of lower respiratory tract disease. The disadvantages of the aerosol route of administration include inability to access obstructed airways, cost, frequency of drug administration, airway irritation by some aerosol preparations, pulmonary contamination with environmental microorganisms, and atmospheric drug pollution. To date, inhalation therapy for horses has predominately focused on administration of bronchodilating agents and corticosteroid preparations for treatment of recurrent airway obstruction (heaves). Aerosolized antimicrobial agents, particularly aminoglycosides, are under investigation for treatment of bacterial infection of the lower respiratory tract in horses.

Aerosol preparations with a particle size of 1–5 microns produce the best therapeutic results and are the target particle size for inhalation therapy. These small particles penetrate deep within the respiratory tract and deposit in peripheral airways. Moderate-sized particles (5–10 microns) frequently settle out by sedimentation in larger, more central airways. Large aerosolized particles (>10 microns) impact in the upper respiratory tract via inertial impaction. The majority (90%) of particles below the target size (<0.5 microns) are inhaled and exhaled freely and rarely impact within the respiratory tract. In addition to particle size, the patient's tidal volume, inhalation and exhalation flow rates, and upper respiratory tract anatomy affect pulmonary drug deposition. Because these physiologic factors affect pulmonary drug deposition, equine clinicians cannot extrapolate data generated from human subjects regarding specific drugs or devices to equine patients.

Several devices have been designed for convenient administration of aerosolized drugs in a metered-dose inhaler (MDI) preparation to horses with recurrent airway obstruction. The advantages of an MDI system include rapid administration, consistent ex-valve dose delivery, minimal risk of pulmonary contamination with environmental microorganisms, ease of cleaning/maintaining equipment, and no requirement for electricity. Pulmonary drug delivery in human patients using MDI devices varies with the specific device, drug preparation, and patient technique. In general, approximately 10–15% of actuated drug reaches the lower respiratory tract and 80–85% of actuated drug

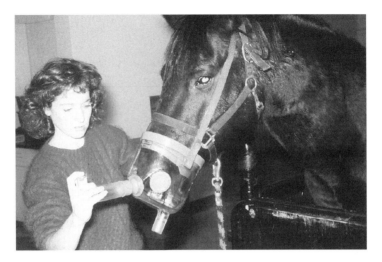

**Fig. 20.4.** Equine AeroMask fits over the entire muzzle and is equipped with a spacer device (AeroChamber attachment) for use with any metered-dose inhaler available for human inhalant administration. Attachments for nebulization of liquid medication and dry powder inhalant delivery are available, but not shown.

is deposited in the caudal pharynx. Propellants containing CFCs are being phased out of most applications due to environmental concerns, and hydrofluoroalkane-134a (HFA) is a nontoxic, ozone-friendly replacement propellant for CFCs.

The Equine AeroMask (Canadian Monaghan, Ontario, Canada) is the most versatile of the delivery systems because it can be used for administration of aerosolized drugs via handheld MDI devices, nebulization solution, or dry powder inhaler (DPI) (Fig. 20.4). This system allows the clinician to administer any drug available for human asthma therapy to horses with heaves. The drug is actuated or nebulized into a spacer device with a one-way inspiratory valve. The mask must fit snugly around the muzzle to ensure adequate negative inspiratory pressure to facilitate drug delivery. Drug delivery to the lower respiratory tract using the Equine AeroMask with an MDI is approximately 6% of actuated drug when using a CFC propellant and approximately 14% of actuated drug when using an HFA propellant. The drug is uniformly distributed throughout all pulmonary fields.

The Equine Aerosol Drug Delivery System (EADDS, Boerhinger Ingelheim Vetmedica, Germany) is a novel, handheld device designed for administration of aerosolized drugs in horses (Fig. 20.5) The EADDS device fits into the left nostril of the horse. The operator actuates a puff at the onset of inhalation, denoted by a flow indicator within the device. The operator must pay particular attention to the timing of drug delivery, because drug delivered during mid- to late inhalation may reach the tracheal lumen only to be exhaled. The advantage of this device is the highly efficient drug delivery. The mean particle size generated using this system with a CFC propellant is 2.3 +/- 2 microns, and approx-

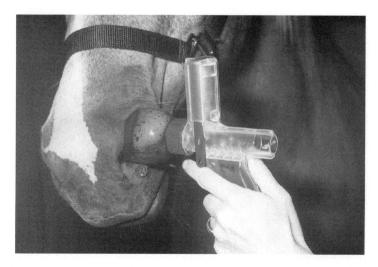

**Fig. 20.5.** Equine Aerosol Delivery Device System fits snugly within the left nostril, is preloaded with one canister of specified drug, and is disposable when the entire canister has been actuated.

imately 23% of actuated drug is delivered to the lower respiratory tract. The mean particle size using an HFA propellant is 1.1 microns, and approximately 43% of actuated drug is delivered to the lower respiratory tract in horses. Ventilation imaging using radiolabeled aerosol confirms that drug is deposited in all pulmonary fields with minimal deposition in the nasal cavity, oral pharynx, or trachea. Currently, the EADDS is commercially available for administration of albuterol sulfate in an HFA propellant (Torpex, Boehringer Ingelheim Vetmedica) and is designed for disposal after the drug has been dispensed.

The Equine Haler (Equine Healthcare APS, Hillerod, Denmark) is a spacer device that fits over the entire left nare of the horse, and is designed for administration of aerosolized drug using any handheld MDI device (Fig. 20.6). The mean particle size generated using the Equine Haler is 2.1 μm with a range of 1.1–4.7 μm (fluticasone/CFC-free propellant). Drug deposition in the lower respiratory tract is approximately 8% of the actuated dose with diffuse pulmonary drug delivery that is adequately distributed to the periphery of the lung. Unlike the AeroMask, the Equine Haler can accommodate any size horse without concerns for ensuring an airtight seal with the mask. Rather, the operator is responsible for maintaining an airtight seal between the device and the muzzle. Poor pulmonary drug delivery can occur if the administrator does not pay particular attention to align the MDI with the spacer and the spacer apparatus with the nasal passages of the horse during actuation.

### Mechanical nebulizers

Ultrasonic nebulizers and jet nebulizers are ozone-friendly delivery systems, used as alternatives to CFC propellant inhalers. Ultrasonic nebulizers produce aerosol particles using vibrations of a quartz (piezo-electric) crystal, and par-

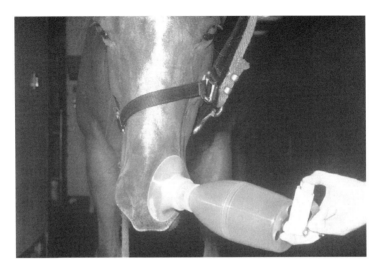

**Fig. 20.6.** The Equine Haler device fits over the entire nostril of the horse and is recommended for use with any metered-dose inhaler designed for human inhalant administration.

ticle size is inversely proportional to the operating frequency. High quality ultrasonic nebulizers are required to produce satisfactory particle size. Jet (pneumatic) nebulizers operate by the Venturi effect (dry air compressor) to fragment therapeutic solutions into aerosol particles. The diameter of particles generated by a jet nebulizer is inversely proportional to the airflow, and minimum gas flow rates of 6–8 L/min are required to generate suitable particle diameter (<5 µm) for pulmonary delivery. Jet nebulizers are readily accessible, inexpensive, and easy to use. The primary disadvantage of jet nebulization is noise generated by the system. Ultrasonic nebulizers are silent; however, they are expensive and fragile. High pressure jet nebulization (Hudson RCI, Temecula, CA) using a delivery system developed for horses (Nebul, Agritronix Int, Meux, Belgium) delivers approximately 7% of the drug to the pulmonary system, and ultrasonic nebulization (Ultra-Neb, DeVilbiss, Somerset, NJ) delivers approximately 5% of the drug to the pulmonary system. Deposition of radiolabeled drug into peripheral pulmonary fields using jet nebulization is superior to ultrasonic nebulization. Pulmonary contamination with environmental bacteria and fungi may occur using these aerosol delivery systems; therefore, rigorous disinfection of the equipment is required to avoid this complication. Aerosol therapy via jet and ultrasonic nebulization requires an administration time of approximately 10–20 minutes.

## Dry powder inhalant (DPI) devices

Dry powder inhalant devices allow rapid drug administration, minimal risk of environmental contamination with drug, and no requirement for electricity. The DPIs are comprised of gelatin capsules containing a single dose of drug and a rotor. The rotor of the DPI device is breath-actuated, and the device punctures the capsule containing powdered drug releasing it into a chamber for inhalation by the patient. This system eliminates the need for the operator to synchronize administration with inhalation. The entire dose from an individual dry powder capsule is delivered during a single inhalation; prolonged duration of inspiration and multiple inhalations do not improve pulmonary drug delivery. Dry powder inhalant devices are designed for use by human patients, but have been adapted for drug administration to horses using a specialized facemask (EquiPoudre, Agritronics Int, Meux, Belgium) or a unique adaptor to the Equine AeroMask. The efficiency of drug delivery can be influenced by relative air humidity, airflow, and head position. The masks used with DPIs must fit snugly around the muzzle to create adequate inspiratory pressure and flow rates (60 L/min), which ensures sufficient inhalant emptying rates. This minimum flow rate is easily generated by healthy and heaves-affected horses. The DPI device and mask must be aligned with the longitudinal axis of the nasal cavities to avoid impacting the powder within the mask or nasal passages. High relative humidity increases retention of drug within the device due to aggregation of powder. If the relative air humidity exceeds 95%, water actually penetrates the DPI and significantly limits drug delivery. Manufacturers recommend administration of DPIs under conditions of low relative humidity to minimize the loss of powder within the device. Ipratropium bromide is the most extensively investigated DPI preparation for administration to horses and has demonstrated effective bronchodilation in heaves-affected horses.

## FURTHER READING

Duvivier D.H., Votion D., Vandenput S., and Lekeux P. 1997. Review: Aerosol therapy in the equine species. *Vet J* 154:189–202.

Hoffman, A.M., Mazan, M.R., and Ellenberg, S. 1998. Association between bronchoalveolar lavage cytologic features and airway reactivity in horses with a history of exercise intolerance. *Amer J Vet Res* 59(2):176–181.

Robinson, N.E. 1992. Tests of equine airway function. *Proc 10th Amer College Vet Intern Med Forum*, pp 284–286.

Rush B.R., and Cox J.H. 1996. Diagnostic use of bronchoalveolar lavage in horses. *Equine Pract* 18(5):7–15.

Savage, C.J., Traub-Dargatz, J.L., and Mumford, E.L. 1998. Survey of the Large Animal Diplomates of the American College of Veterinary Internal Medicine regarding percutaneous lung biopsy in the horse. *J Vet Intern Med* 12:456–464.

Smith, B.L., Aguilera-Terjero, E., Tyler, W.S., et al. 1994. Endoscopic anatomy and map of the equine bronchial tree. *Equine Vet J* 26:283–290.

Sweeney, C.R., Weiher, J., Baez, J.L., et al. 1992. Bronchoscopy of the horse. *Amer J Vet Res* 53(10):1953–6.

Votion D., Ghafir Y., Munsters K., Duvivier D.H., Art T., and Lekeux P. 1997. Aerosol deposition in equine lungs following ultrasonic nebulisation versus jet aerosol delivery system. *Equine Vet J* 29:388–393.

Votion, D., and Lekeux, P. 1997. Scintigraphy of the equine lung. *Equine Vet J* 12:172–183.

# Lower Respiratory Tract Infectious Disease and Diagnostic Techniques

Infectious, noncontagious, lower respiratory tract diseases constitute an important group of diseases in horses of all ages. Although these conditions do not result in epizootics of disease, they are frequently serious and, in many cases, life-threatening.

The defense mechanisms of the lower respiratory tract involve both nonspecific and specific immunological mechanisms. These include the mucociliary escalator, alveolar macrophages, the local (mucosal) immune system based around the bronchial-associated lymphoid tissue (BALT), and the systemic immune system. Damage to any of these mechanisms may predispose to the development of lower respiratory infection.

In many cases, the infective agent will be a commensal or opportunistic agent that would normally be unable to establish infection in the face of normal pulmonary defense mechanisms. Examples of predisposing conditions that may lead to pulmonary infection include the prematurity and failure of passive transfer of immunity, viral-induced damage of the mucociliary escalator, and immunosuppression induced by the stress of traveling or general anesthesia. All of these conditions may allow the pulmonary defenses to become overwhelmed by infection. The failure of the defense mechanisms is also one of the reasons why such infections may respond relatively poorly to treatment. Intensive and aggressive treatment is, therefore, often required to eliminate the infection, but, once achieved, the long-term prognosis of most of the diseases is generally good.

# Juvenile Pneumonia

**21**

Bronchopneumonia is a common cause of morbidity and mortality in foals under 8 months of age:

- The majority of cases of bronchopneumonia are caused by opportunistic pathogens secondary to viral respiratory disease, stress, or parasitic migration.
- Bacterial culture of samples obtained via transtracheal aspiration is indicated to determine appropriate antimicrobial therapy.
- Foals with persistent, low-grade respiratory infection, despite appropriate antimicrobial therapy, may benefit from administration of a nonspecific immunostimulant.

Bronchopneumonia is a common cause of morbidity and mortality in foals under 8 months of age. Most bacterial isolates obtained from suckling and weanling foals with pneumonia are opportunistic pathogens, with the exception of *Rhodococcus equi*. *Streptococcus zooepidemicus*, a normal inhabitant of the upper respiratory tract, is the most common opportunistic pathogen in foals and adults with pneumonia. *Streptococcus pneumoniae*, *Actinobacillus* spp., *Pasteurella* spp., *Bordetella bronchoseptica*, *Klebsiella* spp., and *Escherichia coli* are also frequently isolated from foals with pneumonia. Foals develop bacterial pneumonia secondary to parasitic pulmonary migration, viral respiratory infection, and stress due to transportation, overcrowding, and/or weaning.

Clinical signs of pneumonia in foals include fever, depression, anorexia, cough, and purulent nasal discharge. The absence of fever does not preclude a diagnosis of pneumonia in foals. Advanced cases will demonstrate tachypnea, tachycardia, respiratory distress, and cyanosis. Tracheal and laryngeal palpation may trigger coughing in affected foals, and a tracheal rattle (indicative of mucopurulent exudate in the trachea) is a consistent finding in foals with pneumonia. Crackles and wheezes will be most prominent in the cranioventral lung fields. A rebreathing procedure will accentuate abnormal lung sounds and may induce coughing in some foals. Rebreathing should not be performed on foals that exhibit respiratory difficulty at rest. Pulmonary fields with diminished breath sounds or decreased resonance on percussion are indicative of consolidated lung, pulmonary abscesses, or pleural effusion. Hyperfibrinogenemia and neutrophilic leukocytosis are the most consistent findings on routine clinicopathologic evaluation. Bacterial culture of a transtracheal wash sample is indicated to determine the pathogen(s) and antimicrobial sensitivity. Thoracic radiography documents the extent of parenchymal disease and allows the clinician to monitor the response to therapy. Evaluation of thoracic radiographic patterns may allow differentiation of bronchopneumonia, *Rhodococcus equi* infection, and bronchointerstitial pneumonia. Radiographic findings consistent with bronchopneumonia include cranioventral distribution of consolidation and alveolization characterized by the presence of air bronchograms (Fig. 21.1). *Rhodococcus equi* pneumonia often demonstrates perihilar abscessation and alveolization, and interstitial pneumonia appears as diffuse to caudodorsally distributed interstitial infiltration.

Parasitic migration may play an important role in development of secondary bacterial pneumonia. Peripheral blood eosinophilia may be noted in foals

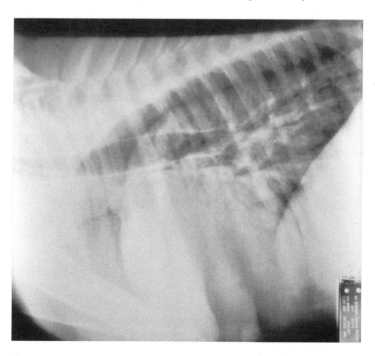

**Fig. 21.1.** Thoracic radiograph of a foal with aspiration pneumonia. Note the cranioventral distribution of consolidation and presence of air bronchograms over the cardiac silhouette.

with heavy parasite loads and may reflect parasitic migration as a predisposing factor. Pulmonary migration of *Parascaris equorum* occurs 7–14 days after larval ingestion, but 10–12 weeks are required for detection of a patent infection via fecal float for ova. Donkeys are the reservoir of *Dictyocaulus arnfieldii*, the equine lungworm. A history of housing foals with donkeys should trigger a suspicion of lungworm as a contributing or primary factor. *Dictyocaulus arnfieldii* may or may not produce a patent infection in foals, and rarely produces a patent infection in adult horses. Determination of parasitic migration or infection as a significant predisposing factor in the development of pneumonia is based on history (insufficient anthelmintic administration), appropriate environmental conditions (overcrowding, presence of donkeys), and an eosinophilic response in secretions from the lower respiratory tract.

Bacterial culture and sensitivity of transtracheal aspirate samples direct appropriate antimicrobial therapy in foals with bacterial pneumonia. However, pending results of in vitro testing, antimicrobial therapy is based on severity of clinical signs, knowledge of common pathogens, and results of Gram stain of tracheal secretions. Because *Streptococcus* spp. are the most common isolates, penicillin (22,000 IU/kg) is often the treatment of choice for uncomplicated, Gram-positive, bacterial pneumonia in foals. If a mixed infection is suspected (i.e., Gram-positive and Gram-negative organisms), gentamicin sulfate (6.6 mg/kg, SID) can be added to penicillin to augment penicillin's predominate Gram-positive spectrum. Trimethoprim-sulfonamide (15 mg/kg, PO, BID) has the advantages of ease of administration, Gram-positive and Gram-negative spectrum for common opportunistic pathogens, and inexpensive cost. Ceftiofur (5 mg/kg, IM BID) has an appropriate antimicrobial spectrum for common opportunistic pathogens, and is often successful as solo therapy for juvenile pneumonia. Antimicrobial therapy for foals with mixed infections or extensive pulmonary compromise may require more sophisticated antimicrobial therapy, as directed by in vitro sensitivity testing.

*Bordetella bronchoseptica* represents a unique treatment challenge. The organism appears to be overlooked as a significant respiratory pathogen in foals, but is frequently isolated and may be associated with herd outbreaks of pneumonia in foals. *Bordetella bronchoseptica* is a potent ß-lactamase producer, which may result in bacterial overgrowth due to death of competing, penicillin-susceptible organisms. Foals with bordetella pneumonia may show an initial favorable response to administration of a ß-lactam antibiotic, followed by deterioration in clinical status due to *B. bronchoseptica* overgrowth. In addition, the organism lives anchored to the epithelial surface of the airway. Many foals with *B. bronchoseptica* pneumonia require prolonged antimicrobial administration for complete resolution of disease, which may result from extensive epithelial injury by bacterial toxins and inaccessibility of the respiratory epithelium by antimicrobial agents. Aminoglycosides (gentamicin and amikacin) are the antibiotics of choice for treatment of *B. bronchoseptica*; however, erythromycin and tetracycline may also be effective. Administration of gentamicin via nebulization provides direct delivery of antibiotic to the respiratory epithelial surface, improving accessibility of the drug to the organism.

Supportive therapy for foals with pneumonia includes provision of a clean, comfortable environment and highly palatable, dust-free feeds. Nonsteroidal anti-inflammatory therapy should be administered, as needed, to maintain rectal temperature below 39.5°C. Bronchodilator therapy may or may not improve arterial oxygenation in foals with pneumonia. In cases of severe consolidation, rapid bronchodilation may exacerbate hypoxemia due to increased dead-space ventilation and potentiation of ventilation-perfusion mismatch. If bronchodilator therapy is indicated, aminophylline has the advantage of delaying fatigue of the muscles of respiration in foals with severe respiratory distress. If aminophylline (5–10 mg/kg PO, BID) is administered, other drugs in the therapeutic regimen should be investigated for potential drug interactions. Nasal insufflation with oxygen is necessary in foals with severe respiratory compromise. Ulcer prophylaxis is indicated in foals that are stressed by respiratory difficulty, frequent handling, hospitalization, and transportation.

Response to therapy can be monitored by physical examination, including thoracic auscultation, complete blood count, and thoracic radiographic examination. Owners should obtain a rectal temperature at least twice daily to monitor response to therapy. If signs of improvement are not observed within 3 days or clinical signs of disease worsen at any time, the therapeutic plan should be reevaluated. Antimicrobial therapy should be continued until all physical examination and clinicopathologic findings are within normal limits. Pneumonia and pulmonary abscessation caused by ß *Streptococcus* in foals has a negative influence on future racing performance.

Foals with opportunistic pulmonary infections may fail to completely resolve clinical signs despite appropriate antimicrobial therapy, or clinical signs may consistently relapse upon withdrawal of antimicrobial therapy. The most common clinical signs that persist in these foals are nasal discharge and cough. Foals with chronic, unresponsive pulmonary infections may have secondary immunosuppression or may be immunotolerant to the pathogen. Nonspecific immunostimulant therapy (see Chapter 19) enhances innate and acquired cytotoxic activity and often improves clinical signs of respiratory disease in weanling foals with persistent, low-grade pulmonary infection. Immunostimulant therapy is not recommended for foals with acute infection and/or clinical signs of depression, anorexia, and fever.

## RHODOCCOCUS EQUI

*Rhodococcus equi* is the most serious cause of pneumonia in foals between 1 and 5 months of age:

- *R. equi* causes life-threatening pneumonia in foals from 1–5 months of age.
- Foals acquire pulmonary infections in the first two weeks of life via inhalation of contaminated soil.

- *R. equi* infection produces chronic progressive pneumonia with acute to subacute onset of clinical signs.
- Colonic/mesenteric abscessation and osteomyelitis are the most common extrapulmonary sites of *R. equi* infection.

*Rhodococcus equi* is not the most *common* cause of pneumonia in this age group; however, it has significant economic consequences due to mortality, prolonged treatment, loss of performance potential, surveillance programs for early detection, and relatively expensive prophylactic strategies. The organism is likely present on all premises to some degree; however, disease incidence may be enzootic, sporadic, or nonexistent for specific farms. Clinical disease is reported in horses over 8 months of age, but is exceedingly rare. It appears that pulmonary infection occurs via inhalation of contaminated environmental sources early in life. Compelling epidemiologic data indicates that pulmonary infection probably originates within the first two weeks of life.

*Rhodococcus equi* is a Gram-positive, facultative intracellular pathogen that is nearly ubiquitous in soil. High-ambient summer temperatures, sandy soil, and dusty conditions favor multiplication and dissemination of the organism in the environment. The optimal environmental temperature for replication is 30°C, and under ideal conditions, one organism can multiply to 10,000 in 2 weeks. Inhalation of dust particles laden with virulent *R. equi* is the major route of pneumonic infection. On dry, windy days, *R. equi* can be isolated from samples of air from endemic farms. It is easily cultured from fecal samples of adult herbivores, but its presence in adult manure is likely contamination from ingestion of soil (passive) rather than active replication within the intestinal tract. In contrast, the organism readily multiplies within the intestine of foals up to 3 months of age. Foals with pulmonary infections swallow *R equi*-laden sputum, which replicates in their intestinal tract. Therefore, manure from pneumonic foals is a major source of virulent bacteria contaminating the environment. Ingestion of the organism is a significant route of exposure, and likely of immunization, but rarely leads to hematogenous-acquired pneumonia.

The pathogenicity is linked to the ability of *R equi* to survive intracellularly, which hinges on failure of phagosome-lysosomal fusion in infected macrophages, and failure of functional respiratory burst upon phagocytosis of *R. equi*. Virulent forms of *R. equi* contain 80–90 kb plasmids encoding a family of virulence-associated proteins (Vap), including Vap-A and Vap-C through Vap-H. Strains without these plasmids fail to replicate and survive in macrophages and are not virulent to foals in vivo. Expression of all of the Vap-like genes may be necessary to maintain virulence of a particular strain of *R. equi*.

## Clinical signs
*Rhodococcus equi* is a slowly progressive infection with acute to subacute clinical manifestation. Clinical signs of disease are difficult to detect until pulmonary lesions reach a critical mass, resulting in decompensation of the foal.

Some foals will present with acute respiratory distress and fever, without previous indication of clinical respiratory disease. Pulmonary lesions are relatively consistent and include subacute to chronic suppurative bronchopneumonia, pulmonary abscessation, and suppurative lymphadenitis. At the onset of clinical signs, most foals are anorexic, lethargic, febrile, and tachypneic. Cough is a variable clinical sign, and purulent nasal discharge is less common. Thoracic auscultation reveals crackles and wheezes with asymmetric/regional distribution. Pulmonary regions with marked consolidation lack breath sounds and exhibit dull resonance on thoracic percussion. Diarrhea is observed in many foals with *R. equi* pneumonia due to colonic microabscessation. Immune-complex polysynovitis is identified in approximately 1/3 of foals with *R. equi* pneumonia. The stifle and tibiotarsal joints are affected most frequently with mild to marked joint effusion, minimal lameness, and little resistance to palpation. Cytologic examination of synovial fluid from foals with immune-complex synovitis reveals nonseptic mononuclear pleocytosis. Less common manifestations of immune complex disease secondary to *R. equi* infection include uveitis, anemia, and thrombocytopenia.

Intestinal and mesenteric abscesses are the most common extrapulmonary sites of *R. equi* infection. Foals with abdominal involvement often present with fever, depression, anorexia, weight loss, colic, and diarrhea. Intestinal lesions are characterized by multifocal, ulcerative enterocolitis and typhlitis involving Peyer's patches with granulomatous or suppurative inflammation of the mesenteric and/or colonic lymph nodes. A single large abdominal abscess, originating from mesenteric lymph node, may or may not be associated with intestinal adhesions and colic (Fig. 21.2). The prognosis for foals with abdominal forms of *R. equi* is less favorable than pulmonary disease, because ap-

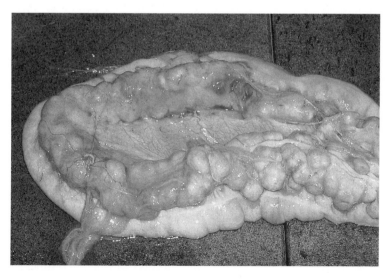

**Fig. 21.2.** Multiple *Rhodococcus equi* abscesses along the mesenteric border of the large colon of a 3-month-old foal.

proximately 50% of foals with intestinal involvement die of their disease despite aggressive therapy.

Septic physitis and osteomyelitis are less common extrapulmonary sites of *R. equi* infection. Foals with *R. equi* osteomyelitis are more painful than foals with immune-mediated polysynovitis. Cytologic evaluation of synovial fluid from septic joints due to adjacent *R. equi* osteomyelitis reveals neutrophilic inflammation. Vertebral osteomyelitis may result in pathologic vertebral fracture and spinal cord compression, and is a devastating manifestation of *R. equi* osteomyelitis (Fig. 21.3). In addition to standard antimicrobial therapy, aggressive local therapy, consisting of debridement and lavage, is necessary to achieve successful resolution of *R. equi* osteomyelitis. Less common sites of extrapulmonary infection include panophthalmitis, guttural pouch empyema, sinusitis, pericarditis, nephritis, and hepatic and renal abscessation.

## Diagnosis
Routine laboratory evaluation of complete blood count and serum chemistry reveals nonspecific abnormalities consistent with infection and inflammation:

* Bacterial culture of transtracheal wash samples provides the definitive diagnosis of *R. equi* pneumonia.
* Identification of perihilar alveolization, abscessation, and mediastinal lymphadenopathy via thoracic radiography is consistent with *R. equi* pneumonia.
* Thoracic ultrasound can identify consolidation and abscessation of peripheral lung, but cannot identify deeper parenchymal lesions.
* Serologic testing results in overdiagnosis of *R. equi* infection.

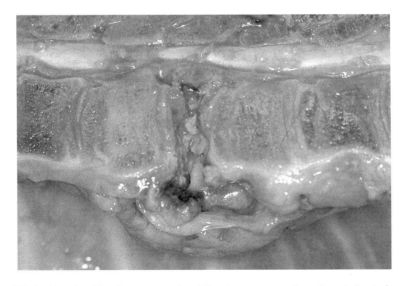

**Fig. 21.3.** Vertebral body osteomyelitis (*Rhodococcus equi*) and pathologic fracture at $T_{11}$–$T_{12}$ from a 4-month-old foal with pneumonia and acute hindlimb paralysis.

The severity of neutrophilic leukocytosis and hyperfibrinogenemia appears related to prognosis. Thrombocytosis (platelets >250,000/µl) is a common clinicopathologic finding in foals with *R. equi* infection. Thoracic radiographic evaluation of foals with *Rhodococcus equi* pneumonia reveals a fairly consistent pattern characterized by perihilar alveolization, consolidation, and abscessation (Fig. 21.4). Identification of nodular lung lesions and mediastinal lymphadenopathy in foals 1–5 months of age is highly suggestive of *R. equi*. If characteristic *R. equi* lesions are identified via thoracic radiography, additional testing may be averted to prevent further stress to a compromised foal. Serial thoracic radiographic examination is valuable to assess severity of pneumonia and monitor response to therapy. Ultrasonographic evaluation may identify consolidation and abscessation of peripheral pulmonary regions (Fig. 21.5), but may not be as useful as thoracic radiography to evaluate the extent of pulmonary lesions. Overlying aerated lung will obscure detection of deep parenchymal abscesses. Nonetheless, ultrasonographic evaluation is often abnormal in affected foals and serves as a valuable screening technique for early detection on endemic farms. A sector scanner equipped with a 7.5 or 5.0 MHz transducer is preferred for evaluation of the thoracic cavity, but linear scanners (commonly used in equine reproduction) can also be used.

Bacterial culture of transtracheal wash samples is a consistent and reliable method for identification of pneumonic foals, and is required for definitive diagnosis of *R. equi*. Bacterial culture of nasal or fecal swabs is unreliable, because these samples are easily contaminated with environmental *R. equi*. Cytologic evaluation of transtracheal wash samples reveals intracellular coccobacilli (Fig. 21.6), identification of which indicates initiation of appropriate antimicrobial therapy pending culture results.

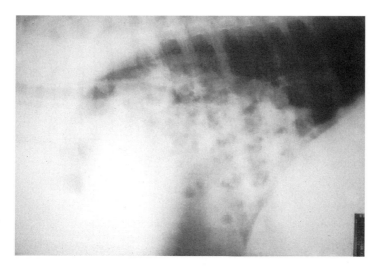

**Fig. 21.4.** Thoracic radiograph from a 3-month-old foal with *Rhodococcus equi* pneumonia. Note the perihilar distribution of pulmonary consolidation and abscessation. Numerous gas pockets are seen within the pulmonary abscesses.

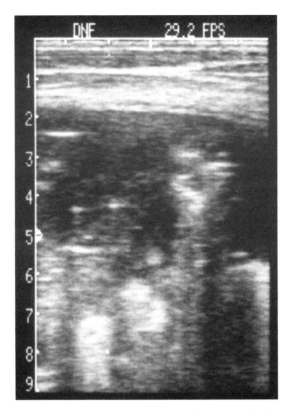

**Fig. 21.5.** Thoracic ultrasound from a 2-month-old foal with *Rhodococcus equi* pneumonia. Consolidation and abscessation of peripheral lung fields were detected via ultrasound in this foal with advanced disease.

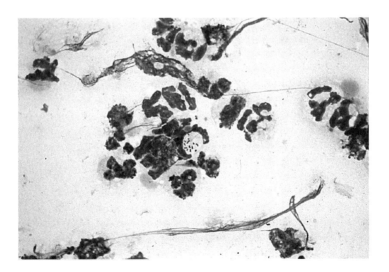

**Fig. 21.6.** Cytologic evaluation of a transtracheal aspirate from a foal with *Rhodococcus equi* pneumonia. Note the Gram-positive, pleomorphic rods within a macrophage. Gram stain, 40x. *(See also color section.)*

PCR amplification, based on the Vap-A gene sequence, is more sensitive than bacterial culture for detection of *R. equi* from transtracheal aspirate samples. PCR amplification can detect a minuscule number of organisms, and the bacteria do not have to be viable to be identified by PCR. Therefore, previous antimicrobial administration will not interfere with detection of the organism. Unfortunately, PCR amplification may increase false positive diagnosis of *R. equi* due to extreme sensitivity of the technique (environmental contamination). Unlike bacterial culture techniques, PCR amplification cannot identify concurrent bacterial infections or determine antimicrobial susceptibility. Therefore, PCR amplification should not replace bacterial culture for evaluation of transtracheal aspirates in foals with pneumonia, but may be used in conjunction.

There are two serologic tests for identification of antibody against *R. equi*: agar gel immunodiffusion (AGID) and enzyme-linked immunosorbent assay (ELISA). The sensitivity and specificity of these serologic tests are not sufficient to reliably differentiate exposure to *R. equi* from clinical disease. Reliance on serology for diagnosis of *R. equi* results in overdiagnosis of disease due to the presence of passively acquired maternal antibody and antibody production due to pathogen exposure. These serologic tests may serve as a screening tool to assess the prevalence of the organism within a herd, but are of little value in the diagnosis of *R. equi* for individual patients.

## Treatment

Routine evaluation of *R. equi* isolates to identify susceptibility to antimicrobial agents is misleading:

- The combination of erythromycin and rifampin has markedly improved survival of foals with *R. equi* pneumonia.
- Adverse effects of erythromycin are relatively common in foals, and antibiotic-induced colitis in the dams of treated foals may be life-threatening.
- Azithromycin is a newer generation macrolide with greater bioavailability than erythromycin and may be administered once a day to every other day as solo therapy.

In vitro, *R. equi* appears sensitive to a wide variety of antimicrobial agents. However, the organism exists intracellularly and within granulomatous masses in the patient; therefore, most antimicrobial agents are ineffective in vivo. The combination of erythromycin (25 mg/kg, q 6 hrs, P.O.; esters or salts) and rifampin (5 mg/kg q12 hr or 10 mg/kg q 24 hr) has become the treatment of choice for *R. equi* infections in foals. These antimicrobials may be bacteriostatic, but their activity is synergistic, and the combination has markedly improved survival of foals with *R. equi* pneumonia. Rifampin is lipid-soluble (able to penetrate abscess material), and is concentrated in phagocytic cells. Erythromycin is concentrated in granulocytes and alveolar macrophages; however, its antimicrobial activity is somewhat inhibited by intracellular pH.

Adverse reactions are relatively common in foals treated with the erythromycin/rifampin combination. Idiosyncratic hyperthermia and tachypnea can occur with erythromycin administration during periods of warm environmental conditions, and anorexia, bruxism, and salivation may be observed. Life-threatening, antibiotic-induced enterocolitis, due to *Clostridium difficile*, has been observed in the dams of nursing foals treated with erythromycin. This is presumably due to coprophagic behavior by the mare, which leads to ingestion of sufficient active erythromycin to perturb the intestinal flora of the mare. Resistance of *R. equi* to erythromycin/rifampin is uncommon, but has been reported.

Azithromycin is a newer-generation macrolide with greater bioavailability than erythromycin. Azithromycin achieves higher drug concentrations in phagocytic cells and tissues, and produces less gastrointestinal side effects in human patients. Azithromycin is administered orally (10 mg/kg), once daily until clinical signs stabilize, followed by every other day until resolution of disease. The safety and efficacy of azithromycin for treatment of *R. equi* pneumonia has not been rigorously investigated in foals. Anecdotally, the duration of treatment appears reduced and the incidence of gastrointestinal side effects appears to be less common than observed with erythromycin.

Supportive therapy for foals with *R. equi* pneumonia includes provision of a clean, comfortable environment and highly palatable, dust-free feeds. Judicial intravenous fluid therapy and saline nebulization facilitates expectoration of pulmonary exudates. Nonsteroidal anti-inflammatory therapy should be administered as needed to maintain rectal temperature below 39.5°C. Nasal insufflation with oxygen is necessary in foals with severe respiratory compromise. Bronchodilator therapy may or may not improve arterial oxygenation in foals with *R. equi* pneumonia. In cases of severe consolidation, rapid bronchodilation may exacerbate hypoxemia due to increased dead space ventilation and potentiation of ventilation-perfusion mismatch. If bronchodilator therapy is indicated, aminophylline has the advantage of delaying fatigue of the muscles of respiration in foals with severe respiratory distress. Prophylactic antiulcer medication is indicated in foals with *R. equi* that are stressed by respiratory difficulty, pain (osteomyelitis), frequent handling, hospitalization, and transportation.

The survival rate of *R. equi* pneumonia is approximately 70–90% with appropriate therapy. The case fatality rate without therapy (or with inappropriate antimicrobial therapy) is approximately 80%. Dyspnea and severe thoracic radiographic changes are poor prognostic indicators. The duration of antimicrobial therapy typically ranges from 4–9 weeks. Parameters for discontinuation of therapy include resolution of clinical signs, normalization of fibrinogen concentration, radiographic or ultrasonographic resolution of pulmonary consolidation and abscessation. Foals suffering from clinically apparent *R. equi* pneumonia are slightly less likely to race as adults. However, the racing performance of *R. equi* foals, that do get to the racetrack and complete their first start, is not different from the United States racing population.

## Prevention

There are three basic strategies to decrease the incidence of R. equi pneumonia on endemic farms: decrease exposure to the organism, early detection of clinical cases, and passive immunity for neonatal foals:

- Exposure to R. equi can be minimized by elimination of environmental conditions that favor dissemination of the organism.
- Surveillance programs allow early detection of clinical cases on endemic farms.
- Administration of hyperimmune plasma to neonatal foals reduces the incidence and severity of R. equi pneumonia in juvenile foals.

Most endemic farms have a mutual history of prolonged use as a breeding facility resulting in progressive buildup of environmental contamination. The primary route of infection is inhalation of R. equi–contaminated dust within the first 2 weeks of age. Neonatal foals should be maintained in well-ventilated, dust-free areas, avoiding dirt paddocks and overcrowding. Pasture rotation will prevent loss of grass and reduce environmental contamination. Grass should be planted in dirt paddocks, and manure should be removed on a regular basis. Pneumonic foals represent a major source for contamination of the environment with virulent organisms; therefore, foals with R. equi disease should be isolated and their manure composted.

Early diagnosis of R. equi pneumonia results in greater treatment success and reduced treatment time. In addition, early detection limits further contamination of the premises by allowing earlier isolation of affected foals. Herd surveillance programs for early detection of pneumonic foals on endemic farms varies, but may include twice weekly physical examination and auscultation, periodic determination of complete blood count and fibrinogen concentration, periodic serologic testing (AGID), or weekly thoracic ultrasonographic examination. Obtaining white blood cell counts on a monthly basis is more sensitive and specific for early detection of R. equi pneumonia than fibrinogen concentration or serologic surveillance. Foals with white blood cell counts greater than 14,000 cells/μl should be subjected to further evaluation or treated for R. equi.

The final strategy to reduce R. equi associated losses on endemic farms is administration of hyperimmune plasma to neonatal foals. Commercially available hyperimmune plasma is produced in horses via vaccination with various R. equi antigens. Surprisingly, vaccination of mares and foals with virulence-associated protein extracted from R. equi does not protect foals from disease and may enhance the severity of R. equi pneumonia. Administration of hyperimmune plasma reduces the incidence and severity of R. equi within the herd, but is not completely effective in preventing disease. Hyperimmune plasma (1 liter) is administered intravenously within the first week of life, followed by a second liter at approximately 25 days of age. The mechanism of the partially protective effect of passively transferred anti–R. equi antibody is not completely understood, but may involve nonspecific factors present in plasma that facilitate opsonization, in addition to *R. equi*–specific antibody.

## PNEUMOCYSTIS CARINII

*Pneumocystis carinii* is a ubiquitous, unicellular eukaryote that causes opportunistic pneumonia in individuals with primary or secondary immunodeficiency:

- *Pneumocystis carinii* pneumonia is associated with primary or secondary immunodeficiency syndromes in foals from 6–12 weeks of age.
- Ante-mortem diagnosis requires cytologic identification of the organism from bronchoalveolar lavage samples.

*Pneumocystis carinii* is the most common pulmonary infection related to human immunodeficiency virus, and has been associated with combined immunodeficiency syndrome, corticosteroid administration, CD4+ lymphopenia, and *Rhodococcus equi* infection in foals. Pneumocystis pneumonia appears to be a clinically relevant, but rarely recognized, respiratory disorder of young foals. The organism exists in trophozoite (2–7 μm) and cyst forms (4–6 μm), and the entire life cycle of *P. carinii* takes place within the alveoli of immunocompromised patients. The cysts contain 4–8 intracystic bodies, which are released when a cyst ruptures. The released intracystic bodies become trophozoites, which reproduce by binary fission or further cyst formation. Genetically distinct forms of *Pneumocystis carinii* infect different mammalian hosts. Interestingly, the strain of *P. carinii* isolated from infected foals is genetically distinct from isolates obtained from other hosts. If horses are the primary host for this strain, subclinical infection and commensal carriage of *P. carinii* is likely more common than currently recognized.

Pneumocystis pneumonia occurs in foals within a narrow age range, with all reported cases between 6 and 12 weeks of age at presentation. Clinical signs of pneumocystosis are nonspecific. Historical complaints of fever, lethargy, and weight loss of several days' to several weeks' duration are common. Clinical examination of foals with pneumocystosis reveals tachypnea, inducible cough, and increased lung sounds. Nasal discharge is a variable finding. Routine laboratory evaluation of complete blood count and serum chemistry profile reveals nonspecific abnormalities consistent with infection and inflammation.

Confirming a definitive diagnosis of *P. carinii* is difficult, and clinical suspicion of pneumocystis pneumonia is crucial to successful diagnosis. The organism cannot be grown in culture and is rarely present in tracheal secretions. Therefore, cytology and culture of transtracheal wash samples are unrewarding for diagnosis of *P. carinii* pneumonia. Ante-mortem diagnosis is typically made by cytologic examination of bronchoalveolar lavage fluid samples stained with Wright-Giemsa. Characteristic oval or crescent-shaped cysts of

*P. carinii* are identified within alveolar macrophages, and the accompanying cytologic profile is neutrophilic inflammation (Fig. 21.7). In human patients, the sensitivity of bronchoalveolar lavage fluid cytology for diagnosis of *P. carinii* pneumonia is 97%, regardless of the results of supportive diagnostic procedures. Bronchoalveolar lavage is rarely performed as a routine diagnostic procedure in 2–3-month-old foals with respiratory disease, which has historically limited ante-mortem diagnosis of this organism. Thoracic radiography may reveal radiographic signs indicative of pneumocystosis, prompting the clinician to perform bronchoalveolar lavage. Radiographic findings consistent with pneumocystis pneumonia include diffuse interstitial to miliary, reticulonodular infiltration extending from the hilar region. The interstitial to reticulonodular radiographic pattern is not present in all foals with *P carinii*,

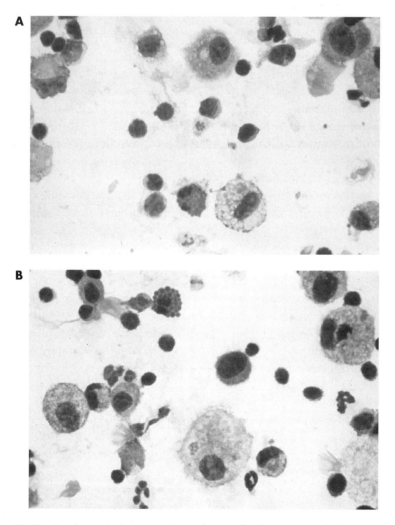

**Fig. 21.7.** Cytologic evaluation of bronchoalveolar lavage sample from a foal with *Pneumocystis carinii* pneumonia. Note the extracellular (A) and intracellular (B) *Pneumoncystis* cysts. Wright-Giemsa stain. *(See also color section.)*

therefore, bronchoalveolar lavage should be performed on foals of this age group with undiagnosed pneumonia. Severe respiratory compromise may preclude bronchoalveolar lavage in some foals. Hypertonic (3.0%) saline nebulization expectorates small airway secretions and improves recovery of pneumocystis organisms from sputum samples by approximately 50% in human patients. Therefore, hypertonic saline nebulization for 10 minutes prior to transtracheal aspiration may be an alternative to bronchoalveolar lavage in dyspneic foals. Because the organism is found primarily in alveoli, lung biopsy or fine needle aspiration has been suggested for ante-mortem diagnosis of *P carinii*. These techniques are relatively invasive, and may be dangerous in foals with respiratory distress.

At gross necropsy examination, foals with fatal pneumocystosis have uniformly meaty lungs that fail to collapse, and cut pulmonary surfaces have diffuse pink and yellow mottling. These findings are similar to necropsy examination of other species with fatal pneumocystis pneumonia. Histopathologic evaluation reveals diffuse alveolar flooding with foamy macrophages and proteinaceous to fibrinoid eosinophilic material. Interstitial spaces are infiltrated with lymphocytes and plasmacytes. Hyaline membrane formation may be prominent with mild to marked type II pneumocytic hyperplasia. The organism is best identified using Grocott's methenamine silver stain or immunostaining using mouse monoclonal antibody to *P. carinii*. Using a silver stain, pneumocystis cysts appear as empty oval or crescent-shaped structures with a brownish-black wall.

Treatment with trimethoprim/sulfamethoxazole (25 mg/kg, PO, q 12 hr) has demonstrated variable success in foals. In some instances of treatment failure, the disease may have been too advanced to respond to appropriate antimicrobial therapy or death may have resulted from a concurrent infection (i.e., *Rhodococcus equi*). Human patients are treated with potentiated sulfa antimicrobials or pentamidine isethionate, an antiparasitic drug. Pentamidine is administered intravenously for active cases of pneumocystis pneumonia and via inhalation as prophylaxis for at-risk patients (CD4+ cells < 200/µl) with acquired immunodeficiency syndrome. In human patients with active pneumocystis infection, gas exchange and survival is superior with trimethoprim-sulfamethoxazole therapy compared to intravenous pentamidine.

## BRONCHOINTERSTITIAL PNEUMONIA

Bronchointerstitial pneumonia is an important cause of acute respiratory distress in foals from 1–8 months of age and may represent a clinical syndrome that is similar to adult respiratory distress syndrome (ARDS) in human patients:

- Bronchointerstitial pneumonia causes respiratory distress in weanling and suckling foals.

- Thoracic radiographs may provide the most useful diagnostic information for distinguishing bronchointerstitial pneumonia from bacterial pneumonia.
- Treatment is nonspecific and may include corticosteroids, NSAIDs, broad-spectrum antibiotics, bronchodilator therapy, supplemental oxygen, and supportive care.

Like the majority of the interstitial pneumonias in adult horses, the incidence of bronchointerstitial pneumonia in foals is sporadic and the etiology unknown. Proposed etiologies include viral respiratory infection, heat shock, pneumotoxin ingestions, bacterial toxins, *Pneumocystis carinii,* and *Mycoplasma* spp. One of the most consistent factors associated with bronchointerstitial pneumonia in foals is warm environmental temperature (25°C and higher). It is likely that a number of different insults, rather than a single factor, initiate a cascade of events resulting in a final common response of severe pulmonary damage and acute respiratory distress. Bronchointerstitial pneumonia of foals is rapidly progressive and may result in sudden death due to fulminate respiratory failure. Although mortality is high, affected foals that receive aggressive medical care have a reasonably favorable prognosis for survival (70%). The long-term pulmonary consequences after recovery from bronchointerstitial pneumonia are variable, ranging from undetectable to persistent exercise intolerance.

The most striking clinical signs of interstitial pneumonia are acute respiratory distress, cyanosis, tachycardia, hyperthermia, and sudden death due to respiratory failure. Thoracic auscultation reveals increased bronchial sounds over central airways and reduced bronchovesicular sounds in peripheral areas of lung. Crackles and wheezes can be detected in the caudodorsal lung fields. Anorexia, depression, cough, and nasal discharge are commonly reported in foals with bronchointerstitial pneumonia; however, these signs are also observed in foals with infectious pneumonia. Approximately half of the foals with bronchointerstitial pneumonia have a history of mild to moderate infectious respiratory disease prior to the onset of respiratory distress, and administration of erythromycin may be one of the precipitating factors.

Baseline clinicopathologic evaluation of foals with acute respiratory distress should include arterial blood gas, complete blood count, serum chemistry analysis, and thoracic radiographic examination. Hypoxemia, hypercapnea, and respiratory acidosis are consistent findings in foals with bronchointerstitial pneumonia. These arterial blood gas findings aid the clinician in quantifying the severity of respiratory impairment and monitoring the response to therapy. The hypoxemia of bronchointerstitial pneumonia is relatively resistant to supplemental oxygen therapy, indicating extreme ventilation-perfusion mismatch with intrapulmonary shunting of blood. Similar to bacterial pneumonia, hyperfibrinogenemia and neutrophilic leukocytosis are observed in the majority of foals with bronchointerstitial pneumonia. Physical examination and clinicopathologic findings may appear similar to foals with severe *R. equi* pneumonia, and thoracic radiographic examination may be the most valuable diagnostic test to differentiate *R. equi* pneumonia from bronchointerstitial pneumonia. *Rhodococcus equi* pneumonia classically demonstrates perihilar abscessation and alveolization, whereas interstitial pneumonia appears as diffuse to caudodorsally distributed interstitial and bronchointerstitial pulmonary opacities (Fig. 21.8). With advanced disease, the radiographic pattern of bronchointerstitial pneumonia progresses to include patches of a coalescing alveolar nodular pattern with air bronchograms (Fig. 21.9). Transtracheal as-

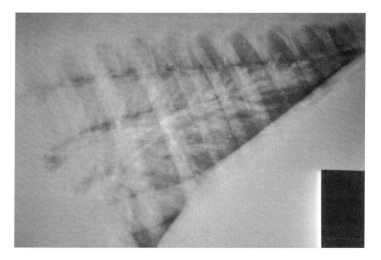

**Fig. 21.8.** Thoracic radiograph from a 4-month-old foal with bronchointerstitial pneumonia of moderate severity. Infiltration of the connective tissue framework of the lungs results in an interstitial pattern, which appears as an increase in background opacity that results in loss of visualization of vascular structures.

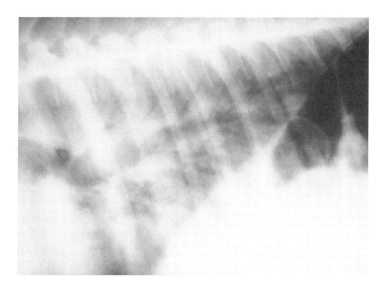

**Fig. 21.9.** Thoracic radiograph of a 5-month-old foal with severe bronchointerstitial pneumonia. In this advanced stage of disease, the interstitial pattern is obscured by transudation of fluid into alveolar spaces, resulting in an alveolar pattern with air bronchograms.

piration may be prohibitively dangerous to perform on a dyspneic foal, but should be performed when the patient becomes more stable to obtain samples for bacterial culture/sensitivity, cytologic evaluation, and virus isolation. Cytologic evaluation of tracheal aspirates reveals acute neutrophilic inflammation with or without evidence of sepsis. Bacterial organisms are often recovered from samples obtained from transtracheal aspiration or necropsy of foals with bronchointerstitial pneumonia, including *Streptococcus* spp., *Klebsiella* spp., *Proteus mirabilis, Enterobacter* spp., and *Escherichia coli;* however, no single organism is consistently recovered from foals with these clinical signs.

Necropsy examination reveals diffusely enlarged lungs that fail to deflate upon opening of the thoracic cavity with rib impressions on the visceral pleural surface. The cut surface of lung is mottled with dark red lung interspersed with more normal-appearing lung tissue, and edematous separation of lobules. The most prominent histopathologic findings are severe, diffuse, necrotizing bronchiolitis, alveolar septal necrosis, and neutrophilic alveolitis. Surviving foals develop a proliferative epithelial and interstital response, including bronchiolar and alveolar epithelial hyperplasia, type II cell hyperplasia, and hyaline membrane formation. Multinucleated giant cells are observed in some cases.

Because the etiology of bronchointerstitial pneumonia is unknown, there is no specific therapy. However, the treatment plan should include a broad range of goals including anti-inflammatory therapy, broad-spectrum antibiotics, thermoregulatory control, bronchodilation, supplemental oxygen, and supportive care. Based on an uncontrolled case series, anti-inflammatory therapy with potent, injectable corticosteroids (i.e., dexamethasone 0.1 mg/kg, IV, q 24 hr) appears to be associated with survival in foals with bronchointerstitial pneumonia. Nonsteroidal anti-inflammatory drugs (NSAIDs), flunixin meglumine (1.1 mg/kg, q 12 hr) and/or dipyrone (22 mg/kg, IV or IM), provide additional anti-inflammatory activity, in addition to antipyretic activity. Techniques for external thermoregulatory control, such as an alcohol bath, an air-conditioned stall, and/or a fan, can be used in conjunction with NSAIDs to maintain rectal temperature below 39.5°C. The suitability of an antibiotic regimen, based on subsequent bacterial sensitivity, appears to have little bearing on the outcome of bronchointerstitial pneumonia. Nonetheless, broad-spectrum antibiotic therapy should be instituted to treat preexisting bacterial pneumonia or prevent secondary bacterial infection. Aerosolized albuterol is a rapid (2–5 minutes) and powerful bronchodilator for horses. Aerosolized albuterol (360 µg) can be administered every 15 minutes for 2 hours to overcome poor pulmonary drug distribution and provide sequential bronchodilation in foals with severe bronchospasm. Long-acting bronchodilators, such as aerosolized ipratropium (2-3 µg/kg, q 8 hr to q 6 hr), aerosolized salmeterol (210 µg, q 12 hr to q 8 hr) or oral clenbuterol (0.8–3.2 mg/kg q 12 hr), should be administered to provide more sustained bronchodilation. Aminophylline (5–7 mg/kg, po, q 12 hr) is a weaker bronchodilator, but has the advantage of delaying fatigue of the muscles of respiration in foals with severe respiratory distress. Additional supportive therapy includes provision of a clean, comfortable environment and highly palatable, dust-free feeds. Ulcer prophylaxis (i.e., omeprazole 4 mg/kg, po, q 24 hr) is indicated in foals with bronchointerstitial pneumonia due to frequent NSAID administration and the stress of respiratory difficulty, frequent handling, hospitalization, and transportation. Clinical improvement in respiratory difficulty should be observed by 48 hours after initiation of therapy.

Preventive strategies to avoid cases of bronchointerstitial pneumonia are difficult to develop, given the sporadic nature of disease and uncertainty of inciting factors. Because heat stress may play a role in the pathophysiology of some cases, foals should have access to shady, well-ventilated areas during periods of extreme summer temperatures. Producers should avoid transporting foals in hot weather, and particular care should be taken to provide a cool environment for foals with an existing pulmonary infection.

## FURTHER READING

Ainsworth, D.M., Eicker, S.W., Yeagar, A.E., et al. 1998. Associations between physical examination, laboratory, and radiographic findings and outcome and subsequent racing performance of foals with *Rhodococcus equi* infection: 115 cases (1984–1992). *J Am Vet Med Assoc* 213(4):510–515.

Ainsworth, D.M., Weldon, A.D., Beck, K.A., et al. 1993. Recognition of *Pneumocystis carinii* in foals with respiratory distress. *Equine Vet J* 25:103–108.

Baverud, V., Franklin A., Gunnarsson, A., et al. 1998. *Clostridium difficile* associated with acute colitis in mares when their foals are treated with erythromycin and rifampicin for *Rhodococcus equi* pneumonia. *Equine Vet J* 30(6):482–488.

Ewing, P.J., Cowell, R.L., Tyler, R.D., et al. 1994. *Pneumocystis carinii* pneumonia in foals. *J Am Vet Med Assoc* 204:929–933.

Flaminio M.J.B.F., Rush B.R., Cox J.H., et al. 1998. CD4+ and CD8+ lymphopenia in a filly with *Pneumocystis carinii* pneumonia. *Austalian Vet J* 76(6):7–10.

Garcia-Cantu, M.C., Hartmann, F.A., Brown, C.M., et al. 2000. *Bordetella bronchoseptica* and equine respiratory infections: A review of 30 cases. *Equine Vet Educ* 2:46–50.

Giguere, S. 2001. *Rhodococcus equi* pneumonia. In *Proceedings of the Amer Assoc Equine Pract* 47, pp 456–467.

Higuchi, T., Taharaguchi, S., Hashikura, S., et al. 1998. Physical and serologic examinations of foals at 30 and 45 days of age for early diagnosis of *Rhodococcus equi* infection on endemically infected farms. *J Am Vet Med Assoc* 212(7):976–981.

Lakritz, J., Wilson, W.D., and Berry, C.R. 1993. Bronchointerstitial pneumonia and respiratory distress in young horses: Clinical, clinicopathologic, radiographic, and pathologic findings in 23 cases. *J Vet Intern Med* 7:277–288.

Lavoie, J-P., Fiset, L., and Laverty, S. 1994. Review of 40 cases of lung abscesses in foals and adult horses. *Equine Vet J* 26(5):348–352.

Peters, S.E., Wakefield, A.E., Whitwell, K.E., et al. 1994. *Pneumocystis carinii* pneumonia in thoroughbred foals: Identification of a genetically distinct organism by DNA amplification. *J Clin Microbiol* 32(1):213–216.

Sellon, D.C. 2001. Investigating outbreaks of respiratory disease in older foals. In depth: Current Concepts in Pediatrics. *Proceedings of the Am Assoc Equine Pract* 47 pp 447–555.

# Pneumonia in Adult Horses 22

Pneumonia in adult horses includes bacterial pneumonia/pleuropneumonia, fungal pneumonia, and pulmonary metacestode infection.

## BACTERIAL PNEUMONIA/PLEUROPNEUMONIA

Bacterial pneumonia is rarely primary in adult horses and more typically occurs after a predisposing event that suppresses pulmonary immunity:

- Bacterial pulmonary infections often occur after events that suppress pulmonary immunity.
- Viral respiratory infection, long-distance transport, general anesthesia, and strenuous exercise are common predisposing factors.
- Race and sport horses, under the age of 5 years, have a higher incidence of infectious pulmonary disease.

Bacterial pathogens isolated from adult horses with pneumonia are opportunistic, environmental, or commensal organisms that are not capable of primary invasion. Pleuropneumonia develops secondary to bacterial pneumonia, with extension of the infection into the pleural space. Penetrating thoracic wounds produce septic pleural effusion without pneumonia; however, extension of the infection to the pulmonary parenchyma can occur, particularly if pulmonary contusions resulted from the traumatic event. Spontaneous pleuritis (without accompanying pneumonia) is uncommon in horses. The differential diagnoses for pleural effusion in horses include neoplastic effusion, congestive heart failure, thoracic hemorrhage, chylothorax, and pulmonary hydatidosis. In the United States, approximately 70% of horses with pleural effusion have pleuropneumonia. In the United Kingdom, where lower respiratory tract infection is less common, approximately 30% of horses with pleural effusion have pleuropneumonia, and the relative incidence of neoplastic effusion is higher.

The history of most horses with pneumonia/pleuropneumonia includes events or factors that suppress pulmonary defense mechanisms. Viral respiratory infection, long-distance transportation, general anesthesia, and strenuous exercise are common predisposing factors that impair pulmonary defense mechanisms, allowing secondary bacterial invasion. Race and sport horses are subject to many of these factors, making this population particularly at risk. The majority of horses with pleuropneumonia are athletic horses less than 5 years of age. Exercise-induced pulmonary hemorrhage may contribute to development of respiratory infection by providing a favorable environment for bacterial replication. The principal pulmonary defense mechanisms are the mucociliary escalator, bronchial-associated lymphoid tissue, and alveolar macrophages.

The mucociliary escalator is responsible for physical removal of particles within the airways and represents a nonspecific pulmonary defense mechanism. The mucociliary blanket extends from the respiratory bronchioles to the pharynx. It is comprised of a double layer of mucus, which is propelled toward the pharynx by ciliated respiratory epithelium. Inhaled particles and debris in the lower respiratory tract become trapped within the upper layer of mucus, and are transported to the pharynx and swallowed. Influenza replicates within and destroys the ciliated epithelium of the mucociliary escalator. Regeneration of the respiratory epithelium requires approximately 21 days after recovery from influenza, even in the absence of secondary bacterial infection. High ammonia concentrations (due to poor sanitation) depress ciliary motility and delay mucociliary clearance. Dehydration increases the viscosity of mucus layer inhibiting ciliary movement and efficiency of the mucociliary apparatus. Smoke inhalation denudes the respiratory epithelium.

Bronchial-associated lymphoid tissue (BALT) is comprised of lymphoid nodules within the submucosa of segmental bronchi and terminal bronchioles. Bronchial-associated lymphoid tissue coordinates antigen-specific pulmonary defense mechanisms and participates in both humoral and cell-mediated immunity. B lymphocytes within BALT produce all classes of immunoglobulin except IgM. Secretory IgA is the predominant immunoglobulin in the upper respiratory tract and blocks adherence of pathogens to the respiratory epithelium. IgG is the predominate immunoglobulin in the lower respiratory tract and acts as an opsonizing antibody to promote uptake and destruction of inhaled pathogens. Equine herpesvirus replicates within BALT resulting in necrosis of lymphoid nodules and secondary immunocompromise.

The mucociliary escalator and BALT do not extend to the respiratory zone; therefore, alveolar macrophages are the predominant immune defense mechanism in the terminal bronchioles and alveoli. The alveolar macrophage is the link between specific and nonspecific defense mechanisms. Particles deposited in alveoli are phagocytozed and cleared by alveolar macrophages. Macrophages that have phagocytozed particles are removed from the lung via mucociliary transport to the pharynx or penetration of the respiratory epithelium to be cleared by the lymphatic system. Alveolar macrophage function is impaired or destroyed by strenuous exercise, long-distance transport, and viral respiratory infection.

In addition to impaired pulmonary defense mechanisms, there are several miscellaneous factors that may contribute to development of pneumonia. Hematogenous seeding of bacteria to the lung from a distant focus of infection (i.e., endocarditis, subsolar abscess) can produce metastatic pneumonia. Lungworms (*Dictyocaulus arnfeldi*) or ascarid migration may damage pulmonary tissue, induce excessive mucus production, and contribute to development of secondary bacterial pneumonia. Dysphagia due to mechanical (choke, laryngeal/pharyngeal mass, laryngeal surgery) or neurogenic (peripheral or central neuropathy) etiologies results in aspiration of feed material, which may overwhelm pulmonary defense mechanisms.

## Clinical signs
Clinical signs of bacterial pneumonia/pleuropneumonia include the following:

- Fever, depression, lethargy, and inappetence are common nonspecific findings in horses with bacterial pulmonary infections.
- Horses with pleuropneumonia may demonstrate clinical signs of pleural pain, endotoxemia, and rapid, shallow respiration.
- Auscultation and percussion of the thoracic cavity can identify regions of dullness consistent with pleural effusion, consolidation, or abscessation.

Most horses will not demonstrate respiratory difficulty at rest unless pulmonary consolidation is extensive. A moist, soft, productive cough may occur spontaneously and can be induced with tracheal manipulation. A tracheal rattle, indicating mucus within the tracheal lumen, will often be detected, particularly after coughing. Nasal discharge is a variable sign, because most adult horses swallow exudate originating from the lower respiratory tract. Crackles and wheezes may be noted at rest or with the assistance of a rebreathing procedure. In most instances, crackles will be prominent in the cranioventral lung fields in horses with bacterial pneumonia.

In addition to the above clinical signs, horses with pleuropneumonia may demonstrate signs of pleural pain (pleurodynia), respiratory difficulty, and endotoxemia. Horses with pleural pain have an anxious facial expression, stand with their elbows abducted, and are reluctant to move, cough, or lie down. Affected horses walk with a stiff, stilted gait, and some will grunt in response to thoracic pressure, auscultation, or percussion. The severity of respiratory difficulty depends on the volume of effusion and the extent of pulmonary consolidation. In most cases, the respiratory pattern is characterized by rapid, shallow respiration due to pleural pain and restricted pulmonary expansion by pleural effusion. A plaque of sternal edema is observed in horses with a large volume of pleural effusion. Horses with endotoxemia will have injected mucous membranes, delayed capillary refill time (>2 sec), and tachycardia.

Nasal discharge is variably present, and ranges from mucopurulent to serosanguinous in character. Bloody nasal discharge is a poor prognostic indicator in horses with pneumonia and is observed in cases with infarcted lung, necrotizing pneumonia, and ruptured pulmonary abscess. Putrid breath or fetid nasal discharge indicates anaerobic bacterial infection.

Auscultation of horses with pleuropneumonia reveals a lack of breath sounds in the ventral lung fields and abnormal lung sounds (often crackles) in dorsal lung fields. Cardiac sounds may be muffled or absent, or may radiate over a wider area. Although uncommon, pleural friction rubs are most prominent at end-inspiration and early expiration, and are detected in horses with peracute disease (prior to development of effusion) or after thoracic drainage. A rebreathing procedure is rarely required for auscultation of horses with pleuropneumonia, and may be too stressful for horses with pleural pain and/or respiratory difficulty. Thoracic percussion is performed by tapping a rubber reflex hammer against the concave surface of a spoon, with the convex surface of the spoon held against the thoracic wall. The examiner slides the spoon down each intercostal space over the thoracic cavity to identify regions of hyporesonance. Identification of dull areas on thoracic percussion indicates pulmonary consolidation, abscessation, or pleural effusion. Horses with pleural effusion typically have a horizontal fluid line, below which all pulmonary fields are dull, and above which resonant sounds are produced. Horses with pleurodynia object to this procedure, and may grunt in response to examination.

## Diagnosis

Clinical pathologic abnormalities will vary with the stage and severity of disease:

- Thoracic ultrasound is indicated in horses with regions of poor to absent breath sounds, thoracic pain, and/or dull thoracic percussion.
- Thoracocentesis is performed for diagnostic and therapeutic purposes, and the ideal site for drainage is determined via thoracic ultrasound.
- Bacterial culture is performed on pleural fluid samples and transtracheal aspirates.
- Thoracic radiographs are obtained after drainage of the pleural cavity.

In horses with peracute pleuropneumonia, laboratory findings will reflect bacterial sepsis or endotoxemia, and will include abnormalities such as leukopenia, neutropenia, left shift, hemoconcentration, and azotemia. Horses with more stable disease will have leukocytosis, mature neutrophilia, hyperfibrinogenemia, hyperglobulinemia (chronic antigenic stimulation), hypoalbuminemia (loss in pleural space), and anemia of chronic disease. Horses with chronic disease may have a normal white blood cell count and fibrinogen concentration, despite persistent pulmonary or pleural infection.

## Thoracic ultrasound

Thoracic ultrasound is the ideal diagnostic tool for investigation of pleural effusion and peripheral pulmonary disease, and is indicated in horses with regions of poor to absent breath sounds, thoracic pain, and/or dull thoracic
percussion. Ultrasound examination can identify gas echoes, fibrin, loculation,
or highly cellular fluid within the pleural space, which provides prognostic information for horses with pleuropneumonia. Transudative pleural fluid (peracute pleuropneumonia, neoplastic effusion) appears anechoic, whereas more
cellular exudate appears echogenic. Gas echoes (Fig. 22.1) represent small air
bubbles within pleural fluid, which may indicate an anaerobic pleural infection (poorer prognosis), a bronchopleural fistula, or iatrogenic introduction of
air. Pulmonary atelectasis (Fig. 22.2), consolidation (Fig. 22.3), and abscessation (Fig. 22.4), can be identified if the lesions are located in peripheral lung
fields. Gas impedes ultrasound penetration; therefore, identification of lesions
below air-filled lung is unrewarding, and deep pulmonary abscesses cannot be
detected. Ultrasonographic evidence of large areas of pulmonary consolidation, in conjunction with serosanguinous suppurative pleural effusion, is consistent with pulmonary infarction and necrotizing pneumonia. Adhesions of
the visceral to parietal pleura (Fig. 22.5) can be visualized using thoracic ultrasound, and these regions should be avoided during thoracocentesis.
Pneumothorax can be diagnosed via thoracic ultrasound, but the severity cannot be determined. In horses with pneumothorax, a reverberated white line is
seen (similar to air-filled lung), however, the white line does not slide back and
forth with respiration. In some instances, mediastinal masses may be imaged
via ultrasound. Ultrasound examination should be performed prior to pleurocentesis to determine the site to provide maximum drainage, and the safest site

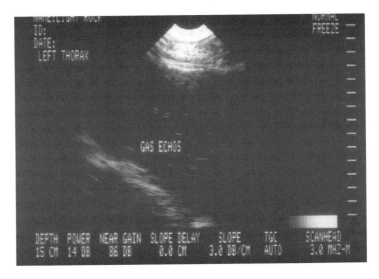

**Fig. 22.1.** Thoracic ultrasonographic image demonstrating gas echoes (bubbles)
within pleural fluid, which may result from an anaerobic pleural infection (poorer prognosis), a bronchopleural fistula, or iatrogenic introduction of air.

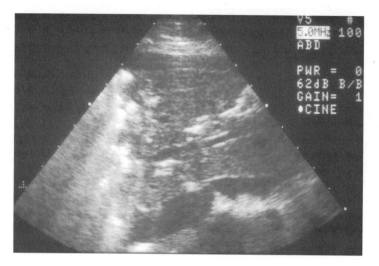

**Fig. 22.2.** Thoracic ultrasonographic image demonstrating pulmonary atelectasis in a foal with septic pleuropneumonia. Note the anechoic pleural fluid surrounding the collapsed lung lobe, fluid-filled airways, and diaphram deep to the lung lobe.

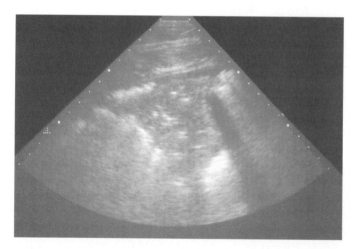

**Fig. 22.3.** Thoracic ultrasonographic image demonstrating pulmonary consolidation in an adult horse with pleuropneumonia. Note the air-filled airways surrounded by fluid-filled parenchyma.

to avoid cardiac or diaphragmatic puncture. Management of horses with pleuropneumonia includes daily ultrasound examination to monitor fluid production, evaluate effective drainage, identify isolated fluid pockets, and assess peripheral pulmonary disease.

### Thoracocentesis

Thoracocentesis is performed for diagnostic and therapeutic purposes in horses with pleuropneumonia. The site for thoracocentesis is determined by ultrasonographic examination to determine the most ventral site for effective

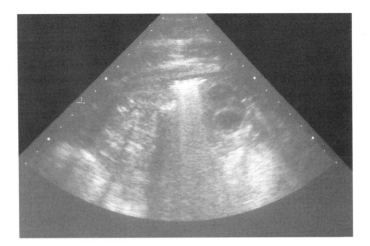

**Fig. 22.4.** Thoracic ultrasonographic image demonstrating peripheral pulmonary abscesses. The abscesses are fluid-filled and have a discrete wall. Although air-filled lung is present adjacent to the abscesses, consolidated lung can be identified in the left half of this image.

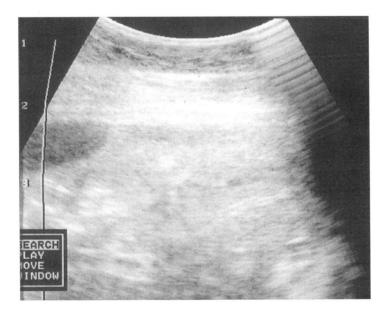

**Fig. 22.5.** Thoracic ultrasonographic image demonstrating an adhesion between the visceral and parietal pleural surfaces in an adult horse with pleuropneumonia. Note the hyperechoic pleural fluid adjacent to the adhesion (total cell count 147,000 cells/µl).

drainage, the position of the heart and diaphragm (may be displaced by a large volume of fluid or mass), and the presence of loculation or pleural adhesions. The technique for thoracocentesis is described in Chapter 23. A large volume of pleural fluid should be drained relatively slowly (over 30 minutes) to avoid hypotension due to third-space loss, and intravenous fluid therapy is indicated during thoracic drainage. Healthy horses do not have an intact mediastinum; however, the communications are relatively small and may be sealed with fibrin in horses with septic pleuritis. The hemithorax that appears to contain the most fluid is drained first, and the opposite hemithorax is reevaluated via ultrasound to determine whether bilateral drainage is necessary. In horses with thoracic neoplasia or peracute pleuritis, bilateral pleural fluid can often be drained via one hemithorax. Bilateral thoracocentesis is usually necessary for thoracic drainage in horses with pleuropneumonia. Intrathoracic pressure changes associated with draining a large volume of effusion may cause rupture of a pulmonary abscess into the pleural space. In this instance, horses may appear toxemic and shocky during, or immediately after, thoracic drainage.

Gross examination of pleural fluid includes evaluation of color, odor, volume, and turbidity. Malodorous pleural fluid is associated with necrotic tissue and anaerobic infection, and indicates a more guarded prognosis. Serosanguinous pleural fluid has been observed in horses with necrotizing pneumonia, pulmonary infarction, thoracic trauma, and thoracic neoplasia. Thoracocentesis samples are submitted for cytologic evaluation (EDTA), anaerobic/aerobic bacterial culture and sensitivity, Gram stain, and biochemical analysis. Cytologic evaluation of septic pleural fluid reveals purulent exudate (>90% neutrophils) with increased cellularity (25,000–200,000 cells/µl) and increased total protein (>3.0 gm/dl). Intracellular and extracellular bacteria may be observed, and Gram stain examination is used to direct initial antimicrobial therapy. Biochemical analysis is performed on pleural fluid samples to differentiate septic from neoplastic effusions. Pleural fluid obtained from horses with complicated pleuronpneumonia is acidic (pH <7.1) with glucose concentrations less than 40 mg/dl and lactate dehydrogenase activity greater than 1000 IU/L.

In addition to pleural fluid, bacterial culture and sensitivity should be performed on transtracheal aspirate samples upon presentation. Transtracheal aspirates yield positive bacterial cultures more frequently than pleural fluid samples, and the bacteria isolated from the airway will differ from those cultured from the pleural space in some cases. The technique for transtracheal aspiration is described in Chapter 23. A Gram stain may provide information to direct initial antibiotic therapy, pending results of bacterial culture and sensitivity. Samples for cytologic evaluation will yield degenerative neutrophils, damaged cells, and bacteria. The presence of squamous epithelial cells on cytologic evaluation indicates pharyngeal contamination of the sample or aspiration of feed and saliva.

Polymicrobial and mixed anaerobic-aerobic infections are common in horses with pleuropneumonia. Fifty to 90% of horses with pleuropneumonia have more than one organism isolated from transtracheal aspirates. Aerobic bacteria are isolated from more than 90% of the cases of pleuropneumonia, and the most common organisms are *Streptococcus zooepidemicus*, *E. coli*, *Actinobacillus* spp., *Klebsiella* spp., *Enterobacter* spp., *Staphylococcus aureus*, and *Pasteurella* spp. Anaerobic bacteria are isolated from 40–70% of horses with pleuropneumonia, and *Bacteroides* spp., *Clostridium* spp., *Peptostrepto-*

*coccus* spp., and *Fusobacterium* spp., are the most commonly isolated anaerobic bacteria. Although fetid breath and malodorous pleural fluid are reliable indicators of the presence of an anaerobic infection, the absence of odor does not preclude an anaerobic pulmonary infection. The etiology of pleural infection in horses is usually bacterial, although fungal, *Mycoplasma felis*, and nocardial agents have been isolated from pleural effusions.

The chest tube may be removed immediately after drainage of the thoracic cavity, or may be secured in place to allow continual drainage. The volume and character of pleural fluid will determine whether single, intermittent, or continual drainage is indicated. Continual drainage is preferable in cases with fibrinous, cellular, malodorous, and/or large volume of effusion. A one-way (Heimlich) valve allows constant drainage of pleural fluid, with minimal risk for development of pneumothorax. An indwelling chest tube should remain in place as long as drainage is productive. Pleural fluid should be recultured at 7–14 day intervals to determine whether the bacterial isolates or sensitivity patterns have changed in response to antimicrobial therapy. The tube can be aspirated with a 60 ml catheter tip syringe if it becomes obstructed with fibrin or inspissated exudate. An ultrasound examination will determine whether an unproductive tube is clogged (fluid accumulating in the thoracic cavity) or whether exudate production has ceased. Cellulitis may develop at the entry site of an indwelling chest tube. Warm compresses should be applied to the site to reduce swelling; however, development of a serious subcutaneous infection will necessitate removal of the tube. In some instances, pleural fluid will accumulate in pockets (identified via ultrasound) that cannot be drained by a single indwelling chest tube. Thoracocentesis is performed at the most ventral aspect of the pocket to drain the accumulated fluid. The thoracic cavity can be lavaged with polyionic fluids to assist with removal of fibrin and exudates. The indwelling tube can be used for infusion and drainage of lavage fluid, or a dorsal tube can be placed for infusion and the indwelling tube can be used for drainage. Five to 10 liters of sterile, warm isotonic fluid is infused into each hemithorax by gravity flow. Infusion should stop to allow drainage of fluid if the horse appears anxious or restless, regardless of the volume administered. Pleural lavage is contraindicated in patients with a bronchopleural fistula. Coughing and nasal drainage of pleural fluid during infusion suggests the presence of a communication between an airway and the pleural space. Continued lavage may result in dissemination of septic fluids to other regions of lung. To confirm the presence of a bronchopleural fistula, flouroscein dye is infused into the pleural cavity, and appearance of the dye at the nares confirms the presence of bronchopleural fistula.

### Thoracic radiographs

Unlike thoracic ultrasound, thoracic radiographs cannot detect small volumes of pleural fluid, distinguish unilateral disease, or identify fibrin, cellularity or gas echoes. However, thoracic radiographs can evaluate deep pulmonary parenchymal lesions, mediastinal structures, and the presence/severity of pneumothorax. Thoracic radiographs should be obtained after thoracocentesis to maximize visualization of parenchymal disease. Serial examination can identify disease progression and response to treatment. Pulmonary alveolization (consolidation) is most severe in the cranioventral pulmonary fields in most cases of bacterial pneumonia. However, horses with hematogenous (metastatic) pneumonia will have caudodorsal distribution of pulmonary disease. Air bronchograms are rarely observed in adult horses.

## Treatment

The keys to successful management of horses with pleuropneumonia are appropriate antimicrobial therapy, effective thoracic drainage, meticulous patient monitoring, and client commitment:

- Broad-spectrum antimicrobial therapy is indicated, because the majority of horses with pleuropneumonia have polymicrobial infections.
- Daily monitoring of the thoracic cavity via ultrasound is necessary to evaluate effective drainage, identify isolated fluid pockets, and assess peripheral pulmonary disease.
- Supportive care consists of intravenous fluid therapy, nutritional support, and NSAID therapy.
- Thoracostomy may be required in refractory cases.
- Clients should be committed to a treatment plan that may be prolonged, expensive, and complex.

Some horses with pleuropneumonia will have uncomplicated effusions, which require thoracic drainage on one occasion (or not at all), and respond quickly to antibiotic therapy. These cases are less common than cases that require indwelling chest tubes or intermittent thoracocentesis. Early intervention reduces the complexity of case management and reduces hospitalization time. Meticulous monitoring of the horse is necessary to determine efficiency of thoracic drainage, appropriateness of antibiotic coverage, and development of complications. Clients should be aware from the onset that treatment of pleuropneumonia is often prolonged and expensive, and complications are common.

Medical therapy for bacterial pneumonia and pleuropneumonia requires broad-spectrum antimicrobial therapy, anti-inflammatory drugs, and supportive care. Most cases of pleuropneumonia have polymicrobial infections requiring combination drug therapy (Table 22.1). The combination of penicillin, gentamicin, and metronidazole is often used for initial therapy in horses with pleuropneumonia. *Streptococcus zooepidemicus* isolates are usually sensitive to beta-lactam drugs such as penicillin or sodium ampicillin, and an aminoglyocoside drug such as gentamicin sulfate provides Gram negative spectrum for organisms such as *E. coli, Actinobacillus* spp., and *Pasteurella* spp. Although penicillin is effective against many anaerobic bacterial infections, *Bacterioides* spp. are penicillin-resistant due to ß lactamase production. Therefore, metronidazole is administered initially to provide more complete anaerobic bacterial

**Table 22.1.** Antimicrobial drug dosages for bacterial pneumonia and pleuropneumonia in horses.

| Drug | Class | Dose | Route | Frequency | Comments |
|---|---|---|---|---|---|
| Procaine penicillin G | β lactam | 22,000 IU/kg | IM | BID | Penicillins have Gram + and anaerobic spectrum, but |
| Potassium penicillin G | β lactam | 20,000–40,000 IU/kg | IV | QID | are not effective against *Bacteroides* or *Staphlococcus* |
| Sodium penicillin G | β lactam | 20,000–40,000 IU/kg | IV | QID | due to b-lactamase production. |
| Ampicillin sodium | β lactam | 15–30 mg/kg | IV | QID to TID | Gram + and limited Gram – spectrum |
| Gentamicin sulfate | aminoglycoside | 6.6 mg/kg | IM or IV | SID | Gram – spectrum; no activity against anaerobes |
| Amikacin sulfate | aminoglycoside | 20 mg/kg | IM or IV | SID | Gram – spectrum; no activity against anaerobes |
| Metronidazole | nitroimidazole | 15–25 mg/kg | PO | QID | Anaerobic spectrum; can be given per rectum |
| Trimethoprim-sulfa | potentiated sulphonamide | 15–30 mg/kg | PO | BID | Bacteriostatic at low doses, bacteriocidal at high doses |
| | | 15 mg/kg | IV | BID | |
| Chloramphenicol | N/A | 25–50 mg/kg | PO | QID | Bacteriostatic; human health (aplastic anemia) concerns |
| Ceftiofur sodium | cephalosporin | 2.5–5.0 mg/kg | IM or IV | BID | 3rd generation cephalosporin |
| Doxycycline HCL | tetracyclines | 3–10 mg/kg | PO | SID to BID | Bacteriostatic; Gram +, Gram –, antiprotozoal spectrum |
| Enrofloxacin | quinilone | 5.0 mg/kg | IV | SID | Excellent Gram – and good Gram + spectrum; effective |
| | | 7.5 mg/kg | PO | SID | against *Mycoplasma*; not effective against Strep |
| Rifampin | rifamycin | 5–10 mg/kg | PO | BID | Gram +, Gram –, and mycobacterial spectrum; resistance |

281

coverage until results of anaerobic culture are negative and clinical signs of anaerobic infection (gas echoes, putrid breath) have resolved. The antimicrobial regimen may require adjustment as the results of bacterial culture and sensitivity become available. Alternative antimicrobial agents for successful treatment of pleuropneumonia include enrofloxacin, ceftiofur, amikacin, trimethoprim-sulfadiazine, doxycycline, chloramphenicol, and rifampin. Intravenous antibiotics are preferable in the early stages of treatment (14–28 days) to ensure adequate drug concentrations. Oral antimicrobial therapy can be instituted as the horse becomes more stable and production of pleural fluid subsides.

Nonsteroidal anti-inflammatory agents are indicated in horses with pleuropneumonia for pyrexia, inflammation, endotoxemia, and pain. Phenylbutazone (2.2–4.4 mg/kg IV or PO q12 hrs) and flunixin meglumine (0.25–1.1 mg/kg every 8–24 hrs IV or PO) are commonly used. Dehydration potentiates the adverse effects of NSAID, and the toxic effects of flunixin and phenylbutazone are additive with concurrent administration. Judicious administration will avoid gastrointestinal (gastric and right dorsal colon ulceration) and renal (papillary necrosis) complications of NSAID administration. Intravenous fluid therapy may be required to correct dehydration, maintain hydration, and replace ongoing losses into the pleural space. Skin turgor, mucous membrane character, and packed cell volume are used to monitor the volume of fluid therapy, whereas the type of fluid administered is determined by serum electrolyte concentrations and acid-base status. Horses with serious pulmonary infections are anorexic and suffer rapid weight loss. Adequate nutrition provides an important contribution to the recovery of these patients. The owner or clinician should offer highly palatable feeds and fresh grass to encourage the horse to eat. In some instances, supplemental enteral or parenteral nutrition may be necessary. In addition, a clean, dry comfortable environment will encourage adequate rest and feed intake.

## Thoracostomy

Some horses fail to clear the pleural infection over the course of weeks to months of antimicrobial therapy and drainage via indwelling chest tubes. Thoracostomy allows manual removal of organized fibrinous material and necrotic lung. Case selection is critical, and this technique should be limited to horses with chronic, stable, unilateral disease with resolving infection in the contralateral hemithorax. Horses should be systemically stable, and must have been treated for more than 1 month to be a candidate for this procedure. Ideally, the abscess pocket will be walled off from the rest of the thorax with a complete visceral-to-parietal seal. Prior to performing a thoracotomy, the clinician must determine that the pneumothorax will remain unilateral (complete mediastinum) and will not compromise the respiratory function of the horse. The one-way valve should be removed from an indwelling chest tube at the prospective surgery site to allow pneumothorax to develop for a minimum of 2 hours. If respiratory distress results, air should be removed from the thoracic cavity and the procedure should be delayed.

There are two options for creating a thoracostomy in horses with pleuro-pneumonia: a rib resection or dissection through the intercostal space (finger-hole). The intercostal approach heals more quickly and usually allows adequate drainage, but manual access to the thoracic cavity is limited and resection of necrotic lung is difficult. Rib resection creates a larger defect for more effective drainage and debridement, but heals more slowly, is more painful after surgery, and may develop a chronic draining tract. Both procedures are performed in standing, sedated horses with local analgesia. A standing procedure avoids complications of general anesthesia, allows the clinician to monitor the response to unilateral pneumothorax, and ensures that the skin incision is directly aligned with the thoracic incision (skin incision may shift caudal to the thoracic incision upon standing if procedure is performed in a recumbent horse). Postoperatively, the pleural cavity can be debrided manually and lavaged (sterile, isotonic fluids) on a daily basis to loosen and remove debris. After adequate granulation of the incision (7–10 days), hydrotherapy of the wound and thorax can be performed with tap water.

## Complications

Complications of pleuropneumonia may directly involve the thoracic cavity or may occur in other body systems. The most common complications directly involving the thoracic cavity include pneumothorax, pleural adhesions, pulmonary abscess, pulmonary infarction, bronchopleural fistula, and cranial mediastinal abscess. Pneumothorax is one of the most common intrathoracic complications of pleuropneumonia and can result from thoracocentesis (iatrogenic) or bronchopleural fistula. In many cases, pneumothorax is self-limiting in horses with pleuropneumonia; however, dorsal pleurocentesis and aspiration of air is indicated in horses with respiratory difficulty due to pneumothorax (Fig. 22.6). Pulmonary infarction results in hemorrhagic necrotizing pneumonia, which is characterized by serosanguinous, malodorous pleural fluid, and ultimately, a poor response to therapy. Bronchopleural fistulas develop in horses with necrotic lung, creating a communication between the pleural cavity and an airway. Bronchopleural fistula does not limit the prognosis for survival, but does prevent thoracic lavage, limits the prognosis for athleticism, and prolongs the duration of hospitalization. Cranial mediastinal abscesses result from organization of septic pleural fluid trapped cranial to the heart. Clinical signs of a cranial mediastinal abscess include pointing of a forelimb, tachycardia, jugular vein distention, pectoral edema, spontaneous jugular vein thrombosis, and caudal displacement of the heart. Diagnosis is confirmed via ultrasonographic identification of an abscess pocket cranial to the heart and caudal displacement of the heart. Some cranial mediastinal abscesses will respond to systemic antibiotic therapy. Abscesses that compromise cardiovascular function by compressing the cardiac chambers and great vessels should be drained via trocharization and lavage, performed under general anesthesia.

The most common complications involving other extrathoracic systems in-

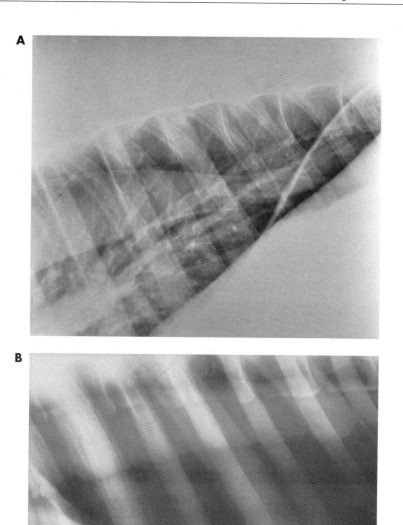

**Fig. 22.6.** Lateral thoracic radiographic image of dorsal lung fields of 2 horses with pneumothorax. A. Mild, unilateral, iatrogenic pneumothorax resulting from thoracocentesis. B. Severe, bilateral, life-threatening pneumothorax resulting from a bronchopleural fistula.

clude laminitis, antibiotic-induced colitis, and jugular vein thrombosis at the catheter entry site. Laminitis may limit the prognosis for return to athletic function, despite a favorable response to therapy for pleuropneumonia. Antibiotic-induced colitis is often life-threatening in this population of horses because they are debilitated and antibiotic therapy cannot be discontinued (but should be changed). If thrombophlebitis occurs in numerous vessels, it may eliminate the intravenous route of drug administration, limiting the options for antimicrobial therapy. Septic thrombophlebitis can be life-threatening, and aspirate samples should be collected for bacterial culture and sensitivity. To minimize the risk of thrombophlebitis, intravenous catheters with low thrombogenicity should be used and repeated venipuncture should be avoided.

## Prognosis

The prognosis for horses with pleuropneumonia has greatly improved over the past 20 years due to early recognition, advancements in diagnostic testing (primarily ultrasound), and aggressive therapy (thoracocentesis, thoracostomy). The duration and expense of treatment varies greatly depending on the severity of disease and development of complications. With owner commitment and clinician experience, the survival rate is reported to be as high as 90% by some investigators with a 60% chance to return to athletic performance. The duration of hospitalization is not indicative of outcome; however, a delay in initiation of appropriate therapy by more than 48 hours does promote development of anaerobic infection, and ultimately, poorer response to treatment. Placement of an indwelling chest tube does not limit the prognosis for return to athletic function, but complications such as cranial thoracic mass and bronchopleural fistula appear to worsen the prognosis for racing. Horses with hemorrhagic necrotizing pneumonia respond poorly to conventional therapy and have a low survival rate.

## FUNGAL PNEUMONIA

Despite constant inhalation of fungal elements from bedding and feed, fungal pneumonia is uncommon in horses:

- The most common isolate obtained from horses with fungal pneumonia is *Aspergillus* spp.
- The most important predisposing factor for the development of fungal pneumonia is gastrointestinal disease and disruption of the intestinal mucosa.
- Heightened awareness of predisposing conditions that contribute to development of fungal pneumonia will improve the probability of ante-mortem diagnosis.

The most common isolate from horses with fungal pneumonia is *Aspergillus* sp., and the majority of cases occur in horses with severe gastrointestinal disease. Chronic debilitation, neutropenia, and immunosuppression are also risk factors. Enteritis, colitis, and typlitis are suspected to predispose horses to fungal pneumonia by disrupting the gastrointestinal mucosa, allowing invasion of fungal organisms and embolic dissemination of fungal elements to the lung.

Nonsteroidal anti-inflammatory drug administration may contribute to mucosal disruption in horses with gastrointestinal disease. In addition, profound neutropenia associated with severe gastrointestinal disease limits the patient's ability to combat the infection. Neutropenia is a substantial risk factor in human patients with fungal pneumonia. In horses, leukopenia and neutropenia are reported in more than half of the cases of fungal pneumonia, however, the role of neutropenia in the pathophysiology is unclear. In support of hematogenous dissemination in horses with gastrointestinal disease, fungal organisms are found in tissues other than the lung (kidney and brain) in approximately 40% of horses with pulmonary aspergillosis. Overwhelming exposure to inhaled spores may be the route of infection for fungal pneumonia resulting from immunosuppression due to prolonged corticosteroid administration, pituitary adenoma, or debilitating disease. Invasive fungal organisms—such as *Coccidioides immitis, Histoplasma capsulatum,* and *Cryptococcus neoformans*—do not require a predisposing condition to establish a pulmonary infection, but are rarely reported in horses.

The clinical signs of fungal pneumonia in horses include tachypnea, fever, nasal discharge, epistaxis, nasal plaques or erosions, abnormal lung sounds, and pleural friction rubs. Most horses have a history of progression of respiratory disease despite aggressive and prolonged antibiotic therapy. Careful examination of the nasal passages may reveal a nasal plaque or ulcer. This clinical sign is present in only 10% of the cases, but is highly predictive of concomitant or future invasive pulmonary aspergillosis. Low-volume pleural effusion may be identified via ultrasound examination, and fibrin plaques have been observed at necropsy on visceral and parietal pleural surfaces. Some horses show no signs of respiratory disease, despite obvious pulmonary disease at post-mortem examination.

Ante-mortem diagnosis of fungal pneumonia is rarely reported. The majority of documented cases were diagnosed post-mortem. Ante-mortem diagnosis depends on the clinician's awareness of predisposing conditions that contribute to development of fungal pneumonia and careful monitoring of the respiratory tract of horses with risk factors. In horses with severe gastrointestinal disease, development of abnormal lung sounds (crackles and wheezes), pleural friction rubs, or pulmonary hemorrhage should alert the clinician to investigate pulmonary aspergillosis.

Observation of fungal spores on cytologic evaluation and/or culture of fungal elements from transtracheal aspirate samples are not strong indicators of a diagnosis of fungal pneumonia in horses. *Aspergillus* spp. are isolated from transtracheal aspirates in 16% of healthy horses and may represent inhaled spores or colonization of the respiratory tract, rather than invasive disease. In human patients, fungal culture and cytologic examination of BAL fluid are more specific and sensitive for diagnosis of pulmonary aspergillosis than culture of tracheal aspirates or sputum samples. Heavy growth of fungus from a BAL sample in horses should be considered supportive evidence of fungal pneumonia. Culture and histologic evaluation of lung biopsy samples provide definitive evidence of fungal pneumonia, but may be too invasive. In addition, the multi-focal distribution of the disease may lead to false negative lung biopsy results. *Aspergillosis* spp. is the most common opportunistic organism in horses with fungal pneumonia; however, *Scopulariopsis* sp, *Phycomycetes* spp., and *Candida* have been isolated. Unlike the opportunistic fungi, organisms capable of primary invasion—such as *Coccidioides immitis, Histoplasma capsulatum,* and *Cryptococcus neoformans*—are best diagnosed from culture and cytology of transtracheal aspirates due to the multifocal distribution of infection.

Thoracic radiographs of horses with fungal pneumonia can demonstrate virtually any radiographic pattern. Patchy bronchopneumonia and miliary/reticulonodular interstitial patterns are common. The distribution of coalescing nodules is multifocal and lesions are visualized in peripheral lung fields (see Fig. 23.11). Abnormalities on thoracic radiographs may be more striking than the clinical signs of disease. Low-volume pleural effusion can be detected by thoracic ultrasound. If pleural effusion is identified, pleural fluid samples should be submitted for cytologic evaluation and culture. Nasal ulcerations or plaques on horses with suspected fungal pneumonia should be biopsied; histologic evidence of fungal organisms in these samples is highly predictive of concomitant or future pulmonary aspergillosis.

Specific antifungal therapy for treatment of mycotic pneumonia is dependent on the isolate. Successful treatment is rarely documented, which may reflect rare ante-mortem diagnosis and/or poor response to therapy. Amphotericin-B is an appropriate therapeutic choice for aspergillosis, but may be cost-prohibitive for many horses. Recommended dosage regimens include the following schedule: 0.3, 0.45, and 0.6 mg/kg on days 1, 2, and 3, respectively, followed by every-other-day administration of 0.6 mg/kg until a cumulative dose of 6.75 mg/kg amphotericin B has been administered. Amphotericin B is mixed in 1 liter of 5% dextrose and administered over 1 hour via an intravenous catheter. Side effects include polyuria/polydypsia (4th week of treatment), intermittent fever (first two weeks), and lethargy (after every treatment). Urinalysis and serum biochemical profile should be obtained weekly to detect evidence of renal or hepatic dysfunction. Ketoconazole (30 mg/kg, intragastric, BID) and oral iodides (20 gm/450 kg, SID) are less expensive, but in general, are less likely to resolve fungal pneumonia. Successful treatment has been described with ketoconazole initially, followed by aerosolized enilconazole (1.2 mg/kg in saline via ultrasonic nebulization, BID) for long-term treatment in a horse with *Scopulariopsis* sp. pneumonia. The horse responded favorably to ketaconazole therapy, and the follow-up treatment with aerosolized enilconazole was an effective, economic, and safe alternative therapy.

## PULMONARY METACESTODE INFECTION

There are few reports of clinical respiratory disease resulting from metacestode infections in horses. In the United Kingdom, hydatidosis (*Echinococcus gran-*

*ulosis*) is generally well-tolerated in horses, and cysts in the liver and lung may be an incidental finding at post-mortem examination. Occasionally, large pulmonary or pleural cysts rupture, resulting in a large volume of pleural effusion. In the United States, *Echinococcus granulosis* and an unidentifiable aberrant, acephalic metacestode have been identified in the liver and lungs of horses. In the U.S., the acephalic metacestode has been the offending parasite in horses with large-volume pleural effusion and clinical disease.

Affected horses may have intermittent fever, depression, rapid shallow respiration, pectoral edema, and nonspecific laboratory findings indicative of in-

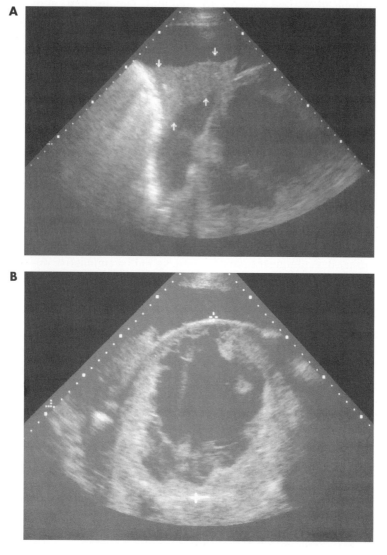

**Fig. 22.7.** Thoracic ultrasound demonstrating pleural effusion (A), pulmonary atelectasis (A), and a large cyst on the surface of the diaphragm (A,B) from an 8-year-old horse with unidentified aberrant, acephalic metacestode infection.

flammation. A large volume of pleural effusion is a consistent finding in horses with pulmonary and pleural metacestode infection. The effusion has low to moderate cellularity (5,000–80,000 cells/μL), 20–80% neutrophils, and markedly increased protein concentration (5.0–8.0 gm/dl). Bacterial and fungal culture of the pleural fluid is negative. The clinical disease is difficult to differentiate from neoplastic effusion. Some tumors of the thoracic cavity are minimally exfoliative; therefore, the absence of neoplastic cells on cytology does not preclude a diagnosis of neoplasia. Ultrasound examination may reveal a large fluid-filled cyst within the pulmonary parenchyma, on the surface of the diaphragm (Fig. 22.7), and/or within the hepatic parenchyma. Metacestodes may be attached to a thickened pleural surface, or hypoechoic cysts (1 x 4 mm) may be seen floating within the pleural or peritoneal fluid.

This author has treated a horse with an unidentified aberrant, acephalic metacestode using albendazole (10 mg/kg, PO, SID x 30d), thoracic drainage, and surgical debridement of the pleura and cyst (10 x 10 x 17 cm) on the surface of the diaphragm. Disruption of a cyst by centesis or surgery may result in an anaphylactic reaction or seeding of daughter metacestodes within the thoracic cavity. Surgical intervention was performed in this case after 2 weeks of antiparasitic therapy. The horse was asymptomatic 6 weeks after treatment, and has remained athletic for 4 years.

## FURTHER READING

Carr, E.A., Carlson, G.P., Wilson, W.D., et al. 1997. Acute hemorrhagic pulmonary infarction and necrotizing pneumonia in horses: 21 cases (1967–1993). *J Am Vet Med Assoc* 210(12):1774–1778.

Chaffin, M.K., and Carter, G.K. 1993. Equine bacterial pleuropneumonia. I, Epidemiology, pathophysiology, and bacterial isolates. *Comp Cont Educ Pract Vet* 15: 1642–1650.

Chaffin, M.K., Carter, G.K., and Byars, T.D. 1994. Equine bacterial pleuropneumonia. III, Treatment, sequelae, and prognosis. *Comp Cont Educ Pract Vet* 16:1585–1589.

Chaffin, M.K., Carter, G.K., and Redford, R.L. 1991. Bacterial pleuropneumonia. II, Clinical signs and diagnostic evaluation. *Comp Cont Educ Pract Vet* 16:362–378.

Nappert, G., Van Dyck, T., Papich, M., et al. 1996. Successful treatment of a fever associated with consistent pulmonary isolation of *Scopulariopsis* sp. in a mare. *Equine Vet J* 28(5):421–424.

Seltzer, K.L., and Byars, T.D. 1996. Prognosis for return to racing after recovery from infectious pleuropneumonia in Thoroughbred racehorses: 70 cases (1984–1989). *J Am Vet Med Assoc* 208:1300–1301.

Slocombe, R., and Slauson, D. 1988. Invasive pulmonary aspergillosis of horses: An association with acute enteritis. *Vet Pathol* 25:277–281.

Sweeney, C.R., and Habecker, P.L. 1999. Pulmonary aspergillosis in horses: 29 cases (1974–1997). *J Am Vet Med Assoc* 214(6):808–811.

# Techniques for Infectious Respiratory Disease

Transtracheal aspiration (TTW) provides a representative sample of the bacterial population from the lower respiratory tract, and is the most appropriate procedure to perform to obtain respiratory secretions for bacterial culture in horses with infectious respiratory disease.

## TRANSTRACHEAL ASPIRATION

Transtracheal aspiration is well-tolerated in most horses, and light sedation and local anesthetic will facilitate completion of this procedure. The procedure should be performed at the junction of the proximal 1/3 and distal 2/3 of the cervical trachea. The ventral aspect of the tracheal rings should be readily palpable. A 10 cm x 10 cm area of skin is clipped and prepared using sterile technique. Approximately 1 ml of local anesthetic is infused subcutaneously, and a 3–5 mm stab incision is made vertically through the skin and subcutaneous tissue using a No. 15 blade. A transtracheal wash trochar is inserted, perpendicular to the skin, between tracheal rings, while manually stabilizing the trachea (Fig. 23.1). Firm, constant pressure, with slight twisting to seat the trochar, will facilitate penetration of the tracheal wall. After penetration, the trochar is removed from the sheath, and the sheath is inserted *down* the trachea. A lavage catheter (i.e., 5–8F tomcat) is introduced through the sheath into the airway to the level of the thoracic inlet (50–60 cm), and 30–50 ml of isotonic crystalline solution is instilled and immediately aspirated from the airway (Fig. 23.2). If no fluid is initially recovered, the catheter can be repositioned in an attempt to locate pooled fluid within the trachea. The flushing/aspiration procedure can be repeated if an inadequate sample is obtained after the first attempt. Coughing may improve

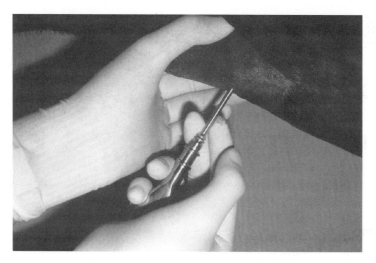

**Fig. 23.1.** Insertion of a transtracheal wash trochar at the junction of the upper 1/3 and lower 2/3 of the neck, perpendicular to the skin, while manually stabilizing the trachea.

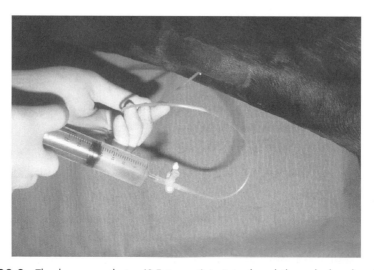

**Fig. 23.2.** The lavage catheter (8-F tomcat) is introduced through the sheath into the airway, and 30–50 ml of isotonic crystalline solution is instilled and immediately aspirated.

recovery of exudate/pathogens from the lower respiratory tract. However, paroxysmal coughing may retroflex the catheter to the pharynx, contaminating the sample. After collection of a satisfactory sample, the catheter should be completely removed prior to removal of the sheath to minimize contamination of the subcutaneous tissues with respiratory pathogens. If the procedure has been performed using a large bore needle to introduce the catheter, the needle must be withdrawn from the tracheal lumen and skin prior to manipulation of the catheter (to avoid shearing the catheter). This technique requires dragging the contaminated catheter through subcutaneous tissues, and may increase the risk of cellulitis. A bandage may be placed over the site for 24 hours or a simple interrupted suture may be used to close the skin.

Tracheal samples for bacterial culture and sensitivity can be obtained through an endoscope using guarded bronchoscopy or with specifically designed guarded catheters introduced via the nasopharyx. These techniques are less invasive than percutaneous transtracheal aspiration. The endoscopic procedure allows the clinician to visual exudate within the airway for sampling. However, contamination of the sample with organisms from the nasopharynx or endoscopy equipment (particulary *Pseudomonas* spp.) makes interpretation difficult. Sterilization of endoscopy equipment and guarded catheter techniques reduce the likelihood of pharyngeal contamination, but do not eliminate the possibility. Samples can be submitted to the laboratory in the syringe or sterile transport media for anaerobic/aerobic bacterial culture and sensitivity. A Gram stain may provide information to direct initial antibiotic therapy, pending results of bacterial culture and sensitivity. Samples for cytologic evaluation should be submitted in EDTA preservative. The presence of squamous epithelial cells on cytologic evaluation indicates pharyngeal contamination of the sample.

Significant care should be exercised during and after the transtracheal wash procedure to avoid iatrogenic complications, such as cellulitis, bleeding, subcutaneous emphysema, tracheal ring damage, and loss of the catheter within the tracheal lumen. Cellulitis results from dragging bacteria (from the lumen of the airway) through the subcutaneous space after completion of the procedure. Untreated cellulitis can be serious and may migrate ventrally to invade the mediastinal space. Serious bleeding occurs with laceration of the carotid artery or jugular vein by the trochar. A firm pressure bandage is applied to reduce blood loss into the subcutaneous space, and prophylactic antibiotics are administered to avoid bacterial infection of the hematoma. Damage to the tracheal rings can occur with overzealous and/or inappropriate trochar placement. Damage to rings on the ventral aspect of the trachea occurs when the operator fails to introduce the trochar between tracheal rings and attempts to puncture through tracheal rings. Overzealous introduction of the trochar can result in traumatic injury to the lumenal surface of the tracheal rings on the dorsal aspect of the trachea. Cartilagenous damage can produce chondromas or stenosis of the tracheal lumen. The catheter may shear off within the tracheal lumen with excessive manipulation of the catheter during infusion or aspiration. This is particularly likely if a large bore needle is used for introduction of the catheter. Horses frequently cough up the catheter within 20 minutes, however, endoscopic retrieval of a severed catheter may be necessary. In some instances, the severed catheter may remain attached to the wall of the trachea at the site of penetration. Damage to the tracheal wall or excessive coughing may result in subcutaneous emphysema, which is usually self-limiting and resolves in 2–7 days.

## THORACIC ULTRASOUND

Thoracic ultrasound is an ideal diagnostic tool for investigation of pleural and peripheral pulmonary disease. Thoracic ultrasound is indicated in horses with regions of poor to absent breath sounds, thoracic pain, and/or dull thoracic percussion. The quality of portable ultrasound equipment has made this diagnostic tool readily accessible for most equine clinicians and relatively easy to interpret. The depth of penetration is inversely proportional and the degree of image resolution is directly proportional to the frequency of sound generation. A 3.5–5.0 MHz transducer should be used to penetrate the pleural space and peripheral pulmonary tissue. Sector and linear-array scanners can be used to image the equine thorax. Sector scanners provide higher quality images than linear-array scanners (typically used for reproductive evaluation), but are more expensive.

Hair is clipped from the region of interest to provide adequate contact for imaging, although this may not be necessary in horses with a short haircoat. Acoustic coupling gel or alcohol should be applied to the skin to maximize contact with the probe. Normal lung tissue is air-filled, and thus reflects the ultrasound beam, producing a thin, white line at the pulmonary surface(Fig. 23.3). As the horse breathes, the reverberation (white) line of the pulmonary surface can be seen sliding back and forth across the parietal pleural surface. Ultrasonographic imaging of each hemithorax should be performed from the dorsal to the ventral lung border, imaging the entire lung field.

Ultrasound examination of the thorax is superior to radiographic examination to identify the location, depth, and character of pleural fluid. Ultrasound examination can identify gas echoes, fibrin, loculation, or highly cellular fluid

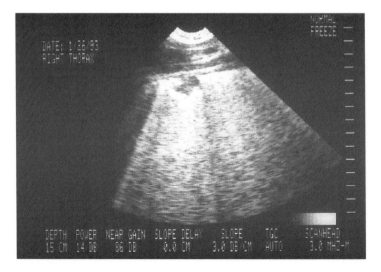

**Fig. 23.3.** Thoracic ultrasonographic image demonstrating the white line generated by ultrasound reflection of air-filled lung at the pulmonary surface. A small area of peripheral pulmonary consolidation is observed.

within the pleural space, which provides prognostic information in horses with pleuropneumonia. Transudative pleural fluid (peracute pleuropneumonia, neoplastic effusion) appears anechoic, whereas more cellular exudates appear echogenic. Gas echoes (bubbles) within pleural fluid may result from an anaerobic pleural infection (poorer prognosis), a bronchopleural fistula, or iatrogenic introduction of air (see Chapter 22, Fig. 22.1). Adhesions of the visceral to parietal pleura can be detected via thoracic ultrasound (see Chapter 22, Fig. 22.5). Pulmonary atelectasis (see Chapter 22, Fig. 22.2), consolidation (see Chapter 22, Fig. 22.3), and abscessation (see Chapter 22, Fig. 22.4) can be identified if the lesions are located on the peripheral aspect of the lung and communicate with the pleural space. Gas impedes ultrasound penetration; therefore, investigation of lesions below air-filled lung is unrewarding, and deep pulmonary abscesses cannot be visualized. Pneumothorax can be detected via thoracic ultrasound, but the severity cannot be determined. In horses with penumothorax, a reverberated white line is noted (similar to air-filled lung); however, the white line does not slide back and forth with respiration. In some instances, mediastinal masses may be imaged via ultrasound. The presence of pleural fluid facilitates visualization of caudal mediastinal masses by displacing aerated lung. Cranial mediastinal masses may be visualized at the 3rd right intercostal space. Thoracic radiographs are superior for investigation of pulmonary parenchymal lesions. The pericardiodiaphragmatic ligament is readily imaged in horses with a moderate to large volume of anechoic pleural fluid. It appears as a continuous, thin tissue-dense structure attached at both ends (no free end), and should not be misinterpreted as a fibrin tag (Fig. 23.4). Ultrasound examination should be performed prior to thoracic drainage to determine the ideal location for pleurocentesis to provide maximum drainage and avoid cardiac or diaphragmatic puncture.

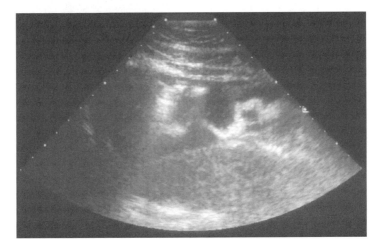

**Fig. 23.4.** The pericardiodiaphragmatic ligament is readily imaged in horses with a moderate to large volume of anechoic pleural fluid. It appears as a continuous, thin tissue–dense structure attached at both ends.

## THORACOCENTESIS

Pleural fluid accumulation occurs in horses with pleuropneumonia, penetrating wounds to the thorax, thoracic neoplasia, and hydatid cyst. Percutaneous sampling of pleural fluid is performed for diagnostic and therapeutic purposes. Ideally, the site for thoracocentesis is determined by ultrasonographic examination. Thoracic ultrasound can determine the most ventral site for effective drainage, the position of the heart and diaphragm (may be displaced by a large volume of fluid or mass), and the presence of loculation or pleural adhesions. The skin is clipped and aseptically prepared. The skin and periosteum of the rib is blocked with local anesthetic solution, and a stab incision in the skin is made to facilitate introduction of the trochar. Care should be taken to avoid laceration of the lateral thoracic vein. A large bore (28–32 French) chest tube with a trochar (Argyle) should be used to drain a large volume of pleural fluid. The trochar is introduced directly into the thoracic cavity, perpendicular to the skin, along the cranial border of the rib (to avoid the vein, artery, and nerve on the caudal aspect) (Fig. 23.5). Upon penetration of the thoracic cavity, the trochar is retracted and the chest tube is advanced to the 6–10 cm marker (Fig. 23.6). A hemostat is used during thoracic drainage to prevent iatrogenic introduction of air into the pleural cavity during inspiration. A large volume of pleural fluid should be drained relatively slowly (over 30 minutes) to avoid hy-

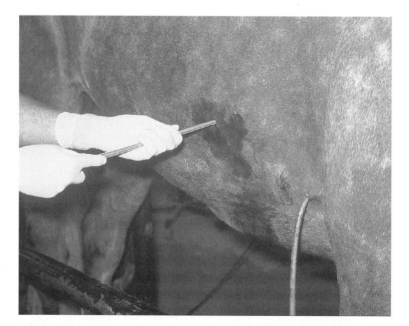

**Fig. 23.5.** A large bore (28F) chest tube with a trochar is introduced directly into the thoracic cavity, perpendicular to the skin, along the cranial border of the rib to drain this isolated pocket of fluid identified via ultrasonography. Note that the first chest tube (cranioventral thorax) remains indwelling, but failed to drain this area of the pleural cavity.

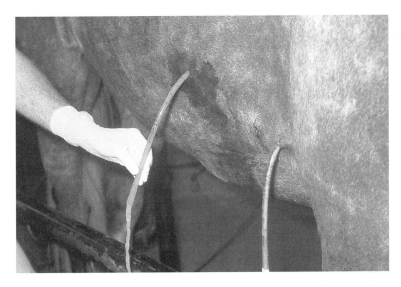

**Fig. 23.6.** A large volume of pleural fluid is allowed to freely drain initially. As the volume gets smaller, a hemostat is used to occlude the drain during inhalation to prevent iatrogenic introduction of air into the pleural cavity.

potension due to third space loss. Intravenous fluid therapy during thoracocentisis is indicated during removal of a large volume of pleural fluid. Horses do not have an intact mediastinum; however, the communications are relatively small and may be sealed with fibrin in horses with septic pleuritis, often necessitating bilateral thoracocentesis. The hemithorax that appears to contain the most fluid is drained first, and the opposite hemithorax is reevaluated via ultrasound to determine if bilateral drainage is necessary. In horses with thoracic neoplasia or peracute pleuritis, bilateral pleural fluid can often be drained via one hemithorax. An indwelling chest tube is sutured in place using a Chinese finger knot, and a one-way (Heimlich) valve allows constant drainage of pleural fluid (Fig. 23.7). If ultrasound guidance is not available, pleurocentesis should be performed at the 6th or 7th intercostal space on the right hemithorax and the 7th or 8th intercostal space on the left hemithorax, 10 cm dorsal to the olecranon (above the costrochondral junction), using a teat cannula, a syringe, and a 3-way stopcock. If aspiration of air is noted after removal of a teat cannula or indwelling chest tube, a suture may be placed to close the skin or a bandage may be placed to prevent development of pneumothorax until the wound heals. A bandage is preferred if cellulitis is present or septic pleural fluid drains from the thoracic wound.

Gross examination of pleural fluid includes evaluation of color, odor, volume, and turbidity. Malodorous pleural fluid is associated with anaerobic bacteria and indicates a more guarded prognosis. Serosanguinous pleural fluid has been observed in horses with necrotizing pneumonia, pulmonary infarction, and thoracic neoplasia. A large volume of clear, yellow pleural fluid with no odor and minimal turbidity is consistent with neoplastic effusion. Differentia-

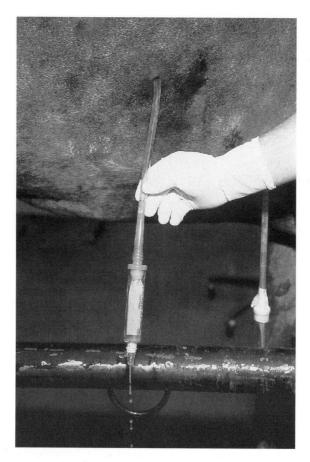

**Fig. 23.7.** A one-way (Heimlich) valve allows constant drainage of pleural fluid with minimal risk of iatrogenic pneumothorax.

tion of septic versus neoplastic pleural effusion is definitively determined by cytologic evaluation. Thoracocentesis samples should be submitted for cytologic evaluation (EDTA), anaerobic/aerobic bacterial culture, and Gram stain. Normal pleural fluid samples contain less than 10,000 cells/μl and 2.5 gm of protein/dl. Cytologic evaluation can be performed on direct smears (high cellularity) or cytocentrifuge preparations (transudates) stained with Diff-Quik or Wright's stain. Cytologic evaluation of septic pleural fluid reveals a purulent exudate (>90% neutrophils) with high cellularity (25,000–200,000 cells/μl) and high total protein (>3.0 gm/dl). Intracellular and extracellular bacteria may be observed, and Gram stain examination may be used to direct initial antibiotic therapy. Neoplastic effusions are typically characterized cytologically as a transudate or modified transudate with low cellularity and mild to moderate elevation in total protein. Neoplastic cells may or may not be identified, depending on the exfoliative nature of the tumor.

Biochemical analysis can be performed on pleural fluid samples to differentiate septic from neoplastic effusions. The most reliable tests for differentiation are pH, glucose, and lactate dehydrogenase. Neoplastic effusions have glucose and pH values similar to venous blood. Septic pleural fluid obtained from horses with complicated pleuropneumonia is consistently acidic (pH <7.1), with glucose concentrations less than 40 mg/dl. Glucose concentrations greater than 60 mg/dl suggest uncomplicated effusion, and concentrations between 40 and 60 mg/dl are inconclusive. Lactate dehydrogenase activity greater than 1000 IU/L is consistent with septic pleural effusion.

The most common complications of thoracocentesis are mild pneumothorax and cellulitis around an indwelling chest tube. Iatrogenic pneumothorax is usually self-limiting unless aspiration of air is allowed to occur unchecked (open-ended tube). Cellulitis at the site of an indwelling chest tube can be treated with warm compresses and may necessitate removal of the tube. Less common (but more serious) complications of thoracocentesis include cardiac puncture, cardiac arrhythmia, pulmonary laceration, diaphragmatic laceration, and damage to liver or bowel. The intrathoracic pressure changes associated with draining a large volume of effusion may cause rupture of a pulmonary abscess into the pleural space. In this instance, horses may appear toxemic and shocky during or immediately after thoracic drainage.

## THORACIC RADIOGRAPHY

An overhead radiograph unit (1000 mA, 150 kV) is required to image the thorax of adult horses. Thoracic radiographs are obtained from standing (perhaps sedated) horses, and 3–4 overlapping lateral radiographic projections are required to visualize the entire thorax. The standard focal-spot to film distance using an overhead radiographic unit is 100 centimeters. The thoracic cavity of foals may be satisfactorily imaged with portable radiographic equipment. Thoracic radiography is superior to ultrasonographic examination to identify pulmonary parechymal lesions, mediastinal structures, and thoracic wall abnormalities. Thoracic radiography is indicated in horses with clinical evidence of bronchopneumonia, aspiration pneumonia, unresponsive heaves, and fractured ribs. Pulmonary abscesses (Fig. 23.8), pulmonary consolidation, interstitial pneumonia, pneumothorax (see Chapter 22, Fig. 22.6), mediastinal lymphadenapathy, and pulmonary fibrosis are preferentially imaged via thoracic radiography. In some horses with exercise-induced pulmonary hemorrhage, regions of pulmonary hemorrhage in the caudodorsal lung fields may be detected for days to weeks after an episode. In horses with pleuropneumonia, thoracic radiographs should be obtained after thoracocentesis to allow visualization of pulmonary parenchymal lesions and mediastinal structures. Serial examination can identify disease progression and response to treatment.

There are 4 basic radiographic patterns for interpretation of thoracic images: alveolar, interstitial, bronchial, and vascular. Identification of these specific radiographic patterns provides insight to the disease process. However, radiographic patterns are not specific for a single disease entity, and more than

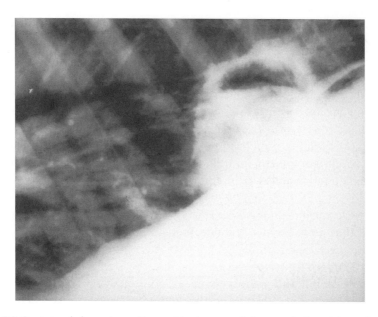

**Fig. 23.8.** Lateral thoracic radiographic image of the caudodorsal lung fields of a horse with a large, fluid and air-filled abscess of the pulmonary parenchyma and diaphragm.

one pattern may be present in a given patient. Modifications or descriptors for the basic radiographic patterns may provide further evidence of the disease process, such as bronchointerstitial, peribronchial, miliary, linear, reticular, nodular. Interpretation of radiographic patterns is intended to assist the clinician in formulating a list of differential diagnoses, rather than providing a pathognomonic sign.

The interstitial pattern is the most common thoracic radiographic pattern observed in veterinary medicine. Inflammation or infiltration of the connective tissue framework of the lungs results in an interstitial pattern, which appears as an increase in background opacity that results in loss of visualization of fine vascular structures typically seen in well-aerated lung (Fig. 23.9). This pattern may be observed in the early stages of most pulmonary diseases, including infectious, neoplastic, cardiogenic, and allergic. A reticular or nodular interstitial pattern suggests that a cellular infiltrate is present in the interstitial space (Fig. 23.10), and the most severe form may indicate metastatic neoplasia or fungal disease (Fig. 23.11). Most pulmonary diseases begin in the interstitium, prior to involving alveoli, so the presence of this pattern is rarely indicative of a specific disease process.

The alveolar pattern appears as patchy, poorly marginated, opaque areas that coalesce and obliterate pulmonary vessels and bronchi. The hallmark of the alveolar pattern is the air bronchogram, which is defined as visualization of a small (<3rd generation) airway. An air bronchogram appears as a branching lucency without visible walls within an opaque pulmonary field (Fig. 23.12). The tubular lucency represents an air-filled bronchus, and the bron-

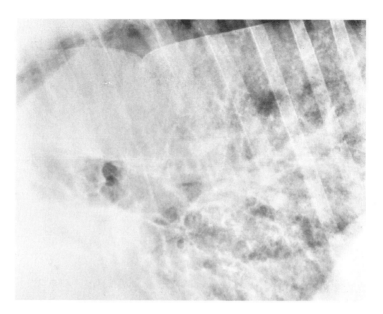

**Fig. 23.9.** Lateral thoracic radiograph of the lungs of an aged horse with a marked interstitial pattern due to granulomatous pneumonitis and pulmonary fibrosis. This radiograph was obtained 20 minutes after pulmonary biopsy was obtained. Note the notch in the dorsal aspect of the lung and the small amount of unilateral pneumothorax.

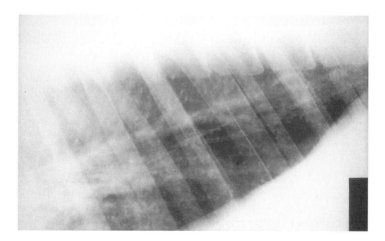

**Fig. 23.10.** Lateral thoracic radiograph of the caudodorsal lung fields of a 5-year-old horse with a miliary interstitial pattern due to eosinophilic pneumonitis. At necropsy, numerous eosinophilic granulomas were observed in the pulmonary interstitium.

chial walls are obscured by fluid-filled (water dense) alveoli. The alveolar pattern is observed in patients with pulmonary edema, hemorrhage, consolidation, and atelectasis. The pulmonary distribution of an alveolar pattern will aid in determining the differential diagnosis (i.e., cranioventral = bronchopneumonia; caudodorsal = cardiogenic, hemorrhagic, septicemic).

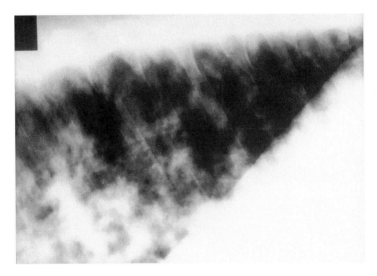

**Fig. 23.11.** Lateral thoracic radiograph of the caudodorsal lung fields of an 8-year-old mare with a reticular nodular pattern due to fungal pneumonia.

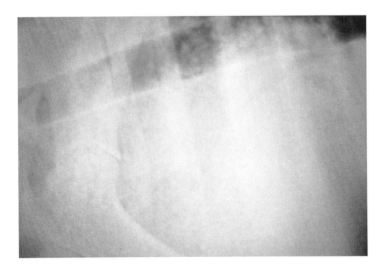

**Fig. 23.12.** Lateral thoracic radiograph of a 4-year-old horse with a marked alveolar pattern because of acute pulmonary edema due to ruptured chordae tendinae. Note the patchy, poorly marginated, coalescing opaque areas and the air bronchogram projecting forward from the hilus.

The bronchial pattern represents disease of the conducting system and appears as increased thickness of bronchial structures and increased numbers of visible bronchi. Well-circumscibed end-on bronchi may be visualized in peripheral lung fields. Opacity of the bronchial wall may be due to peribronchial infiltration or intraluminal exudate (diphtheritic membrane). This linear pattern can be further differentiated on the basis of whether the bronchi appear sharply defined (bronchial) or ill-defined with apparently thickened walls (peribronchial pattern). A bronchial pattern is more indicative of chronic disease with changes in the bronchi themselves (mineralization), whereas a peribronchial pattern is indicative of inflammation around bronchi, which may represent acute (early bronchopneumonia) or chronic (allergic) disease processes.

The vascular pattern is rarely observed in adult equine patients. It is characterized by variation in the size, shape, and number of pulmonary vessels. The vascular pattern is most often observed in patients with pulmonary overcirculation due to left-to-right cardiac shunts.

## FURTHER READING

Ainsworth, D.M., and Biller, D.S. 1998. Respiratory system. In *Equine Internal Medicine*, 1st ed. S.M. Reed and W.M. Bayly, eds.Philadelphia: W.B. Saunders, pp 253–257.

Schott, H.C., and Mansmann, R.A. 1990. Thoracic drainage in horses. *Comp Cont Ed Pract Vet* 12(2):251–261.

# Index